PRACTICAL PSYCHIATRY OF OLD AGE

Practical Psychiatry of Old Age

Fifth edition

JOHN P WATTIS MB ChB DPM FRCPsych
Professor of Old Age Psychiatry, University of Huddersfield

and

STEPHEN CURRAN BSc (Hons), MB ChB, MRCPsych, MMedSc, PhD
Consultant in Old Age Psychiatry, South West Yorkshire Partnership,
NHS Foundation Trust
Professor of Old Age Psychiatry, University of Huddersfield

Foreword by
WENDY BURN

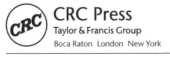

CRC Press
Taylor & Francis Group
Boca Raton London New York

CRC Press is an imprint of the
Taylor & Francis Group, an **informa** business

CRC Press
Taylor & Francis Group
6000 Broken Sound Parkway NW, Suite 300
Boca Raton, FL 33487-2742

First issued in hardback 2017

© 2013 by John P Wattis and Stephen Curran
CRC Press is an imprint of Taylor & Francis Group, an Informa business

No claim to original U.S. Government works

Version Date: 20151016

ISBN-13: 978-1-908911-98-8 (pbk)
ISBN-13: 978-1-138-44581-9 (hbk)

Visit the Taylor & Francis Web site at
http://www.taylorandfrancis.com

and the CRC Press Web site at
http://www.crcpress.com

Contents

Foreword to the fifth edition

I am delighted that there is now a fifth edition of *Practical Psychiatry of Old Age* and that I have been asked to write an introduction.

I first came across this book very early in my professional life when I worked for John Wattis. This was in the early days of old age psychiatry as a specialty, and John was one of those who inspired me to make my career in it. I can still remember my excitement on recognising a patient who had been the subject of one of the case vignettes in the book.

Practical Psychiatry of Old Age has stayed with me throughout my working life and I have used it more than any other reference book. As its title suggests it contains practical and accessible advice for the busy clinician, backed by a solid knowledge of the research literature. Each new edition has reflected the changes in the specialty that have occurred in assessment, treatment and the way that services are organised. I return to it again and again, sometimes to check basic facts, sometimes to help in the preparation of teaching or assessment and sometimes purely out of interest. I always find understandable, lucid explanations and the information is clearly and helpfully set out.

Stephen Curran became involved from the third edition. I have known him since he was a trainee and had the pleasure of being his trainer at one point. Apart from his clinical experience and natural wisdom, Stephen brings an excellent knowledge of psychopharmacology in practice and experience gained in his role as chair of the Royal College of Psychiatrists' Memory Services National Accreditation Programme advisory group. He also has a particular interest in resistant depression in old age and forensic work with the elderly.

The fifth edition has been updated to include modern NICE advice on the tiered approach to managing depression, with an expansion of information on psychological approaches and an update on psychopharmacological matters. Care pathways are covered, and the recent changes to the way in which services are organised are included.

This is a book light enough to be read for pleasure but heavy enough to be used as a clinician's main textbook. I recommend it to anyone of any discipline who works with the elderly and wants their knowledge to be sufficient to ensure that they provide the optimum care for older people with psychiatric problems.

Wendy Burn BM MMedSc FRCPsych
Dean, Royal College of Psychiatrists
January 2013

Foreword to the fourth edition

Not many books make it to a fourth edition. This is a commendation in itself. Of those that do, the epithet 'classic' is likely to be attached. So it is my privilege to undertake the foreword to this classic textbook.

The specialty of psychiatry as applied to older people may be a relative newcomer compared with other branches of medicine, but it has enjoyed vigorous growth over the past 20 years, spurred on by demographic changes in most developed societies. New technologies, such as medication for dementia, have not only helped patients directly but have had an important impact on the seriousness with which conditions like dementia are regarded. In an interesting reversal of dualistic thinking which has pervaded medicine, new concepts such as 'vascular depression' have brought together findings from brain imaging with those from observations of mood, behaviour and psychosocial experience. Around the globe, organisations such as the International Psychogeriatric Association and the Section of Old Age Psychiatry of the World Psychiatric Association are championing service development, teaching and research. There has probably never been a better time to practise in this specialty.

Integral to this endeavour is dissemination of the knowledge base that constitutes the specialty. *Practical Psychiatry of Old Age* is a major contributor to this. If I had to emphasise one word in the book's title it would be 'practical'. The two authors are clinicians who have devoted their professional lives to the practical care of older people with mental ill health. I can picture them returning after an assessment in a patient's home thinking 'that will make a great case history for the book'. Paradoxically, the term 'practical' can have slightly negative connotations – the mere fixing of problems, unacademic, not having much depth. It is important then to note that the immensely practical approach of this book is underpinned by a strong evidence base which the two authors, both of whom have robust academic credentials, have clearly weaved throughout the fabric of the contributions.

In a textbook which is comprehensive in scope, it is vital that the authors have a grip on 'quality control'. Not only is this apparent but they have made clear from the earliest chapter and throughout the book that they are serious about treating the whole person. So theory and practice are expertly melded but there are also important insights regarding ethical dilemmas, societal values and spiritual concerns. The overall 'feel' of this book then is one of expert knowledge within a compassionate, humane and holistic framework.

This book will appeal to a wide readership – from those who want general information on the major mental health problems of later life to specialists who want to refresh and update their knowledge.

Robert Baldwin DM FRCP FRCPsych
Consultant Old Age Psychiatrist and Honorary Professor
at the University of Manchester
Manchester Royal Infirmary
March 2006

Preface

When the first edition of this book was published, old age psychiatry in the UK was in its infancy and the senior author was a newly appointed consultant. Now, 30 years on, things have changed almost beyond recognition. Some of the changes have been welcome. There are many more old age psychiatrists and many more multidisciplinary teams. Other changes have been less welcome, including the virtual abolition of NHS-funded long-term care for people with severe dementia. Some things have, despite changes in the organisation of services, remained depressingly familiar, like the still too frequent examples of neglect and abuse in the care of old people.

One thing remains certain: old people with mental health problems require compassionate and competent services. This edition seeks to bring up to date our clinical primer for doctors and others caring for old people with mental health problems. We have incorporated many changes in clinical and organisational areas. We hope we have retained the emphasis on good diagnosis, care and management combined with an emphasis on the importance of showing old people that we value them by relating to them in a respectful way.

John P Wattis
Stephen Curran
January 2013

About the authors

John Wattis was appointed Visiting Professor of Psychiatry for Older Adults at Huddersfield University in 2000. Before this he was responsible for pioneering old age services in Leeds, where he worked as a Consultant and Senior Lecturer for nearly 20 years. He completed his psychiatric training in Birmingham and Nottingham, where he was lecturer in the Department of Health Care of the Elderly, which combined psychiatric and medical teams. He has management experience as Medical Director of a large community and mental health trust. He is a former Chairman of the Faculty for Psychiatry of Old Age at the Royal College of Psychiatrists, and the committee that advises on the higher training of doctors in general and old age psychiatry. He has published research on the development of old age psychiatry services, alcohol abuse in old age, the prevalence of mental illness in geriatric medical patients, and outcomes of psychiatric admission for older people. He has written or edited a number of books and contributed numerous chapters in the area of old age psychiatry.

Stephen Curran works as Consultant Old Age Psychiatrist in Wakefield, and was appointed a Visiting Professor at Huddersfield University in 2001. He graduated in psychology before studying medicine and then worked as a Research Fellow and Lecturer in Old Age Psychiatry at the University of Leeds. His research interest is in psychopharmacology in older people with mental illness, particularly the pharmacological management of depression and early detection of Alzheimer's disease. He has numerous research publications to his credit, and has co-authored and co-edited a number of books.

Together, John and Stephen have contributed to undergraduate and postgraduate teaching both of doctors and of those in other disciplines. Their approach to healthcare for older people is founded on three principles:
1 recognition of the importance of *good relationships* between individuals and between different health and social care providers
2 firm commitment to the need to develop and integrate evidence-based practice
3 an emphasis on the need for creativity in improving treatment and services.

They are committed to a multidisciplinary and inter-agency approach to healthcare of the elderly that sees mental health and illness in the context of physical health and social pressures.

Acknowledgements

We gratefully acknowledge the work undertaken by Mike Church and Carol Martin, co-authors of the first two editions, some of which is retained or reflected in this fifth edition. We are also indebted to Shabir Musa, Arun Devasahayam and Jayanthi Devi Subramani, for allowing us to use part of their contribution to *Practical Management of Dementia (2nd edition)* as the basis for the section on legal issues in Chapter 10.

We would also like to thank Gill Nineham for help and advice given over many years, and Jenny Monk for her work on the revised manuscript for this edition.

To our families –
for their patience with us whilst we have been working on this book.

Setting the scene

INTRODUCTION

This chapter sets the scene for the whole book. Those who are eager to address some practical problem such as what to do with a confused or depressed patient in the consulting-room can safely skip it and return to it later.

The pace of change in medicine and society is accelerating. We are in a period of confusion as the 'industrial age' gives way to the 'information age'. We may move into a period of *relative* stability once this has occurred. In the mean time, the busy clinician and the educated consumer have to learn to work *with* constant change. The following are among the most relevant:

➤ technical progress – molecular medicine, new scanning techniques, new drugs (medications) and new classes of drugs, and new information technology
➤ the need to develop good practice based on the best available evidence, meeting the challenge of changing the behaviour of clinicians and patients
➤ improving the interpersonal aspects of clinical practice
➤ frequent reorganisation as politicians 'modernise' the way services are delivered.

Our understanding of ageing and the issues that surround it has also moved on. In particular, our understanding of the dementing illnesses such as Alzheimer's disease has developed in a number of ways, from the molecular biology to the 'science of the art' of diagnostic practice[1] and interpersonal care.[2] Social and political trends are also influencing *how* services are delivered. These include the following:

➤ a move from quantitative to descriptive standards of service provision
➤ a move from public to private funding and provision
➤ a move from medical dominance to 'stakeholder' or even consumer power (potentially leading to neglect of weaker consumer groups such as old people)

➤ a move from hospital to community services
➤ rising inequality in Western societies (especially the USA and the UK).[3]

The changes in the population structure continue. These include not only the 'greying' of the population but also other social and cultural changes with regard to marriage, divorce and parenting. The political context is also changing. In the UK we are moving away from the post-war welfare state, which was dominated by monolithic (some would say 'neolithic') public services, towards a 'mixed economy' of health and welfare provision. This is more able to cope with rapid change, but there may be more risk of vulnerable groups being neglected. Mental health services for older people are a relatively new development both around the world and in the UK.[4] They are children of change, and should be able to thrive in the changing world, though increased emphasis on private provision and consequent fragmentation of services may not serve old people well.

In this chapter we intend to give a brief overview of some of these issues. In particular, we hope to cover the following areas:
➤ what ageing is – a biological and psychological understanding
➤ ageing in society – social, cultural and political aspects
➤ a developmental viewpoint on ageing and its challenges
➤ the impact of technical advances and 'evidence-based medicine/evidence-based practice' (EBM/EBP)
➤ the epidemiology of mental disorder in late life
➤ the development of specialist services for old people with mental disorder and their interface with other services for old people, especially memory services.

WHAT IS AGEING?

Age can be measured in various ways, including the following approaches:
➤ chronological
➤ biological
➤ psychological
➤ developmental
➤ social.

A particular individual may well be at different stages on these and other dimensions. These various aspects of ageing are not independent of each other. Psychological and biological ageing interact with each other and with the social and physical environment to produce the complicated picture that we recognise as ageing. We shall now, for the sake of simplicity, describe some of these areas separately.

Biological ageing

Biological ageing can be considered at the level of molecular, cellular, organ, organ-system or whole-organism ageing.

Despite the Bible's 'threescore years and ten', human life expectancy is scientifically indeterminate. We can discuss the average age of populations and the known limit of longevity, but individuals may (and probably will, in due course) survive beyond that apparent limit. However, we are here more concerned with present reality than with any theoretical limit. In the UK in 2011 a man aged 65 years could expect on average to live to 83 years, and a woman of the same age to 85.6 years (*see* Age UK website). Even within the UK there are marked geographical differences in life expectancy.[5]

What determines the age of death and what processes are important? Usually death occurs as a consequence of the inability of the body to deal with some disease process, rather than as a direct effect of ageing. Indeed, one definition of ageing is that it is a progressive change in the organism that leads to an increased *risk* of disease, disability and death. At the *genetic* level, some argue that lifespan is 'pre-programmed', although no direct evidence of this has yet been found. Others argue that errors in protein synthesis, damage to DNA (the genetic coding material of the cell) or chromosomal mutation in tissues that renew themselves may play a part. Certainly cell cultures grown in the laboratory seem to survive for a long but limited time unless they undergo a mutation (e.g. into cancer-like cells) whereby the normal cellular mechanisms that control growth and cell division are no longer active.

Another type of genetic mutation, in the immune system, might result in it starting to attack healthy cells. External factors such as ionising radiation may be responsible for damaging the DNA and producing mutations. Even at this level, attempts to separate internal and external factors may be in vain. At the *cellular and tissue level* some cells (e.g. nerve cells) are not replaceable if they die. However, even nerve cells are able to generate new connections and so, to a limited extent, 'bypass' problems caused by cell death. Other cells are replaced with varying degrees of rapidity in processes that are sensitive to internal feedback mechanisms. Pigments and other products of metabolism may accumulate in cells and extracellular tissue and may potentially cause harm, as may certain heavy metals.

Whatever the underlying mechanisms, we know a great deal about the changes that normally occur in different *organ systems* of the body as they age. Heart disease accounts for most deaths over the age of 65 years. Muscle fibres in the ageing heart are reduced and the pigment lipofuchsin, which first appears in the heart at around 20 years of age, represents over 5% of the muscle fibres in those aged over 80 years. Within wide individual variation there is an average reduction in the pumping performance of the heart. Each individual contraction is slower, probably as a result of changes in the cellular enzymes that facilitate this action. The reserve capacity of the heart to cope with the stress of vigorous exercise is reduced with increasing age, but is generally still considerable. Changes also occur in the blood vessels, with decreased elasticity in the vessel walls, compounded in virtually all cases by the deposition of fatty atheromatous plaques in the lining of arteries. This loss of elasticity may be one of the reasons why blood pressure tends to increase with increasing age. However, another reason may be only indirectly age related, as obesity tends to be more common in middle age, and is itself a risk factor for high blood pressure, and possibly for later onset of Alzheimer's disease.

In the digestive system, apart from wear and tear on teeth, there are no major consistent changes with ageing. The loss of neurons in the brain is probably only marginal, and although nerve cells do not generally regenerate in humans, they are capable of growing new connections to other nerve cells (synapses). Sensory input to the brain may be reduced by ageing and disease. The eye becomes less able to shift focus, and night vision declines with increasing age. High-frequency hearing loss develops gradually over the age of 50 years. Reflexes are more slowly reactive, and the capacity of the brain to make decisions in complex situations is slightly reduced, apparently largely as a result of intrinsic changes.

Skin shows reduced elasticity and adherence to subcutaneous tissues. With the exception of the female menopause, relatively few changes occur in the endocrine system. There is no decrease in thyroid activity, although there may be reduced utilisation of thyroxine by other cells. Corticosteroid hormones, produced by the adrenal cortex, may show a slight reduction in levels, but the adrenals retain their capacity to react to stress. The production of insulin by the pancreas is undiminished in health, but may be less reactive to changes in blood sugar levels. Male sex hormones gradually decline between the ages of 50 and 90 years, and male sexual activity decreases from around four episodes weekly at age 20 years to around once weekly at 60 years. The majority of this decline appears to occur by the age of 45 years. Of course, the extent to which this is hormonally determined and the extent to which it is a result of social and psychological expectations is not easily determined.

The *body as a whole* changes partly as a result of less effective feedback and control systems. It also changes in composition, with less lean body mass and relatively increased fat and fluid levels. Some of the loss of lean body mass may be due to reduced muscle mass resulting from reduced physical activity. This again emphasises the problems of distinguishing biological ageing from social and psychological factors.

Expectations about health have an important part to play in old people's satisfaction. For example, one study suggested that older people describe themselves as sufficiently fit if they can carry out the tasks of daily living, even though these may require minimal activity. Levels of fitness in the general population may be much lower than optimal, and many people may be accepting restrictions on their lifestyle unnecessarily.

Psychological understanding of normal ageing

There are many false beliefs about the psychology of human ageing. However, there are some well-established facts. In the area of cognition, for example, research shows that response time slows – that is, it takes longer for older people to process new information. The size of the change is small, but in some circumstances even that may be critical, especially in combination with sensory or motor changes or stress, or when complicated decisions are involved. Many older people compensate by developing skills and strategies. For example, older typists look further ahead when typing and have extra time for processing, thereby maintaining their speed. The slowed reflexes and greater difficulty in decision making in older people, coupled with sensory changes, should make older people less safe drivers. However, again they use experience to compensate (and more than compensate), as the actuaries who set insurance premiums so high for young people clearly understand.

The differences that are found between groups are *statistically* significant, but there are older individuals whose performance matches or exceeds that of younger people. Training older people to use their memories and asking them to perform in areas of special competence allows them to perform as well as younger individuals. Memory for events in the distant past is not necessarily better than memory for recent events, and some of the stories that are retained by individuals may be over-learned and told in an automatic, repetitive way. In normal ageing, the ordinary tasks involving memory (e.g. sending someone a birthday card or remembering that the bath is running) do not decline. Where levels of motivation are high, older people may be better at telephoning someone at a set time, for example, but apparently perform less well when tasks are not regarded as vital. Certainly older people have a tendency to complain that they are more forgetful, particularly of names and the last place in which they put something. Their 'working memories' often have less capacity than those of younger people. However, there is a suggestion that the thinking of old people becomes more context bound and more expertise related, and intuitive, because it is *more* efficient to proceed in this way, thus compensating for reduced capacity.

Chronological age is an inadequate but necessary marker for more important but less easily measured phenomena of biological and psychological ageing.

AGEING IN SOCIETY

Social and legal construction of ageing

In the UK, there was until recently a statutory retirement age of 65 years. This is still often seen as the age at which people are defined as 'old' in terms of public services. However, things are changing. Pensions are increasingly deferred to a later age, and age discrimination has become illegal. 'Old' and 'young' are comparative terms, and individuals change their opinion about when old age starts as they themselves get older. Perhaps a better question to ask than 'When am I old?' is 'When am I too old for what?'. For everybody, getting older is an issue even during childhood, as it seems clear then that birthdays bring advantage and privileges. However, concerns about ageing start early in adulthood, with worries about reaching the milestones that we have planned. For example, ageing becomes a prominent issue for some women in their twenties and thirties when they try to balance the demands of relationships, career and children. Most people are taking active notice of the process of physical ageing by this point in their lives, and mid-life is an accepted point for review, if not crisis.

The National Service Framework (NSF) for older people in England and Wales[6] described three broad groups as follows:

➤ entering old age (which may be 'retirement age' or as young as 50 years)
➤ transitional phase – in transition between healthy active life and frailty (commonly in the seventh or eighth decade)
➤ frail older people – people who are vulnerable as a result of health problems, social care needs or a combination of both.

On average about half of life expectancy over age 65 fits into the transitional phase. The last years for men and women are often lived with significant disability.[5]

Demography: some key facts

At the start of the 20th century it was estimated that there were about 600 million people over 60 years of age alive, and about two-thirds of them were living in Third World countries. The UK now counts (or discounts, if you prefer) 16% of its population as elderly. This adds up to over 10.3 million individuals over 65 years of age, of whom around 1.4 million are over 85 years old.[5] The role of this group is therefore likely to have important implications for the whole of the population.

The increase in numbers of old people has been due to improvements in public health, reductions in the number of child deaths, and increased quality of life. Dementia increases almost exponentially with age, rising from less than 1% in the under-65 years age group and doubling approximately every five years to 2–3% in the 65–70 years age group, 4–6% in the 70–75 years age group, 8–12% in the 75–80 years age group and over 20% in the over-80 years age group.

In 2002, almost two-thirds of people aged 75 years or over (and almost three-quarters of those aged 85 years or over) were female. At age 95 years or over there are about five times as many women alive as men. This, too, has implications for the possible contributions and needs of old people. At the most concrete end of the spectrum, the financial resources of women have historically been lower than those of men. They earned less when they worked, so they have less at retirement.

Overall, 50% of people aged over 75 live alone. The Age UK Factsheet referred to above gives many more details about demography, poverty, housing and other issues that affect the quality of life in old age.[5] These issues directly affect all health and social services for old people. Increasingly there will be a need for support for old people suffering from dementia that cannot be supplied by the family. With rising standards of living and expectations among the population as a whole, and with the cohort effect as the 'consumer generation' grows old, there may be higher levels of dissatisfaction among old people and their younger relatives with regard to their life circumstances and health and social services provision.

Politics, ageism and sexism

Service provision for old people is largely related to the needs of elderly women, many of whom live alone. Women have been relatively excluded from public life, and the current cohorts of elderly women include fewer highly educated and professional people than are found in their male peer group or among younger women. Many older women were brought up with an ideal of womanhood as passive or receptive. This suggests that at present some old people may be restricted in their expectations and capacity to campaign on their own behalf. This situation is changing, and it is likely to change ever more rapidly as younger women who have had greater access to education, careers and a range of role models grow old.

Pensioners who are mainly dependent on a state pension and who are living alone (mostly women) are much less likely to have a car or a washing-machine, and slightly less likely to have a telephone or central heating, than the rest of the population. Poor public transport selectively penalises this group. Yet decisions on public spending and service priority, many of which influence provisions for older people, are made by people under retirement age, even if the views of older people are (sometimes) researched and taken into account. Hopefully this imbalance of means and needs will not be tolerated by future generations of old people (by which we mean us!).

Images of old age have a continuity across recent history and Western culture. There is a balance between the value accorded to young and old, which shifted towards youth with the post-war baby boom, and which may return as that cohort ages. Whatever the particular images of old age, each contains an implicit comparison with youth, so that people are approved for ageing well (i.e. looking young), or castigated for impersonating youth ('mutton dressed as lamb').

Positive images of several types have been created as old people are developed as a consumer group. Commonly there are images of the 'youthful old person', linked to anti-ageing products and the image of retirement as leisure lifestyle, linked to leisure goods and activities. While these may raise the consciousness of both old and young, the risk would be an increase in dissatisfaction among those who see opportunities but cannot attain them.

Ageism is the expression of disadvantage due to age, and it can be found everywhere, psychiatric services not excepted! Like sexism, it may be difficult to uncover and it is highly reinforced. It is reflected in the very language we use – for example, when general psychiatrists call themselves 'adult' psychiatrists, unconsciously implying that those over 65 years old are no longer adult! It is reflected in the ambiguous attitudes to older people of government documents such as the National Service Framework for Mental Health.[7] It is built into the social networks and institutions in which we work and live, and its effects start in youth. In the UK, as in many other societies, images of beauty and goodness are associated with youth. Our definitions of old age are bound up with our views of other phenomena, including infirmity, dependency, aesthetics, moral and social ideals, gender attributes, independence, competence and employment. Culturally, younger people play a significant role in the definitions and experience of ageing. The healthy under-65s write the soaps and the newspapers, deliver conference papers, treat old people in hospital and serve them in shops. Despite this, old people are much more likely to exercise their democratic right to vote than younger people.[5]

To describe someone as 'old' is often regarded as abusive. The idea of old age as a handicap remains prevalent even among trained psychiatric staff. In a teaching exercise, nurses were asked to think of and describe an old person known personally to them. In each session, virtually everyone who described someone old in positive terms agreed that they thought that the individual was exceptional for their age.

A DEVELOPMENTAL VIEWPOINT

A helpful way of understanding individual ageing in an ageing society is the developmental approach. Development is a dynamic process, and may occur when an individual has to face a new situation and learn new skills, resolve internal conflicts or take on a new role. Some of these are the normal transitions of life, such as retirement, while others are idiosyncratic changes, such as disability, divorce, or loss of a child. The human potential for creative solutions to dilemmas and problems leads to wide variation in skills, lifestyles and coping strategies by the time people grow old.

The developmental approach sees each stage of life as having its own particular and appropriate aspirations and challenges, with none of these being intrinsically 'better' than the others.

Life aspirations

The majority of people have a rough plan for their life. Generally, they want a partner and family, friendships, productive and interesting work and leisure activities. These aspirations develop through childhood along with the characteristics and skills that may enable them to be realised. Fairy tales may owe some of their popularity to the reassurance they offer to children that they may reach adult goals. Some people's lives approach their aspirations, while others do not. Later opportunities and experiences depend to some extent on the degree of satisfaction with life in earlier stages, and the decisions that were made then.

Developmental tasks of late life

Although there is immense variety, at a deeper level there do seem to be issues common to people of particular ages and generations. Erikson suggested that each developmental stage has a 'core conflict' to be resolved.[8,9] He suggested that a dominant conflict for old people is that of 'integrity versus despair', as they struggle to come to terms with the limits of their existence, their achievements and the loss of a future. Erikson's model is based on psychoanalytic theory, and implies that personal growth is achieved through successful resolution of psychosocial conflicts which are brought about by maturational processes and external conditions. Our understanding of these 'core conflicts', based on Erikson's model, is summarised in Table 1.1.

Erikson's model suggests that all of the conflicts he defines are being continually renegotiated. For example, if in adult life someone is betrayed by a partner, the balance of trust may be changed towards mistrust. The degree of the change and its permanence will be dependent on past experiences. If the person's own background was stable and loving, this may allow for the repair of the relationship or reinvestment in another one. If, on the other hand, the person had been severely let down or abused by a parent, it might be difficult or impossible to overcome the adult trauma constructively. A supportive family or friends may help, as may therapy. If it is not overcome, such mistrust may increase in old age as the person faces reductions in strength and independence while fearing that carers will behave in an untrustworthy manner.

Table 1.1 Erikson's model of psychosocial development

Developmental stage	'Core conflict'
First year	Basic trust vs. mistrust
'Toddler'	Autonomy vs. shame and doubt
'Pre-school'	Initiative vs. guilt
Early school years	Industry vs. inferiority
Puberty and adolescence	Identity vs. role confusion
Young adulthood	Intimacy vs. isolation
Middle adulthood	Generativity vs. stagnation
Maturity	Ego integrity vs. despair

This theory may go some way towards explaining the occurrence of distress and severe symptomatology in late life. In younger adult life, people may not develop the skills necessary for intimate relationships and dependency, or for enabling them to act autonomously without excessive anxiety. The changes that are brought about by ageing, such as frailty or bereavement, may then bring them face to face with the problem and their failure.

Personality development in late life

There is evidence for the importance of both change and continuity in personality throughout adult life. Although people's characters tend to remain stable over long periods, stressful life events may require adaptations and promote change. In particular, it seems that some events, such as separation by divorce or bereavement, may set in motion a series of changes and decision making with long-term and profound effects. However, personality types seem to remain stable throughout adult life, while the level of life satisfaction is related to personality type rather than to age. Some researchers have sought to identify common strategies for dealing with ageing itself. One such strand is the reclaiming of opposite-gender characteristics.[10]

Adaptation to stress is important for life satisfaction and depends on the external stressors, the coping abilities of the older person and the social support that is available. Older people tend to view stress in a wider context, so are sometimes less bothered by minor stresses. Changes are often forced on the lifestyle of the older person by events such as disability or bereavement. One change may precipitate others – for example, the death of a partner may necessitate moving from the marital home.

Wisdom and spirituality

Old people are sometimes said to develop wisdom. Wisdom can be defined as the capacity to exercise good judgement when important issues are complex and uncertain. Perhaps the relative slowness of older people's decision making in complicated situations is actually *appropriate* learned behaviour rather than an inevitable concomitant of slower neural processing! Wisdom requires the integration of thought and emotion, and reflexivity, in order to take into account ambiguity and context. Wise people allow that there might be a number of possible solutions to a problem. For many people, interpersonal and spiritual concerns become more important in the second half of life, and this is partially recognised in Erikson's formulation of *ego integrity vs. despair*. However, this formulation does not emphasise the interpersonal aspects of spirituality.

The interface between science and religion is an uneasy one. There are fears about clinicians imposing their religious viewpoints on patients. A useful distinction in this area is that between spirituality, defined as the search for meaning in life, and religion, defined as *one way* of conducting that search. For some old people, spirituality, religion and prayer are important healing resources. Religious beliefs can provide a useful framework for important debates on ethical problems, such as the thorny issue of euthanasia. Some good work on interpersonal (spiritual) care for people with dementia comes from secular sources working in collaboration with religious organisations.[11] The churches are beginning to awaken to the spiritual needs of an ageing population,[12] and particularly the needs of people with dementia.[13] Interested readers are referred to the work of Tournier,[14] an early pioneer in this area, and of Koenig,[15] a more recent author who has attempted to bridge the gap between science and spirituality in relation to ageing.

Transitions and stress

The passage into old age requires an individual to adapt to a number of transitions, which range from retirement or having grandchildren to taking an educational course post-retirement, or experiencing bereavement or late divorce. Many old people adapt well to these changes, whether they are crises or not. Others may experience difficulties even with the predictable events. Sometimes it is possible to see how the problems have arisen in retrospect. For example, a man who has difficulties with intimate relationships but who remains happily bound up with his work may retire to find that he and his wife have different expectations. If the couple cannot resolve these in a satisfactory way, it is possible that one of them might present with symptoms of depression, anxiety or somatic complaints. Psychiatric services might in this case be called in to offer help in negotiating the transition. Bereavement counselling, groups for individuals suffering from isolation or interpersonal difficulties, family therapy and individual therapy may all be helpful to individuals who are coping with transitions.

One of the psychological tasks of old age is that of maintaining self-esteem in the face of the negative images of ageing that we all carry. The success with which an individual may achieve this task is related to earlier experiences of self-acceptance. If these have gone well, the old person will have developed sufficient confidence to enable them to adapt in a flexible and assertive manner. Without this confidence, individuals may resist changes even if this means suffering isolation or loss. An example might be the person who refuses a hearing-aid or a day centre place because this would be felt to be humiliating. One of the tasks facing the professionals in psychiatric services for old people is that of helping vulnerable people to accept help which in no way makes up for what has been lost, but which can make adaptation possible.

Control, autonomy and power

Some of the changes that occur in old age make it more difficult for people to exercise choice or control over their lives, or even over themselves. Physical changes, institutional settings, dementia and restrictive beliefs can all have this effect, often impairing an old person's mental health as a result. Although it is sometimes impossible to proceed without reducing a person's choice, it is an important task within health and social services for old people to attempt to reverse this trend, enabling them to decide on their own lifestyle as far as is possible and appropriate. Langer showed that there were differences in several psychological dimensions and even rates of mortality between a group of old people in institutional care who were encouraged to take responsibility for their own lives and a group who were encouraged to look to staff for the satisfaction of their needs.[16]

Gender, racial, cultural and economic influences operate throughout life, and the resources and influence accrued over the years can buffer some of the effects of ageing. A small group of wealthy older women control a large proportion of privately owned wealth in the USA, often through having survived their husbands. Some senior positions in the professions and important social and political positions are occupied by older people.

As well as material constraints, there are psychological ones. Not only is there the view that old age is a time for leisure rather than for active involvement in social and familial activities, but many older people experience anxiety about becoming dependent on others for help. When such anxiety is troubling, it may lead to inappropriate attempts at avoidance or control.

Sexuality

Myths about sexuality and ageing abound. Older people are thought to be no longer interested in sex, post-menopausal women are believed to be incapable of sexual enjoyment, and old men are thought to be incapable of sustaining an erection. As we have seen, the frequency of sexual activity does decline with ageing, but older people can and do have active and enjoyable sex lives, albeit lived at a slower pace than when they were younger. Sometimes worries about sexual prowess and self-esteem lead to defensive manoeuvres. The middle-aged man who leaves his wife for a younger woman is an example of the abuse of sexuality for the maintenance of self-esteem and protection against anxieties (about failing powers and infirmity or eventual death). For women, sexuality in old age is not only affected by beliefs, but is also pre-dated by the menopause. The sexual politics of the menopause have been explored by Greer.[17] She suggests that HRT is offered, in part, as a 'cure' for ageing. Older women, perhaps unsurprisingly, view the menopause more favourably than younger ones, and do not regard it as a major transition. In most cases where heterosexual couples give up sexual activity, such activity is stopped by the male partner. If this is seen as a problem, it may be amenable to pharmacological or psychological therapy. For many women there are difficulties in maintaining sexual activity, partly because of the substantial proportion who live without partners. Again it may be useful to have the opportunity to talk about this situation, and to consider the options. Unfortunately, however, the opportunities remain limited, partly because older men are often concerned to find younger partners. Some women, it must be said, welcome the freedom that living alone brings, and avoid relationships in case they are restricted or are required to provide care for an older man.

Death and bereavement

Old age requires people to face death. It is in late adulthood especially that individuals have to come to terms with the meaning of their existence and decide for themselves whether their life has been worthwhile. This experience can be seen in Erikson's last stage. It is often presaged by an increased awareness of time limits and reduced opportunities. From the successful resolution of this evaluation emerges the traditional quality attributed to old age, namely wisdom. Fear of death seems to become less common as people age.[18] This is partly perhaps because they have survived frightening or stressful life events by which the experience of death can be estimated. However, preparation for death (e.g. leaving a will) is relatively uncommon, perhaps indicating a more or less healthy denial. Kubler-Ross classically described a series of reactions that individuals tend to experience if faced with the prospect of their own death.[19] These include denial of death and isolation from others (due to difficulty in communicating meaningfully), depression and despair, anger, attempts to bargain and control, and acceptance and hope. It is difficult to predict which feelings a particular individual may experience, or in what order.[19]

Most older people find that their time is still meaningful, but a common clinical problem is that of the demoralised and desperate old person who seems to feel that life is already over or is passing them by. They have difficulty in finding a reason to carry on, or indeed any meaning for their experience. Retirement, losses and discontinuities can lead up to such states of mind, and bereavement can be a cause of such feelings for some. If clinical depression is present it should be treated (see Chapter 5).

The impact of bereavement should not be underestimated in old age, even though it is an almost inevitable crisis. Loss through death may have various meanings, and the mourning process will be greatly affected by this. For example, loss of a partner may bring about loss of a companion, loss or change in material resources and conditions, or even changes in self-definition. Beliefs about self may be important in surviving a loss. For example, if a person believes that they cannot cope without their partner, or that it is awful to be old and alone, there may seem to be no incentive to make new contacts or even to take on the household tasks that were previously done by the other person. People complain more to their doctors, and there is increased risk of mortality, after bereavement.

Models of grieving, like those of facing one's own death, have been conceptualised as stages. The perception of loss has to take place first, and is followed by protest or searching, despair and grief, and then evolves into detachment from the lost person and reinvestment in other relationships or activities. However, these models simplify the reality of a person's experience. In fact, it seems that individuals reiterate their grief with each reminder of their loss. Some individuals find their loss so painful that they protect themselves from grief in a variety of ways, which leads to prolonged states of depression or unconstructive action.

On the other hand, older adults are showing an increasing interest in psychological therapies, including psychoanalysis, and they may bring certain advantages to therapy. These include an awareness of the pressure of time (which can increase motivation), stability, and increased financial resources compared with younger adults. Some adults seek psychotherapy as they approach old age. They are concerned to make the best of their later years, after perhaps recognising the emptiness inside themselves, the failures they have experienced in developing their potential, or the difficulties they have encountered in relationships. Such people wish for therapy to help them to make the best of the time and resources available to them, and they use therapy well. From a position where psychotherapy was perceived to be largely irrelevant to old people, we have moved on to a situation where it is viewed as increasingly relevant,[20] although still hard to access on the NHS.

TECHNICAL ADVANCES

Technical advances in two fields can be described. The first is innovation in scientific understanding, including understanding of the basis of disease, its investigation and treatment. The second has been described as advances in the 'science of the art' of medicine, perhaps best understood through developments in clinical epidemiology and behavioural science related to medicine.

Innovations in technology

So far, innovations in technology have borne relatively little fruit for old age psychiatry. However, the potential arising from a better understanding of human genetics and molecular biology is enormous. Limited gains have occurred in the diagnosis of the dementias, because of advances in expensive imaging technology.[21] New classes of antidepressants and antipsychotics with different side-effect profiles (and often lower toxicity) have also had an impact on the management of depression and psychosis in old age. The arrival of the cholinesterase inhibitors for the management of dementia (principally Alzheimer's disease at present) marks only the beginning of a long road to control or prevention of these disorders, although some potentially beneficial treatments have proved disappointing on further study. At the same time, the new understanding of the genetics of Alzheimer's disease and research on early detection offer the hope that, when a more potent treatment arrives, we shall be able to use it at a very early, possibly pre-clinical stage.

Scientific advances have also enabled developments in information technology which offer hope of increased efficiency and effectiveness by making clinical information and the scientific knowledge base of clinical practice more readily available to both clinician and patient.

Advances in the 'science of the art' of medicine

This term is used to refer to the way in which clinicians, sometimes unwittingly, use logical strategies to increase the probability of correct diagnosis and management of disease. Sackett and colleagues, in their extremely influential texts entitled *Clinical Epidemiology*[1] and *Evidence-Based Medicine*,[22] show how we can systematically use the accumulated knowledge from scientific research to improve the diagnosis and management of disease. They warn us to be suspicious of dogmatic 'authority' and to be prepared to look at the evidence for ourselves. For many this will only be appropriate in a particular specialist field or with a particularly difficult patient. However, for all of us the rational application of scientific knowledge utilising guidelines reliably developed from the available evidence by experts using declared, open and valid methodologies will become an increasingly important part of practice. The development of techniques such as integrated care pathways[23] for the management of common conditions on a team basis will also encourage more rigorous application of the knowledge base in team clinical practice.

Qualitative studies of clinician–patient interactions also help us broaden the 'science of the art'. This was memorably applied in a seminal study of psychotherapy which found that certain characteristics of the therapist predicted success regardless of the psychotherapeutic theory of the therapist.[24] These characteristics included the following:

➤ empathy
➤ respect (unconditional positive regard)
➤ concreteness
➤ genuineness (congruence)
➤ confrontation
➤ immediacy.

Much more recently, similar person-centred ideas have been very successfully applied to dementia care by Kitwood.[2] More recent work, addressing similar areas, is found in the values-based approach to clinical practice.[25]

EPIDEMIOLOGY AND CLASSIFICATION OF MENTAL HEALTH PROBLEMS IN LATE LIFE

Epidemiology is the study of the distribution of disease and its management in populations. It forms the basis for assessment of population needs and the rational planning of health services. When its techniques are applied to individuals (clinical epidemiology), it forms the framework for evidence-based practice.

In order to describe diseases in populations and individuals, we have to be able to describe them in a valid and reliable way. Classification can be based on a knowledge of causative agents, underlying pathology or – more often in psychiatry – the symptoms and natural history of disorders. The science of naming diseases is sometimes called nosology, and it is a bedrock on which both health service planning and the individual management of patients should be based.

Nosology in psychiatry has come a long way, and the World Health Organization's *International Classification of Diseases (ICD-10)*[26] and the related American Psychiatric Association's *Diagnostic and Statistical Manual (DSM-IV)*[27] provide reliable and detailed descriptions of psychiatric disorders which will be discussed further in appropriate sections of this book. We will use ICD-10 mainly, but a useful cross-tabulation is provided in Appendix H of DSM-IV.

The epidemiology of individual disorders will also be considered at an appropriate point. Here we shall describe the most prevalent psychiatric disorders in late life, and their influence on service planning. The mood disorders (ICD-10 F30-F39) are most prevalent in older people at least up to the age of 75 to 80 years, when the dementias take over as the commonest psychiatric disorders. Depending on the definitions used, depressive disorders sufficient to interfere with daily life affect perhaps 11–12% of the elderly population, with about a quarter of these being seriously affected, and a much larger group of older people experiencing transient depressive symptoms. Dementia of sufficient degree to come to clinical attention affects about 7% of the population over 65 years of age, but a much larger proportion of those who are even older. There is an association between chronic physical ill health and disability on the one hand and depressive disorder on the other. Depression and dementia were the main conditions considered in the NSF for Older People.[6] They are also more common in certain populations (e.g. elderly medical inpatients and residents of care homes). Other disorders, such as phobias, are relatively common in the elderly population but rarely come to medical attention. They form a hidden reservoir of disability and distress. One of the main serious psychiatric disorders of younger adulthood, namely schizophrenia, persists into late life, and new cases arise. However, because of the special needs of elderly depressed and demented people, schizophrenia forms a smaller proportion of the work of old age psychiatrists. Other conditions, such as alcohol and drug abuse and personality disorder, are relatively rare but still need to be recognised and managed when they occur.

IMPLICATIONS FOR SERVICES

The last 30 years or so have seen the evolution of specialist multidisciplinary community-focused teams in the UK and elsewhere.[28-30] The previous sections of this chapter help us to consider how an ideal service might be designed. For example, the different ways of understanding ageing highlight the difficulties in defining a service or the target population by birth date alone. In recent years this has been recognised by old age psychiatrists increasingly offering services to younger people with dementia (who, however, face special problems because of their relative physical fitness and family circumstances). It is also clear that expectations and beliefs about what is normal, desirable or pathological in terms of age may affect the nature and usefulness of any service. The philosophy of ageing that is held (whether explicitly or implicitly) by the developers, commissioners and providers of a service will affect its priorities, aims and the range of treatments offered. The initial refusal of some service comissioners in the UK to authorise the use of the anti-dementia drugs demonstrated the importance of these hidden prejudices. However, beliefs and attitudes can be discussed and revised in the light of evidence.

Those working in psychiatric services for old people need to take into account their own ideas and definitions of ageing. Often we, like others, may be satisfied with too little because 'after all, what else can you expect at this age?'. Research on normal ageing (e.g. on the nature and extent of cognitive change in late life, and on the life cycle) can give a more optimistic view of the potential of old people.

For many older people, their use of the services may be relatively straightforward. Physical illness and psychiatric conditions can be diagnosed, and some conditions treated successfully, while others, such as dementia, can be managed in order to improve quality of life. Even this requires a specialised knowledge of ageing, and of the issues relevant to coping with disability. These issues may be similar for people of all ages, but old people have to face a different set of implications and life circumstances. When a man's wife dies at 30 years of age, he will have to deal with an event that is unusual and unexpected among his peers, but he may have more opportunity to remarry than a man whose wife dies when he is 70 years old, even though this is a more 'normal' event. Under these circumstances, the young man might grieve and then seek a new partner, while the older man might have to adapt to living alone and satisfying his emotional needs through friendships and family. If they were referred for depression to a service, both might benefit from a range of approaches, ranging from cognitive behavioural therapy through antidepressants to bereavement counselling or social skills training. The older man will probably be provided with help in the home and day care, yet his problem is likely to be only partially practical. It is important to consider why both he and service providers consider practical support satisfactory. In fact, he may need help to develop new skills. These may be both practical (enabling him to run his own household and perhaps develop an interest in cooking) and psychological (enabling him to identify his needs for companionship and set about satisfying them).

The real needs of old people with mental health problems must be recognised. Recognition does not, of course, mean that we can always help, but this holds true for all age groups. It is better to try to meet real needs than to waste money on irrelevant services that may even increase dependence and disability. Older people often face problems that cannot easily be solved, such as poverty and physical disability. Staff need support to understand and deal with tough situations, for without it they may end up discouraged and liable to avoid the patient's pain. Staff support and good training are essential parts of any service.

There have been massive changes in the way health services are organized in the UK. Responsibility for healthcare has been devolved to Wales and Scotland, and English health services are about to be reorganized in a way more radical than ever before. In the midst of all this change we do well to remember the importance of a culture of 'intelligent kindness'.[31] The full potential for general practitioners to shape services may at last be realised, and new ways of working at the primary/secondary care interface need to be developed and researched, perhaps through the use of devices such as integrated care pathways for the more common conditions. Mentally ill old people are often unable to protest effectively and, in the absence of advocacy, may suffer unnecessary hardship.

Mobility, mental well-being and even mortality are affected by the milieu in which an old person lives.

Opportunities abound for adventurous old age psychiatry services. This is a time of continued upheaval in the health service, and those who have the will also have the opportunity to shape emerging services. Some potential key areas include the following:

➤ developing the primary/secondary care interface

➤ agreeing integrated care pathways for common disorders in old age

➤ developing and quality assuring 'memory services' for the diagnosis and management of dementias

➤ adapting new ideas about how mental health services should be organized to meet the needs of older people

➤ making use of the opportunities arising from 'new ways of working' and changing roles

➤ (in England) learning to work effectively in a service where private providers and social enterprises may take on some or all of the work previously done exclusively by NHS organisations.

We can also expect changes in the ways in which ageing is seen to lead to an increase in the expectations of older people, so that they look after their own health better, feel more able to influence the communities in which they live, and assert themselves more. Under such circumstances they themselves will let service providers know more clearly what they need.

CONCLUSION

These are exciting times for old age psychiatry services. The increasing knowledge base, technical innovations and political change all make it possible to achieve a great improvement in psychiatric services for older people. Political changes, especially the marketisation of healthcare, also carry risks for older people. We not only need to keep up to date with current knowledge, but we also need to apply it in well-designed services where patients are valued as individuals and to learn to influence service commissioners to purchase the best services for older people with mental health problems.

REFERENCES

1 Sackett D, Haynes B, Guyatt GH and Tugwell P (1991) *Clinical Epidemiology: A Basic Science for Clinical Medicine.* Lippincott-Raven Publishers, Philadelphia, PA.

2 Kitwood T (1997) *Dementia Reconsidered: The Person Comes First.* Open University Press, Buckingham.

3 Wilkinson R and Pickett K (2010) *The Spirit Level: Why Equality is Better for Everyone.* Penguin Books, London.

4 National Health Service (1982) *The Rising Tide: Developing Services for Mental Illness in Old Age.* NHS Health Advisory Service, Sutton.

5 Age UK. *Later Life in the United Kingdom.* www.ageuk.org

6 Department of Health (2001) *National Service Framework for Older People.* DoH, London.

7 Department of Health (1999) *National Service Framework for Mental Health.* DoH, London.

8 Erikson EH (1965) *Childhood and Society.* Penguin Books, Harmondsworth.

9 Erikson EH, Erikson JM and Kivnick HQ (1986) *Vital Involvement in Old Age: The Experience of Old Age in Our Time.* Norton, New York.

10 Gutmann D (1989) *Reclaimed Powers: Towards a New Psychology of Men and Women in Later Life.* Basic Books, New York.

11 Kitwood T, Buckland S and Petre T (1995) *Brighter Futures: A Report into Provision for Persons with Dementia in Residential Homes, Nursing Homes and Sheltered Housing.* Methodist Homes for the Aged, Derby.

12 Treetops J (1992) *A Daisy Among the Dandelions: The Churches' Ministry with Older People. Suggestions for Action.* Faith in Elderly People Project, Leeds.

13 Froggatt A and Shamy E (1994) *Dementia: a Christian Perspective.* Christian Council on Ageing, Derby.

14 Tournier P (1972) *Learning to Grow Old.* SCM Press, London.

15 Koenig HG (1994) *Aging and God.* Howarth Pastoral Press, Binghampton, NY.

16 Langer EJ (1983) *The Psychology of Control.* Sage, Beverley Hills, CA.

17 Greer G (1992) *The Change.* Penguin Books, Harmondsworth.

18 Bengston VL, Cuellar JB and Ragan PK (1977) Stratum contrasts and similarities in attitudes towards death. *J Gerontol.* **32**: 76–88.

19 Kubler-Ross E (1969) *On Death and Dying.* Macmillan, New York.

20 Garner J (1999) Psychotherapy and old age psychiatry. *Psychiatr Bull.* **23**: 149–53.

21 Krüger S, Bertoni MA and Curran S (2011) Early detection of dementia. In Curran S and Wattis J, editors. *Practical Management of Dementia.* Radcliffe Publishers, London. pp. 49–76.

22 Strauss SE, Glasziou PP, Richardson WS and Haynes RB (2010) *Evidence-Based Medicine* (4e). Churchill Livingstone, Edinburgh.

23 Hall J and Howard D (2006) *Integrated Care Pathways in Mental Health.* Churchill Livingstone, Edinburgh.

24 Carkhuff R (1960) *Helping and Human Relations: A Primer for Lay and Professional Helpers.* Holt, Rinehart and Winston, Austin, TX.

25 Fulford KWM, Peile E and Carroll H (2012) *Essential-Values-Based Practice.* Cambridge University Press, Cambridge.

26 World Health Organization (1992) *The ICD-10 Classification of Mental and Behavioural Disorders: Clinical Descriptions and Diagnostic Guidelines.* World Health Organization, Geneva.

27 American Psychiatric Association (1994) *Diagnostic and Statistical Manual of Mental Disorders: DSM-IV.* American Psychiatric Association, Washington, DC.

28 Snowdon J, Ames D, Chiu E and Wattis J (1995) A survey of psychiatric services for elderly people in Australia. *Austr NZ J Psychiatry.* **29**: 207–14.

29 Wattis J, Macdonald A and Newton P (1999) Old age psychiatry: a specialty in transition – results of the 1996 survey. *Psychiatr Bull.* **23**: 331–5.

30 Draper B, Melding P and Brodaty H (2005) *Psychogeriatric Services: An International Perspective.* Oxford University Press, Oxford.

31 Ballatt J and Campling P (2011) *Intelligent Kindness: Reforming the Culture of Healthcare.* Royal College of Psychiatrists Publications, London.

FURTHER READING

➤ Bond J, Peace S, Dittmann-Kohli F and Westernof G (2007) *Ageing in Society: European Perspectives on Gerontology.* Sage Publications, London.

2

Assessment

INTRODUCTION

The skills needed to make an assessment and develop treatment and care plans for older people with mental health problems can best be developed in supervised clinical practice. Training should include regular reviews of the process and outcome for individual patients. The discipline of careful assessment, problem formulation and review of outcome is the foundation on which professional development is built. This is recognised in the importance attached to case-based discussions in psychiatric training and appraisal of consultants. Assessment of patients is often undertaken over a period of time, and it usually involves several different disciplines with different insights into the needs of old people. All relevant assessments must be taken into account. The care plan should be modified if necessary as new assessments are made.

This chapter will deal with the assessment of older people and the development of care plans as a framework for service delivery and professional education. Although the focus will be on mental health problems, physical, social and other forms of assessment will also be covered briefly. The self-discipline of good practice with regard to record keeping and review can be improved by the practice of regular peer group audit, which depends on careful record keeping. The use of standardised assessments can facilitate audit. Assessment of the patient is not a 'one-off' event. It should be repeated throughout treatment in order to evaluate progress and, if necessary, to modify treatment and care plans. This creates a 'feedback loop' which should result in high-quality care that is matched to the patient's current needs. It also provides a context for continuing professional development.

PSYCHIATRIC ASSESSMENT

Most elderly patients who are referred for psychiatric assessment should be seen initially in their own homes. This practice has the following advantages.

➤ The patient is seen in the situation with which he or she is familiar.
➤ The confusion and disorientation which may be caused by a trip to hospital, general practice surgery, social services offices or consulting rooms are avoided.
➤ The environment can be assessed as well as the patient (see Box 2.1).
➤ The patient's function in his or her own environment and the level of social support can be assessed.
➤ Neighbours and relatives are often readily available to give a history of the illness and its impact on them.

Box 2.1   Assessment of the home: some important factors

➤ General level of repair and tidiness of the property
➤ Who does the cooking/cleaning/shopping?
➤ Heating, lighting and ventilation
➤ Water supply
➤ Toilet and bathing facilities
➤ Cooking arrangements and food stocks
➤ The stairs
➤ Accident hazards
➤ Sleeping arrangements (has the bed been slept in?)
➤ Bottles or other evidence of alcohol abuse
➤ Tablets and medications (as expected or not?)

Set against this are the disadvantages from the assessor's point of view of time spent travelling and the difficulties of performing physical examinations and tests in the patient's home.

Older people who have to be assessed in hospital should be interviewed in a quiet, distraction-free environment, and every effort must be made to put them at ease. This is particularly important when assessing 'liaison' referrals on medical wards, otherwise any confusion will be compounded and a falsely pessimistic impression of function may result.

The introduction of 'new ways of working'[1] (NWW) means that fewer initial assessments are conducted by senior medical staff. Instead, initial assessments in the patient's home are undertaken by other (predominantly nursing) staff. Patients are then often brought to clinic to see the doctor. Doctors need to be able to trust these initial assessments if they are to work effectively and efficiently. From the patient's point of view there is nothing so tedious as having to answer the same questions every time they see a different member of the team. There is therefore a need for quality-assured standardised assessments that are shared by all the relevant members of the clinical team. It is now the responsibility of the employer to make sure that employees have the necessary skills and support to discharge their duties. However, doctors need to take a lead or at least be intimately involved in ensuring that assessments are adequate and carried out in a way that ensures high-quality care.

The patient's family and neighbours often have a key role to play in assessment and continuing management, and it is important to establish a good relationship with them. At the first interview, the patient and family will have many anxieties, some of which may be founded upon their own ideas about the purpose of the assessment. Time is well spent listening to the problems as they are seen by the patient and relatives. A still popular misconception is that the doctor, nurse or social worker has come to 'put away' the patient in some local institution. (The elderly patient's idea of what institutional care involves may also be quite different to that of the assessor.) Older people sometimes find it difficult to conceive that an admission to hospital or a residential home could be anything other than permanent. We need to take time to listen to these fears and to explain why we are visiting and the scope and limitations of any help that we can offer. Anxiety may inhibit the patient's and relatives' ability to grasp and remember what is being said. It may therefore be necessary to repeat the same information several times and to ask questions in order to clarify whether explanations have really been understood. Although an assessment may be commonplace to us, for the patient and their relatives it is often taking place at a crisis point in their life. An empathetic manner, acknowledging the patient's and relatives' concerns, will help them to realise that their worries have been taken seriously. This will help to establish a good relationship which will form the basis for further treatment.

Assessment instruments of varying lengths[2,3] combine some or all of the areas that follow in a systematic way, and such forms will increasingly be used as the core assessment document in multidisciplinary, multi-agency working.

History

The psychiatric history starts with the presenting complaint (or complaints), including how long it has been present and how it developed. Quite often the patient lacks insight and believes that nothing is wrong. In these circumstances, careful probing is appropriate. Sometimes, when it is difficult to obtain a clear history of the time course of an illness, the situation can be clarified by using 'time landmarks' such as the previous Christmas or some important personal anniversary. Often a proper history of the presenting complaint can only be obtained by talking to a friend or relative before or after seeing the patient. In other cases, information may have to be pieced together from a variety of sources (e.g. home care staff, the social worker, and friends and neighbours).

Usually it is best to follow the history of the presenting complaint with an account of the personal history. Most of us enjoy talking about ourselves, and it is quite easy to introduce the subject. A useful opening line is 'Tell me a bit about yourself – were you born in this area?'. Memory can be unobtrusively assessed while going through the history by reference to important dates (e.g. the date of birth of children and the date of marriage). The family history and the history of past physical and nervous complaints can be woven into this brief account of the patient's lifetime, and an assessment can be made of the patient's values, personality and characteristic ways of dealing with stress. Older people, like young ones, respond well to those who show a genuine interest in them. It is essential to ensure that the patient can see and hear the interviewer. Courtesy is vital, and talking 'across' patients to other professionals or to relatives generates anxiety and resentment, as does lack of punctuality.

The content of the history will vary according to time and circumstances, but should generally include the following:
➤ the presenting complaint and its history
➤ personal and family history (including illnesses and longevity)
➤ past illnesses and operations (including current illnesses and medication)
➤ previous personality
➤ alcohol and tobacco consumption
➤ current social circumstances and support.

Mental state examination

Level of awareness

At an early stage in the interview, the patient's level of awareness should be assessed. The patient may be drowsy as a result of lack of sleep or because of physical illness or medication. A rapidly fluctuating level of awareness is seen in acute confusional states, and a level of awareness that fluctuates from day to day is one of the clues to the diagnosis of chronic subdural haematoma and/ or diffuse Lewy body disease. Impaired awareness can lead to poor function on tests of cognition and memory and, if it is not recognised, can lead to an underestimation of the patient's true abilities. It is especially important to consider this if the patient has a recent-onset physical problem. The patient's ability to concentrate and pay attention is closely related to their level of awareness, but it may be affected by more mundane things. For example, if the patient is in pain, it may be very difficult for them to understand the relevance of giving an account of their mental state. Disturbance of mood and abnormal perceptual experiences can also impair attention and concentration.

Behaviour (and general appearance)

On a home visit, the patient's general appearance, behaviour, dress, personal hygiene and attitude to the interviewer can be observed directly, and their behaviour can also be deduced indirectly from the state of the house (see Box 2.1). Incontinence can often be detected by smell, and mobility can be checked by asking the patient to walk a few steps. Especially if the patient lives alone, inconsistencies between the patient's appearance and behaviour and the state of cleanliness and organisation of the household indicate either that there is a good social support network or that the patient has deteriorated over a relatively short period of time. Various schedules enable the systematic assessment of behavioural 'problems'. These are best seen as a function of the interaction between the patient and their environment, and not as intrinsic characteristics of the patient. The Neuropsychiatric Inventory (NPI)[4] and a shortened form of the Crichton Royal Behavioural Rating Scale (CRBRS)[5] (see Table 2.1) are useful examples. A scale has also been developed for the rating of behavioural symptoms by caregivers.[6] Scales that measure activities of daily living (ADL) concentrate on patients' ability levels (as opposed to concentrating on 'problem' behaviours). At least one scale has been developed specifically to assess this domain in people with dementia.[7]

Behavioural and ADL scales enable numerical values to be attached to a person's needs, abilities and problems in various important areas of behaviour.

Table 2.1 Modified Crichton Royal Behavioural Rating Scale (CRBRS)

Dimension		Score
Mobility	Fully ambulant, including stairs	0
	Usually independent	1
	Walks with minimal supervision	2
	Walks only with physical assistance	3
	Bed-fast or chair-fast	4
Orientation	Complete	0
	Orientated in ward, identifies individuals correctly	1
	Misidentifies individuals but can find way about	2
	Cannot find way to bed or toilet without assistance	3
	Completely lost	4
Communication	Always clear, retains information	0
	Can indicate needs, understands simple verbal directions, can deal with simple information	1
	Understands simple information, cannot indicate needs	2
	Cannot understand information, retains some expressive ability	3
	No effective contact	4

Dimension		Score
Cooperation	Actively cooperative (i.e. initiates helpful activity)	0
	Passively cooperative	1
	Requires frequent encouragement or persuasion	2
	Rejects assistance, shows independent but ill-directed activity	3
	Completely resistant or withdrawn	4
Restlessness	None	0
	Intermittent	1
	Persistent by day	2
	Persistent by day, with frequent nocturnal restlessness	3
	Constant	4
Dressing	Correct	0
	Imperfect but adequate	1
	Adequate with minimum supervision	2
	Inadequate unless continually supervised	3
	Unable to dress or retain clothing	4
Feeding	Correct, unaided, at appropriate times	0
	Adequate, with minimum supervision	1
	Inadequate unless continually supervised	2
	Needs to be fed	3
Continence	Full control	0
	Occasional accidents	1
	Continent by day only if regularly toileted	2
	Urinary incontinence despite regular toileting	3
	Regular or frequent double incontinence	4
Sleep	Normal – no sleeping tablets	0
	Occasional sleeping tablet or occasionally restless	1
	Regular sleeping tablets or restless most nights	2
	Sometimes disturbed despite regular sleeping tablets	3
	Always disturbed at night despite sedation	4

Such scales remind the assessor of important areas and enable discrepancies between different areas of performance to be highlighted, and potentially treatable problems are more easily seen and dealt with. Standardised scales also enable a rough comparison to be made between different patients and between different points in time for the same patient, even when the assessment is made by a different person. Finally, they provide an overall rating of disability which can be used as a guide to the patient's future needs for care. There are many such scales[8] and they are all imperfect, but they do at least provide a quick and systematic approach to the assessment of behaviour and abilities. The numerical values ascribed to such scales are, of course, arbitrary. For example, a patient who is disturbed all night may not be manageable at home, despite the fact that this factor only contributes a score of 4 to the total CRBRS score. Scores must therefore be interpreted skilfully, taking into account the amount of support available and the peculiar impact of certain behaviours.

Affect (mood)

Mood in the technical sense used by psychiatrists is more than just how we feel. It has been described as 'a complex background state of the organism', and it affects not only how we feel but also how we think and even the functioning of our muscles and bowels. Old people are not always used to talking about their feelings, and it can sometimes be quite difficult for them to find the right words. This is particularly true for men, who may not have the words to describe feelings ('alexothymia'). Especially where there are communication difficulties, one may have to resort to direct questioning (e.g. 'Do you feel happy?').

Although patients should always be asked to give an account of their mood, it cannot always be relied upon. Some elderly patients who are quite depressed do not confess to a depressed mood. This is often accompanied by somatisation – that is, the presentation of physical (hypochondriacal) complaints. It may also signify a more or less deliberate 'cover-up' due to fear of hospital admission. 'Anhedonia' (loss of the ability to take pleasure in life) is a useful indicator of severe depression. Psychomotor retardation (the slowing of thought and action) can be so profound that patients are unable to report their mood, or may even say 'I feel nothing', although their facial expression, tears, sighs, slowed movement or agitation may reveal depression. Specific questions should be asked about guilt feelings, financial worries, and concerns about health.

In cases where there is depressed mood, careful enquiry should be made about suicidal feelings. This can be introduced in a non-threatening way by using a question such as 'Have you ever felt that life was not worth living?'. If the patient responds positively to this, further probes can be made about present ideas of self-harm. If psychomotor retardation is present, the answer will take some time to emerge, and it is very easy to rush on to the next question before the patient has had time to respond to the previous one. Risk factors for suicide which should always be borne in mind include the following:
➤ male gender
➤ depression
➤ living alone
➤ bereavement

➤ long-standing physical illness or disability
➤ alcohol abuse.

Being aware of such risk factors complements but does not replace individual questioning.

One group of symptoms is often associated with severe 'biological' depression. This includes early-morning wakening, lower mood in the morning, and profound appetite loss and weight loss. Some self-rating scales have been designed to avoid the confusion caused by the use of 'somatic' symptoms in other scales. They include the following:
➤ the Geriatric Depression Scale (GDS)[9]
➤ short forms of the GDS[10]
➤ the Brief Assessment Scale for Depression Cards (BASDEC);[11] Even Briefer Assessment Scale for Depression (EBAS-DEP)
➤ the Cornell Scale for Depression in Dementia is also useful.[12]

These scales can provide indications of possible mood problems and, together with other scales (especially the Hospital Anxiety and Depression Scale, HAD),[13] can be useful for measuring the severity of depression, response to treatment and outcome. However, the frequent somatisation of depression in old age may cause 'false negatives' on such scales.

The opposite of depressed mood is elated mood, which is seen in mania and hypomania. In older patients, as in younger ones, decreased sleep, hyperactivity, flight of ideas, thought disorder, irritability and hypersexuality may be prominent symptoms.

Anxiety is common in old age, sometimes in response to the stresses of ageing in our society. The patient may be so worried about falling that, in order to avoid anxiety, they restrict their life severely. Thus a patient who has had one or two falls may, instead of seeking medical help, restrict him- or herself to a downstairs room in the house and never go out. As long as the patient continues to restrict their life, they experience little anxiety. Whereas in a young person such behaviour would almost certainly immediately lead to the patient being defined as 'sick', and a call for medical attention, in the elderly patient such restriction is all too easily accepted as 'normal'. When assessing anxiety, attention should therefore be paid not only to how the patient feels during the interview (which may in itself provoke anxiety!), but also to whether they can engage in the tasks of daily living without experiencing undue anxiety. Anxiety is an affect with physiological accompaniments, including a racing pulse, 'palpitations', 'butterflies in the stomach', sweating and diarrhoea. Patients not infrequently use the term 'dizziness' to describe not true vertigo, but a feeling of unreality associated with severe anxiety. Sometimes the physiological changes induced by over-breathing, such as tingling in the arms and even spasm of the muscles of the hand and arm, may make matters worse. The anxiety subscale of the HAD[13] provides an easy patient-related measure of the intensity of anxiety problems.

Panic attacks involving rapidly mounting anxiety, usually with physiological symptoms, may occur as a part of a phobic disorder, in isolation, or (perhaps most commonly in old age) in the context of a depressive disorder.

Phobias occur when the patient is afraid of particular objects or situations. Specific phobias (e.g. of spiders or heights) are relatively uncommon in old age, but generalised phobias (e.g. fear of going out or of social situations) are relatively common and can be crippling.[14]

Perplexity is the feeling that commonly accompanies delirium, and it may also be found in some mildly demented patients. The patient with delirium may experience visual or auditory hallucinations. If they need to be admitted to hospital, they may also be subjected to a whole series of confusing changes in their environment. People always try to make sense of their surroundings, so it is not surprising that patients in this kind of position feel perplexed. Perplexity is a useful diagnostic pointer for acute confusional states. The puzzlement ('delusional mood') experienced by some patients early in a schizophrenic illness in some ways resembles the perplexity that is found in acute confusion, but the other characteristics of acute confusional states (e.g. fluctuating awareness and physical illness) usually make the distinction clear.

Thought (and talk)

The form, speed and content of thought are all assessed. Formal thought disorder occurs in schizophrenia and includes thought blocking (when the patient's thoughts come to an abrupt end), thought withdrawal (when thoughts are felt to be withdrawn from the patient's head), thought broadcasting and thought insertion.

For a fuller description of these phenomena, the reader is referred to a standard textbook of psychiatric phenomenology.[15] Slowing of the stream of thought (thought retardation) is found in many depressive disorders. Slow thinking is also characteristic of some of the organic brain syndromes that are caused by metabolic deficiencies. Thought is speeded up in mania, often leading to 'flight of ideas' where one thought is built upon another in a way that is founded upon tenuous associations. In dementia, spontaneous thought is often diminished (so-called 'poverty of thought'). The patient with an acute confusional state has difficulty in maintaining a train of thought because of their fluctuating awareness. In dementias of metabolic origin, and in some cases of multi-infarct dementia, slowing of thought processes may be accompanied by difficulty in assembling the knowledge necessary to solve particular problems. The observer gets the impression that the patient grasps that there is a problem but is frustrated in trying to cope with it.

Content of thought is influenced by the patient's mood. The depressed patient will often have gloomy thoughts, with ideas of poverty or physical illness. The anxious patient's thoughts may be focused on how to avoid anxiety-provoking situations, and there may be unnecessary worries about all aspects of everyday living. The patient who feels persecuted may think of little else. Every noise or event will be fitted into the persecutory framework. Talk generally reflects the patient's thought, unless suspicion leads to concealment. Speech is also influenced by various motor functions. Slurred speech may be found in the patient who is drowsy or under the influence of drugs or alcohol, and it sometimes also results from specific neurological problems such as a stroke. Patients with multiple sclerosis may produce so-called 'scanning' speech in which words are produced without inflexion and with hesitation between words. Patients with severe parkinsonism may have difficulty in forming sounds at all (aphonia). Some difficulty in finding words and putting speech together is found in many patients with dementia, particularly those with Alzheimer's disease. This is one form of dysphasia. A stream of apparent nonsense (so-called fluent dysphasia) may occur in dementia, but is also sometimes associated with a stroke. The general behaviour of the patient, which is not 'demented', the sudden onset of the dysphasia and, sometimes, associated neurological signs and symptoms of stroke-related dysphasia, provide important diagnostic clues. Occasionally, fluent dysphasia, especially when it includes new words 'invented' by the patient (neologisms), may be mistaken for the so-called 'word salad' produced by some schizophrenic patients. The sudden onset and the absence of other signs of schizophrenia aid diagnosis. An assessment by a speech therapist who is experienced in this area may also help not only in diagnosis but also in suggesting management strategies that build upon the patient's residual (sometimes non-verbal) communication skills.

Hallucinations (false perceptions)

These can be defined as perceptions without external objects. Visual hallucinations are usually found in patients with acute confusional states or dementia, although occasionally they occur in patients with poor eyesight without measurable organic brain damage, especially if they are living alone in a relatively under-stimulating environment. In dementia they are more often found in diffuse Lewy body disease, and their presence may correlate with neuropathological findings.[16] Auditory hallucinations (hearing 'voices' or sometimes music or simple sounds) occur in a variety of mental illnesses, especially schizophrenia, where they may consist of a voice repeating the patient's thoughts or voices talking about the patient in the third person. They also occur in severe depressive illness and mania, when they are often consistent with the patient's mood. Hallucinations of touch (tactile), smell (olfactory) and even taste (gustatory) also occur. Hallucinations of being touched (especially those with sexual connotations) occur in schizophrenia, and hallucinations of smell (especially of the patient believing him- or herself to smell 'rotten') occur in severe depression.

Experiences similar to hallucinations sometimes occur in bereavement, and vary from 'hearing the footsteps' of the lost person to complex phenomena occurring in more than one modality. People explain these experiences in different ways. Some regard them as spiritual and comforting, while others may be afraid that they are 'going mad'.

Delusions (false beliefs)

A delusion is a false unshakeable belief that is out of keeping with the patient's cultural background. Delusions occur in fragmentary forms in organic mental states, but well-developed delusions are usually found only in schizophrenia and severe affective disorders, when ideas of poverty, guilt or illness may develop into absolute convictions. Ideas of persecution are also sometimes found in patients with depression of moderate severity, and these too can develop into full-blown delusions. Delusions of grandeur (e.g. that the patient has extraordinary powers of perception or is fabulously rich) are found in manic states. In paranoid schizophrenia, the delusional content is often very complicated and may involve persecutory activities by whole groups of people. These delusions may be supported by hallucinatory experiences.

Obsessions and compulsions

Obsessions occur when the patient feels compelled to repeat the same thought over and over again. They can be distinguished from schizophrenic phenomena such as thought insertion by the fact that obsessional patients recognise the thoughts as their own and try to resist them. Sometimes such thoughts may result in compulsive actions (e.g. returning many times to check that the door has been locked). Although they are characteristically a feature of obsessive-compulsive disorder, obsessional symptoms also occur in depressed patients, and apparently compulsive behaviour can also be a result of memory loss (e.g. when a patient repeatedly checks that the door is locked because they have forgotten that they have already done so). Many people without psychiatric conditions will experience a mild degree of compulsive checking (e.g. that they have locked their car doors), especially when under stress.

Illusions (misinterpreted perceptions)

Illusions occur when a patient misinterprets a real perception. Some somatic (hypochondriacal) worries can be based on this. For example, many older people have various aches and pains, but sometimes patients may become over-concerned about these and may begin to worry that they indicate some physical illness. Such misinterpretations of internal perceptions are not usually described as illusions, although the term would be quite appropriate. Acute confusional states also produce illusions when the patient, seeing the doctor approaching, misinterprets this as someone coming to do him harm and strikes out. This type of misinterpretation can often be avoided by appropriate management (see Chapter 9).

Orientation/memory/concentration and attention

These will be considered together because they are so interdependent. Orientation with regard to time, place and person should be recorded in a systematic way. The degree of detail would depend on the time available and the purpose of the examination. Orientation for time can easily be divided into gross orientation (e.g. the year or approximate time of day – morning, afternoon, evening or night) and finer orientation (e.g. the month, day of the week and hour of the day). Orientation for person depends on the familiarity of the individual chosen as a point of reference. Orientation for place also depends on familiarity. A useful brief scale which includes some items of orientation as well as some items of memory testing is the Abbreviated Mental Test (AMT) score, developed by Hodkinson[17] from a longer scale which has previously been correlated with the degree of brain pathology in demented patients[18] (see Box 2.2). A slightly longer related scale has been developed for community use,[19] although many people 'adapt' the AMT (e.g. by asking for the patient's home address rather than the hospital name). Like most short scales, the AMT is not always well used.[20]

Box 2.2   Ten-item Abbreviated Mental Test (AMT) score[17]

➤ Age
➤ Time (to nearest hour)
➤ Address for recall at end of test – this should be repeated by the patient to ensure that it has been heard correctly (e.g. 42 West Street)
➤ Year
➤ Name of hospital (place where patient was seen)
➤ Recognition of two people
➤ Date of birth
➤ Years of First World War
➤ Name of present monarch
➤ Count backward from 20 to 1.

Orientation is to a large extent dependent on memory, although it should never be forgotten that the patient may not know the name of the hospital in which they are staying, simply because they have never been told. Memory for remote events can be assessed when taking the patient's history. The ability to encode new material can be assessed by the capacity to remember a short address or to remember the interviewer's name. Many patients with dementia will have great difficulty in encoding and storing new memories. Sometimes, especially in the metabolic dementias, one can form the impression that the patient is encoding and storing new material but that they are having great difficulty in retrieving the memory when asked to do so. This has been described as 'forgetfulness'.

Drawing apraxia (the inability to copy simple drawings) and nominal aphasia (the inability to remember the names of common objects) can also be simply tested. A popular and relatively brief assessment of organic mental state is the Standardised Mini-Mental State Examination (MMSE),[21] which examines memory and a variety of other functions. However, the MMSE has been criticised because it is sensitive to educational attainment, its 'parallel' forms are not truly parallel, it suffers from floor and ceiling effects, and it is not sufficiently sensitive to change. Longer scales such as the CAMCOG[22] are probably too lengthy for routine clinical use. A variety of measures are used to evaluate outcomes in drug trials, especially the ADAS-COG,[23] but these are also generally too lengthy for routine use. They include the Cambridge Cognitive Examination (CAMCOG), the Alzheimer's Disease Assessment Scale Cognitive Subscale (ADAS-COG) and the Informant Questionnaire on Cognitive Decline in the Elderly (IQCODE).

Scales designed to elicit changes in the patient's memory from relatives and carers, such as the IQCODE,[24] were initially promising but have not been widely used.

A useful brief test which assesses a variety of cognitive functions is the 'clock test', in which the assessor presents the patient with a circle and asks them to fill in the numbers as on a clock face and set the time (e.g. to ten to two). This test is a useful screening tool for a broad range of cortical functions.[25] In more severe dementia, where other tests are disabled by 'floor' effects, the Hierarchic Dementia Scale (HDS)[26] may be of use.

More detailed descriptions of organic mental state examination can be found in Lishman's *Organic Psychiatry*.[27]

Insight and judgement

In severe psychiatric illness, insight (in the technical psychiatric sense) is often lost. Depressed patients may be unable to accept that they will get better, despite remembering previous episodes which have improved with treatment. Manic and paraphrenic patients may act on their delusions with disastrous consequences. Patients with severe dementia often do not fully realise their plight, which is perhaps fortunate. Patients with milder dementia may have some insight, especially in the metabolic and multi-infarct types of dementia where mood is (not surprisingly) also often depressed. Judgement is related to insight. This can be a particularly difficult problem with a moderately demented patient who is living alone or living with relatives but left alone for a substantial part of the day. Such patients may leave gas taps on and be dangerous to themselves and others, but at the same time they maintain that they are looking after themselves perfectly well and do not need any help, much less residential or nursing home care. They may also have a mistaken image of the care that they are refusing. Common sense, professional judgement and inter-disciplinary consultation are needed to make decisions in these cases. Consent and legal provisions are discussed further in Chapter 10.

A brief summary of mental state evaluation is given in Box 2.3. It has been put into a mnemonic form for ease of use ('a bath – o man – joe').

Box 2.3   Summary of mental state evaluation

➤ Awareness – level of consciousness (fluctuation), attention and concentration
➤ Behaviour – general appearance of the patient and their house; behaviour during interview
➤ Affect – depression (anhedonia), elation, anxiety, perplexity, suicide risk. Somatic changes – sleep pattern, constipation, appetite and weight in depression. Palpitations, tremor and churning stomach in anxiety
➤ Thought and talk – form, speed, content, dysarthria, dysphasia, perseveration
➤ Hallucinations, delusions, obsessions and illusions
➤ Orientation – with regard to time, place and person
➤ Memory – remote, ability to encode new information, forgetfulness
➤ Apraxia/dyspraxia – constructional, in daily activities
➤ Nominal dysphasia – everyday objects in order of increasing difficulty
➤ Judgement and insight
➤ Other cognitive functions (e.g. arithmetic, proverbs)
➤ Educational level and intelligence – make due allowance!

The psychiatric history and examination of the elderly patient take time, and must be tailored to the patient and approached in a sympathetic way.

Firing seemingly random questions in order to test memory and orientation is unlikely to get the best result from the patient. Time taken to conduct a proper assessment is not wasted; it avoids treatable illness going untreated or a potentially independent old person being forced into dependency in an institution.

Screening

Screening is used to detect illness at an early stage to enable early intervention. Dementia and depression are common conditions in old age and there are reasonable grounds for screening for them, especially in selected populations such as repeated attenders, those admitted to hospital with physical illness and residents in care homes. The AMT has been used to detect cognitive impairment. For depression, the Geriatric Depression Scale or one of its shorter forms may be useful. Certainly the low level of detection of depression in old age in general practice needs to be improved, given the exciting prospect of reducing distress and disability opened up by psychological therapies, as well as by the newer, less toxic antidepressants.

NEUROPSYCHOLOGICAL ASSESSMENT

Neuropsychological assessment is an extension of the type of brief clinical assessment of memory and other cognitive functions described above. Techniques for neuropsychological assessment are more standardised and time-consuming than the brief neuropsychiatric examination described above. They may be justified to assist in a variety of ways. For example, they may perform the following functions:

➤ delineating problems precisely in order to plan a psychological intervention
➤ providing a measure of current status so that the outcomes of interventions may be measured
➤ assisting with difficult diagnoses (although the CT or MRI scans are perhaps more often used these days).

Similarly, behavioural assessment in psychology is more detailed and specific, and more focused on planning interventions than on diagnosis. Because of this, the illustrative case histories used in this section include some details of treatment. The problems that arise from a primary neuropsychological dysfunction are often increased by the personal or interpersonal reaction to the problem, and both types of assessment are necessary to formulate the patient's problems accurately.

Assessment for cognitive, behavioural, psychodynamic and family therapies is not covered here, but is similar to the assessment of a young person. Particular issues relevant to psychotherapy with old people are discussed in more detail in Chapter 3.

In elderly people a number of factors alter the interpretation of assessments, including the effects of ageing on cognitive ability as well as emotional state, vocational opportunities and educational level. One study looked at drawing disability as a measure of constructional apraxia in elderly people with dementia,[28] and found that the drawing of a cube, sometimes used clinically, was not a useful discriminative test, as many non-demented elderly people also performed poorly.

Increasingly, general measures of intelligence and personality have been discarded because they do not define specific dysfunction, predict response to treatment or help in planning management. The need to develop normative data for neuropsychological tests with older individuals has been partly mitigated by the production of a number of tests and screening batteries specifically for use with older people. More attention has been paid in recent years to the assessment of dementia and of specific symptoms, such as poor memory. Neuropsychological assessment provides a detailed picture of a person's cognitive strengths and a definition of deficits which is valuable in planning intervention. In many areas expert neuropsychological assessment may not be available, but some of the basic information and methods can be used by other professionals. The main areas of neuropsychological deficit are outlined in Box 2.4. The Hierarchic Dementia Scale[8,26] covers these and others.

Practical issues

Careful selection of candidates for assessment is vital because of the time-consuming and sometimes stressful nature of neuropsychological tests. As with psychiatric assessment, careful preparation, explanation and attention to the setting are essential. Test results can be affected both by internal (emotional) factors, including fatigue, anger and anxiety, and by external (environmental) factors, such as the expectations and behaviour of others. More detailed descriptions can be found in standard texts.[29]

Standard tests

In the past, standard intelligence tests such as the Weschler Adult Intelligence Scale were used to test the cognitive functioning of older adults. The pattern of scores on each scale was compared for adults of different age bands, so that an individual's performance could be compared with that of a group of subjects of similar age. Some psychologists now use a more qualitative and informal approach, which relies on clinical experience, and which approximates more closely to psychiatric assessment.

Observation of the patient's behaviour and language in the initial interview is the starting point. The interviewer takes the history of the patient's problems and listens for difficulties in understanding questions and directions, word-finding problems, wandering off the point, repetitiveness, and so on. The history also provides information about memory, orientation and cognitive functions such as sequencing. An ordinary magazine can be used as an unthreatening way of testing reading, object and colour recognition, and the use of appropriate words to describe objects.[30] In this way, the stress and inevitable fatigue of the standard 'battery' can be minimised. If the patient is not able or willing to undertake even basic testing, observation can still provide valuable information. One psychologist, faced with a hostile response from a severely disabled and depressed woman, did not attempt formal testing, but instead just talked and listened to her. The woman not only struggled to converse with him, but rewarded him by remembering his name when he saw her again two days later. Observation during ordinary activity, such as dressing or eating, often provides information about spatial abilities, communication skills and apraxia. When specific deficits appear to be present, appropriate formal or informal assessments can be used to delineate them more clearly.

Box 2.4   Areas for neuropsychological assessment

Aphasia/dysphasia
➤ This refers to a difficulty in the use of language.
➤ Nominal aphasia – the person is able to recognise an object, but has difficulty in naming it appropriately.
➤ Receptive dysphasia – the person may have relatively normal speech, but has difficulty in understanding what is being said to them.
➤ Expressive – this is an impairment in the production of speech, which can range from complete loss to shortened sentences and mild word-finding problems.

Agnosia
➤ This refers to an impairment in the ability to recognise things.
➤ Visual agnosia – the person is not only unable to name an object, but will not be able to recognise it for what it is (unless they use another sense, e.g. touch).
➤ Spatial agnosia – the person is unable to find their way round familiar surroundings. There may also be distortion in the memory of spatial relationships of their surroundings.

Apraxia/dyspraxia
➤ This is impairment of the ability to carry out voluntary and purposeful movements (excluding other causes such as muscle weakness and failure of comprehension).

> ➤ Constructional apraxia – there is difficulty in putting together parts to make a whole (e.g. when making a simple drawing).
> ➤ Dressing apraxia – there is a particular difficulty in dressing (e.g. in fastening buttons or tying shoelaces).
>
> **Frontal**
> ➤ Deficits in this area result in a variety of qualitative signs, such as perseveration and emotional lability.
>
> **Memory**
> ➤ One simple distinction that is made is between short-term memory (memory for recent events) and long-term memory. Impairment of short-term memory is identified by assessing a person's ability to learn and recall new material over short time intervals.
>
> **Acquired knowledge**
> ➤ Difficulties with reading (dyslexia), writing (dysgraphia) and arithmetic (acalculia), which are all acquired abilities, can arise from particular cerebral lesions.
>
> **Subcortical**
> ➤ This is characterised by forgetfulness, slowness of thought, personality change and an impaired ability to manipulate acquired knowledge.

Sometimes specific deficits are put down to 'confusion' or are concealed. A woman was referred who appeared to be inconsistently orientated, with limited but coherent speech. She refused to take part in a formal interview. Brief observation and interaction showed that she was grossly receptively impaired, and was covering up her impaired understanding of speech with a repertoire of stock phrases and responses to social cues. Previously no one had considered receptive dysphasia, partly because ordinary assessment procedures did not allow for the possibility, and partly because the woman herself tended to conceal the extent of her problems.

The Middlesex Elderly Assessment of Mental State (MEAMS)[31] is a short test of overall cognitive ability, and the Rivermead Behavioural Memory Test[32] assesses memory. Both instruments are designed to assess practical, 'everyday' aspects of function. They produce less exact and comprehensive information than the longer test batteries, but this is often outweighed by the ease and speed with which they can be administered, and by their obvious practical relevance.

The environment and assessment

The environment is a major influence on behaviour (*see* Figure 2.1). Where particular neuropsychological deficits exist, based on permanent organic

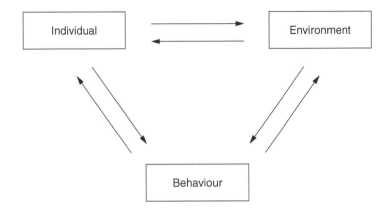

Figure 2.1 The effect of environment on behaviour.

damage, a change in behaviour and improvements in quality of life can still be achieved by offering strategies to compensate for impairments, or by changing the environment. Both physical design and modifying interactions with other people can reduce handicap. The analogy of a deaf person can be used here. If the physical environment is changed by providing a hearing-aid, and persuading other people to talk more loudly and clearly, the level of handicap can be reduced considerably. Strategies of this type include instruction on the use of lists, notices, prompts and diaries for managing the effects of memory problems, or providing information to the patient and their carers on the effects of the deficit, and helping carers to judge how and when to offer assistance. In future technology is likely to play an increasing part in prompting impaired memory.

Planning behavioural intervention

Single-case experimental design allows us to measure the extent of a problem and the effects of a treatment. This is easiest with discrete symptoms. A baseline measurement of the behaviour is taken – for example, information on the number of times a patient is incontinent during one week. If the frequency is fairly stable (say twice a day most days), the planned intervention can be put into action. If there is no pattern, so that the patient is incontinent several times a day during the first few days and then not at all for the last few, more information is collected. The frequency of incontinence can then be measured either consistently throughout the period of the intervention, or after an interval. Ratings should be continued for each intervention and for a period afterwards, so that the effects of the treatment itself, and of stopping the treatment, can be seen. Another example would be a patient with dementia shouting in a residential home, and a patient with this common behaviour is described in Case History 2.1.

Neuropsychological assessment highlights the limitations of some psychiatric diagnoses. Two individuals with the diagnosis of dementia may show different patterns of deficits. One may have a relatively mild impairment of short-term memory, but great difficulty in understanding speech, whereas another may have a severe impairment of short-term memory, but a relatively preserved ability to understand what is being said. In the former patient, the most helpful approach might be to speak in short sentences containing single ideas. In the latter case, the patient would probably benefit more from being regularly orientated with regard to time, person and place in a relaxed and non-threatening manner. An example that illustrates this is summarised in Case History 2.2 and Table 2.2. This case shows how an understanding of the deficits combined with simple behavioural strategies can help to reverse a potentially difficult situation. Attempts to focus on either alone would have been inadequate.

Case History 2.1

Mrs AO suffered from dementia and was referred by the staff of her residential home because of continuous shouting. On observation, it became clear that she was shouting out names. The other residents ignored Mrs AO, or occasionally shouted back at her, and she seemed to be isolated. The staff thought that she was calling them, but the psychologist noticed that the shouts became worse after one of her daughters visited. The daughter confirmed that the names her mother called had belonged to her sisters, who were now either dead or infirm and unable to visit. The psychologist felt that Mrs AO was lonely and that her shouts had resulted not in the company she had wanted, but in rejection by the other residents. Staff were asked to make contact with Mrs AO on a regular basis, by chatting to her as they passed by. They were helped to set up and run a reminiscence group, of which Mrs AO became a member. With established contact, first from staff and then from residents, Mrs AO's need to shout decreased, resulting in permanent improvement.

Case History 2.2

Mr GB was 77 years of age and lived at home with his wife. He was admitted to a medical ward suffering from a suspected occipital stroke. We were consulted about the advisability of discharging him home to his wife after he attacked nursing staff. It turned out that he was both frightened by the stroke and its effects on his perception, and frustrated by his impairment. He returned home on our advice with an agreement to attend day hospital once a week. The management plan shown in Table 2.2 considerably reduced his behavioural problems. After several months, he transferred to a day centre, and although he initially improved, over the next few months he showed an intermittent decline, probably indicative of a vascular dementia. He and his wife needed increasing support to manage at home, but despite the difficulties they appreciated the flexibility with which help was offered, were confident that they could cope, and retained their sense of humour.

Table 2.2 Mr GB's management plan

Neuropsychological and behavioural findings	Management implications
Right visual field defect	Staff to approach from the left at all times
Poor short-term memory	Routine provision of reality-oriented information and cues (e.g. 'My name is Sheila, it is 12 o'clock and lunch is being served. Can I show you the way?')
Visual agnosia and tactile agnosia (astereognosis)	Avoid activities that depend on visual and tactile cues, and concentrate on other activities, such as music
Inappropriate behaviours	Reinforce acceptable behaviour with staff time and interest, and reduce reinforcement of inappropriate behaviour
Insight retained (still applies when insight is lost)	Treat him as an adult; allow him choice
	Listen and respond to his requests; empathise about his loss of abilities
Preserved humour and social skills	Make use of his dry sense of humour

Dysfunction of the frontal lobes and related structures may produce a wide range of behavioural consequences, many of which are difficult to identify or quantify. The tearfulness of emotional lability may be misconstrued as depression, whereas the presence of disinhibition can lead to a misdiagnosis of hypomania or schizophrenia. An example that illustrates this is summarised in Case History 2.3 and Table 2.3.

Case History 2.3

Mrs SG, a 71-year-old woman, was referred when her husband complained that she was acting out of character. She had begun to swear, seemed more impulsive, and her husband said that he found it difficult to reason with her. A psychiatric diagnosis could not be made easily. Frontal signs were found in the absence of global impairment of intellect or other deficits (*see* Table 2.3). A CT scan confirmed the presence of changes in the frontal area. Mr SG was offered a session in which he explained the situation at home in detail and was helped to work out strategies for managing the problems that were identified. When alone, he was able to admit just how infuriating and problematic his wife's behaviour had become. She seemed to be unable to imagine the effects of her behaviour, nor could she stop herself from doing whatever came into her mind. She perseverated in some actions, and was unable to carry through a series of actions, so that she had become unable to bake or make a bed. He was advised to offer her prompts at the relevant point in a sequence, and to distract her if she showed signs of restlessness, perseveration or impulsivity. He was also advised on how to do this in a way that would be unlikely to annoy his wife. After trying these measures, he reported that he found it helpful to distract his wife from carrying out some of her impulsive ideas. Distraction also worked when she continued a behaviour inappropriately (perseveration). Giving step-by-step instructions proved more difficult, and Mr SG discussed more diplomatic ways of offering guidance. These steps improved the quality of the couple's relationship, and some of the more hostile behaviours (including the swearing) subsided. Occasional appointments remained necessary to reinforce and modify the strategies and to support the couple.

Table 2.3 Results of Mrs SG's neuropsychological investigation

Neuropsychological findings	Implications
Premorbid IQ = present IQ	No intellectual deterioration; failure on sequencing tasks; perseveration
Frontal signs	Difficulty in inhibiting actions; difficulty with abstract thought; lack of insight; emotional lability

Detailed assessment of neuropsychological functioning and appropriate management measures can produce marked improvements in the behaviour and quality of life of individuals who might otherwise be 'written off' as beyond help.[33] A further example that illustrates this is summarised in Case History 2.4 and Table 2.4.

One important aspect of Mr DN's management was to make staff aware of his slowness in carrying out tasks, which seemed to be organic in origin, possibly due to subcortical involvement. If this slowness had been interpreted as an inability to carry out or complete the task, the staff might have intervened inappropriately and effectively 'untrained' his self-care skills, making him highly dependent and institutionalised. Because staff at the old people's home were fully informed about the nature and extent of his deficits, they were able to offer care appropriate to his needs, ensuring that he was given sufficient time to act independently.

Case History 2.4

Mr DN was a 66-year-old living at home, supported by relatives who lived next door. He was admitted for assessment following increasing self-neglect. His relatives reported 'slowness rather than silliness'. He had suffered from epilepsy since he was 18 years old. A comparison of the degree and extent of these deficits (*see* Table 2.4) with his score on the Modified Crichton Rating Scale indicated that his behaviour and general functioning were better than might be expected. However, it was still thought that he would not be able to cope with living alone. With his agreement, he was eventually discharged to an old people's home.

Table 2.4 The degree and extent of Mr DN's deficits

Neuropsychological deficit	Management implications
Nominal aphasia	Staff to use cueing (e.g. to say first letter or syllable of word he cannot find)
Receptive dysphasia	Requests and conversations to include only simple, short sentences with one idea at a time
Subcortical involvement (slowness and occasional irritable outbursts)	Allow him time to complete tasks

PHYSICAL ASSESSMENT

The importance of working together

Specialists in the psychiatry of old age need to work closely with their medical colleagues, since psychiatric illness in the elderly is often complicated or precipitated by physical illness. Figure 2.2 illustrates how treatment for psychiatric disorder can cause physical illness, and vice versa.

No psychiatric examination, particularly in the elderly, is complete without a physical examination. Even in the patient's home a selective examination may be carried out, although it may be more appropriate to bring the patient to the clinic or the surgery for a more thorough examination. For a fuller account of assessment from the point of view of geriatric medicine, the reader is referred to *Assessing Elderly People in Hospital and Community Care.*[34]

Sensory impairment

Diminished sensory input, one of the techniques used in 'brainwashing', is often inflicted on old people by our slowness in recognising and correcting defects of sight and hearing. Sensory deprivation may be instrumental in producing paranoid states and in precipitating or worsening confusion. Poor hearing is also associated with depression. An estimate of visual and auditory acuity is part of the examination of every old person. Wax in the ears is an easily remedied cause of poor hearing. Other forms of deafness may require a hearing-aid. A great deal of patience may be needed to learn to use such an aid properly, especially if poor hearing has been present for some time. Look out for flat batteries or other faults in hearing-aids. For assessment purposes, more powerful portable amplifiers are useful. Even the inexpensive amplifiers linked to simple headphones (advertised in popular magazines) can be surprisingly effective. Visual defects range from those that are easily corrected by spectacles and other aids to those such as cataract and glaucoma that require more complicated surgical or medical intervention.

Medication

Medication for physical and psychiatric disorders is particularly likely to produce side-effects in old people and, unless a careful drug history is taken,

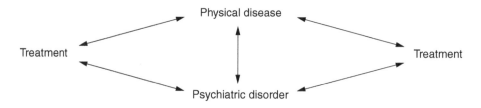

Figure 2.2 Relationships between physical disease and psychiatric disorder.

these side-effects may be mistaken for a new illness. Antihypertensives, digoxin and diuretics may be responsible for depressive symptoms, and all drugs with anticholinergic effects (including many antidepressants and antipsychotics) may produce confusion and constipation, among other side-effects. Box 2.5 gives a fuller list of drugs that produce confusion. The list is constantly expanding and the only safe advice is to assume that any medicine can potentially cause a wide range of unwanted effects.

Box 2.5   Drugs that have been reported to cause or increase confusion in older people

➤ Digoxin
➤ Diuretics
➤ Barbiturates
➤ Non-steroidal anti-inflammatory drugs
➤ Some antibiotics
➤ Benzodiazepines
➤ Tricyclic antidepressants
➤ Anti-parkinsonian drugs
➤ Antipsychotics
➤ Analgesics
➤ Antihistamines
➤ Anticholinergic drugs
➤ ACE inhibitors
➤ Calcium-channel blockers
➤ Histamine-2 blockers
➤ Anticonvulsants
➤ Corticosteroids

Benzodiazepines often have a 'hangover' effect and may accumulate over many days to produce confusion. When benzodiazepines are used as hypnotics, they should only be used in short courses. The same applies to the newer hypnotics. Benzodiazepines should not normally be used for depression, although occasional short-term use is justified in anxiety. Postural hypotension induced by tricyclic antidepressants or antipsychotics and other drugs may be mistaken for histrionic behaviour, and may be dismissed as part of the symptoms of an underlying depressive illness. Many drug interactions occur in older people, who are often on a number of different medications. When an elderly patient presents with a new symptom, their present medication should always be considered as a possible source of the symptom before further drugs are added.

Investigations

Investigations may be planned in the light of findings from the history and examination. There is still a need for conclusive research into the cost-effectiveness of investigations for potentially reversible dementia. The National Institute for Health and Clinical Excellence[35] recommends the following blood tests:

➤ routine haematology
➤ biochemistry tests (including electrolytes, calcium, glucose, and renal and liver function
➤ serum vitamin B_{12} and folate levels
➤ thyroid function tests.

Blood tests for syphilis and HIV are listed as optional. A midstream urine test should always be carried out if delirium is a possibility. An electrocardiogram (ECG) or chest X-ray is recommended only if there are specific indications.

Structural imaging is recommended in people with suspected dementia to exclude other cerebal pathologies and help to establish the subtype of diagnosis. Magnetic resonance imaging (MRI) is preferred, although computed tomography (CT) is acceptable. Perfusion hexamethyl-propylenamine oxime (HMPAO) single photon-emission computed tomography (SPECT) is recommended to help to differentiate Alzheimer's disease, vascular dementia and frontotemporal dementia if the diagnosis is in doubt. Electroencephalography (EEG) is only recommended if Creutzfeldt–Jacob disease is suspected or if there is coincidental epilepsy.

SOCIAL ASSESSMENT

Quantitative assessment

The quality and quantity of relationships need to be considered. The quantity of relationships can easily be summarised in a social network diagram.[36] In our adaptation of this (*see* Figure 2.3), a box is drawn which contains the name of the patient and members of their household, together with a brief note of the type of accommodation in which they live.

Down one side of the box the timing of visits by friends and family who live outside the household is noted, and down the other side the timing of services such as home care, warden, meals-on-wheels service, etc. is listed. The base of the box is used for visits out of the household by the patient.

Case History 2.5 illustrates how the social network diagram can be used not only to summarise current arrangements, but also to plan their improvement.

Qualitative assessment

The quality of relationships can be assessed both indirectly from the past history of the patient and their family, and more directly during a joint interview.

Case History 2.5

Mrs T, a 73-year-old widow who was living alone, presented to the physicians in geriatric medicine with repeated falls. Investigations showed no cause for the falls, and the patient was managed symptomatically. About 18 months after the initial assessment it became evident that she was abusing alcohol and that this was the cause of her falls. Her nephew discovered a cache of empty brandy bottles under the sink with a number of different brand names, which had been unwittingly supplied by a number of helpers, each of whom thought he or she was the patient's only source of supply! Psychiatric assessment revealed that the patient had started to abuse alcohol for the first time in her life in a misguided attempt to relieve depression following the loss of her husband. After a period of inpatient withdrawal and treatment for nutritional deficiency and depression, her social network was reorganised in a way that helped her successfully to fill her life with activities other than drinking alcohol (*see* Figure 2.3).

It is worth trying to assess what each member of the family is aiming for, and how open family members are in their communication with each other. Sometimes there is a pathological attachment between family members which results in a maladaptive pattern of caregiving.

The growing physical and psychological dependence of old people with progressive illnesses such as Parkinson's disease and Alzheimer's dementia can put extraordinary stress on family relationships that will reveal previously carefully disguised 'fault lines'. Skill in family therapy can best be developed in supervised practice, and there are now a few units in the UK which take an interest in this work. Traps for inexperienced workers include collusion in the pattern of family relationships, or ill-timed, unproductive confrontation. Because services are sometimes only made available when a crisis has occurred and family members are at the end of their tether, we do see relatives who may be labelled as 'rejecting'. This happens less frequently than it used to, as the development of more effective services now leads to earlier intervention before a crisis has occurred. Even when a crisis has occurred, it may be possible to manage it in such a way that the relatives realise that they can continue to cope, with the help of appropriate services.

(a)

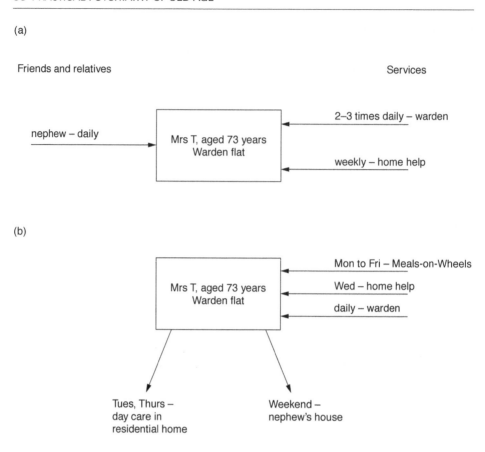

Figure 2.3 The social network diagram. (a) Before intervention. (b) After intervention.

The carer's right to assessment

Recently, the role of family carers and friends in improving the quality of life of disabled people has been recognised in the UK, and carers now have a statutory right to have their own care needs assessed by social services.

Making allies of the family

An important factor here is a prompt response, usually in the form of a home visit. This is the first step in impressing upon the family the fact that help is available. Carers are relieved to find someone who has time and is willing to listen to the problems they are facing, and to provide practical help. This can cause family members to re-evaluate their attitudes and avoid premature decisions to put an elderly relative into a care home. Family members' understanding and assessment of a situation may be quite different to the professional viewpoint, and must be 'heard' and respected by the team that is planning help. The appropriate use of short-term care home or hospital admission, day care, family care and home care services to relieve perceived strains can enable the family to cope. Although the medical members of the team should include social and support needs in their initial assessment, where these are complicated further, expert assessment by another team member is justified, whether this is a social worker, an occupational therapist or a community psychiatric nurse.

The need for 24-hour care

When an old person lives alone and suffers from moderate or severe dementia, it may be impossible to provide adequate supervision without admitting them to a long-stay care facility. This should not be viewed as a 'failure' to keep the person 'in the community', but as the appropriate use of one of a range of options for providing care. Management depends on psychiatric and medical diagnosis as well as the family and social situation, and the skill of the psychogeriatric team lies in understanding the various components of the situation and how they interact in order to produce the best possible management plan.

THE BALANCING ACT

The old person living at home can be considered to be performing a delicate balancing act (*see* Figure 2.4). The old person in this illustration is balancing on a three-legged stool. The legs are her physical, psychological and social 'health'. If any of the legs are taken away, the person becomes subject to ill health in a manner which may not appear to be directly related to the underlying cause.

Case History 2.5 illustrated this well. The underlying problem was unresolved grief and loneliness, leading to depression and excessive drinking, but the initial presentation was to the medical services with falls. Case History 2.6 provides a further illustration.

Case History 2.6

An elderly widow who was living alone suddenly became breathless. Her family doctor thought that she might have had a mild heart attack a few days previously and decided to manage her at home. Two days later she became acutely disturbed, barricading herself in her room and hurling abuse (and small items of furniture) at those who tried to help her. The family doctor made a correct diagnosis of acute confusional state secondary to her physical illness. The doctor was unable to secure a medical admission because of the patient's confusion, but managed to admit her to a psychiatric unit for old people where medical treatment of her heart failure produced a rapid improvement in her mental state.

Hopefully, the closer cooperation that now exists between medical and psychiatric services for old people means that today this patient would be accepted for medical admission.

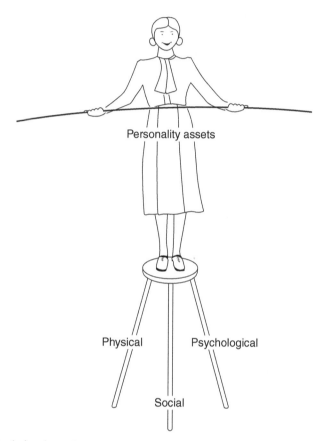

Personality assets

Physical   Psychological

Social

Figure 2.4 The balancing act.

PROBLEM FORMULATION AND MANAGEMENT: 'CARE PLANNING'

Each patient needs a 'tailor-made' care plan of medical, psychological, nursing and social management. This will often need to be agreed on a multidisciplinary basis after assessments by several different members of the team. General practitioners and general hospital doctors usually refer to Mental Health Services through a 'single point of access'. Initial assessments are made at home by appropriately trained staff, usually nurses, backed up by home visits or outpatient consultations with psychiatrists or other team members as appropriate. Patients who are referred chiefly for memory problems are often assessed through a separate but linked memory services pathway. It is essential that the initial assessment includes an overall view of medical, psychological and support needs and social factors, and that the family are given some idea of the likely management and the help available at that first assessment. This includes at least an outline knowledge of local home care, day care, voluntary groups, financial allowances and other relevant sources of help. The care plan will usually evolve and develop as the patient's condition and circumstances change.

Care planning procedures[37] provide a framework for this process in the UK. They introduced a more carefully monitored procedure to replace the informal approach that previously prevailed. The advantages of a more formal procedure are that all stakeholders are more likely to get a 'say' in producing the plans, and that there is less likelihood of poor communication leading to failure. The disadvantages are that the new procedures can be time-consuming and impose a bureaucratic burden on overworked clinicians. This in turn can lead to a slower and less flexible team response, where the central purpose of caring for the patient is obscured by the necessity to fill in forms. Ideally, a synthesis of the personal clinical approach and methodical documentation and process can be achieved, but not without supporting clerical resources and information technology. Care management is a related philosophy which social services departments introduced. This approach potentially allowed a more flexible deployment of resources, although there is also a danger that it could simply become a crude mechanism to control costs and transfer blame. A review of research into care management suggests that approaches in which the care manager is a clinician who is actively involved with the patient work better than those where the care manager is a 'broker' not directly involved with the patient.[38]

Timing and teamwork

A medical, psychosocial and nursing 'diagnosis' is only the beginning of patient management. Because of the multiplicity of problems faced by patients, a haphazard approach to management is time-wasting, inefficient and potentially dangerous. For example, arranging long-term home care support for people who are suffering from undiagnosed and untreated depressive episodes may 'keep them going' in the community, but does not permit them to have the best possible quality of life, and may lead to a treatment-resistant depressive illness or even to suicide. Arranging nursing home care for people whose confusion is due to an undiagnosed medical condition denies them proper treatment, reduces their independence, wastes resources and may also have fatal consequences. On the other hand, a narrowly medical approach to people's problems will also reduce their prospects of independent living. If the patient in Case History 2.5 had not been managed with attention to the social and emotional factors underlying the alcohol abuse, it is much more likely that the abuse would have recurred, producing permanent physical or mental damage.

Teamwork is therefore essential, and it is most important that case management, care planning and single assessment procedures do not detract from the tradition of multidisciplinary teamwork that has been built up in many psychogeriatric services.

The traditional psychiatric formulation of a patient's problems has always included not only the psychiatric diagnosis but also all relevant medical, psychological and social factors. Care plans do the same by listing the patient's needs, planning interventions to meet those needs, and agreeing responsibility between professionals and agencies for different components of the plan. Although these plans are ideally agreed at a meeting of the patient, caregiver(s), health service and social services staff, in practice we have found this too time-consuming to be accommodated within the available resources. Now we reserve full meetings for difficult cases, and we use an abbreviated (although still firmly multidisciplinary) procedure for the majority of cases. Community team members review patients regularly in a multidisciplinary forum, but only arrange formal meetings as and when circumstances demand them.

RISK ASSESSMENT AND MANAGEMENT

Assessing risk is an important aspect of any psychiatric assessment. Risk can be to self or others and may arise from a variety of causes. The risk of self-harm is high in older people with depression (*see* Chapter 5). Risk can also arise from self-neglect or inability to self-regulate in dementia, delirium (*see* Chapter 4) and mood disorders (*see* Chapter 5). Various standardised risk assessments are used in different organisations. The important thing is to assess and document risk appropriately and to make clear plans to reduce risk as far as is possible.

OUTCOME MEASUREMENT, FEEDBACK AND AUDIT

The emphasis on accountability, and in the UK the emphasis on clinical governance, add a new imperative to the need to measure outcomes.[39] Ideally outcomes should be assessed from a variety of perspectives (e.g. patient, carer, provider, commissioner), and measures should be found which will reflect a broad consensus on 'good' and 'bad' outcomes between different viewpoints. A distinction should also be made between overall measures of outcome (e.g. the HoNOS 65+), individualised measures focused on each patient, and specific measures designed for use in particular diagnostic groups. HoNOS 65+ belongs to the HoNOS family (Health of the Nation Outcome Scales), the usefulness of which as tools in routine practice has recently been questioned.[40] In one small study of outcomes on an acute psychiatric ward for old people, the HAD completed by the patient emerged as a good overall measure for the outcome of depression, and it correlated closely with a variety of 'viewpoints'.[41]

Measures such as this, which can 'summarise' outcomes in specific disorders and settings, ideally need to be combined with the less sensitive but more global measures. Building such measures into care pathways would enable routine audit of performance. This could produce feedback to the clinical team and enable comparisons of performance both between teams and within teams over time. As well as increasing accountability, this type of measure should encourage reflective practice and improve clinical quality. The drawback is that researching *and applying* such measures requires time and money. The time that is needed can be reduced by increasing efficiency through good information technology, but this also requires investment.

CONCLUSION

This chapter has dealt with the various aspects of assessment in psychiatric disorder in old people and how these can be brought together to formulate an overall care plan for the patient. It has advocated a flexible team approach to individual patients. However, we recognise that some standardisation of information collection and use can help to foster cooperation between different agencies and professions. In addition, it can provide a framework for routine audit of clinical performance designed primarily to improve quality rather than to feed a bureaucratic machine. However, this framework should be properly supported and should improve practice, which it cannot do if it takes clinician time away from patient care.

REFERENCES

1 Department of Health (2005) *New Ways of Working for Psychiatrists*. Department of Health, London.
2 InterRAI™ www.interrai.org
3 Morgan SC (2000) *Clinical Risk Management. A Clinical Tool and Practical Manual*. The Sainsbury Centre for Mental Health. www.centreformentalhealth.org.uk/pdfs/clir (accessed 9/5/12).
4 Cummings JL, Mega M, Gray K *et al* (1994) The Neuropsychiatric Inventory; comprehensive assessment of psychopathology in dementia. *Neurology*. 44: 2308–2314.

5 Cole MG (1989) Inter-rater reliability of the Crichton Geriatric Behaviour Rating Scale. *Age Ageing.* **18**: 57–60.

6 Rabins PV (1994) The validity of a caregiver-rated brief behaviour symptom rating scale (BSRS) for use in the cognitively impaired. *Int J Geriatr Psychiatry.* **9**: 205–10.

7 Bucks RS, Ashworth DL, Wilcock GK and Siegfried K (1996) Assessment of activities of daily living in dementia: development of the Bristol activities of daily living scale. *Age and Ageing.* **25**: 113-120.

8 Burns A, Lawlor B and Craig S (2004) *Assessment Scales in Old Age Psychiatry.* Informa Healthcare, London.

9 Yesavage J, Brink T, Rose T *et al* (1983) Development and validation of a geriatric depression screening scale: a preliminary report. *J Psychiatr Res.* **17**: 37–49.

10 Yesavage J (1986) Geriatric Depression Scale (GDS): recent evidence and development of a shorter version. *Clin Gerontol.* **9**: 165–73.

11 Adshead F, Daycody D and Pitt B (1992) BASDEC: a novel screening instrument for depression in elderly medical inpatients. *BMJ.* **305**: 397.

12 Alexopoulas GS, Abrams RC, Young RC and Shamolan CA (1988) Cornell scale for depression in dementia. *Biol Psychiatry.* **23**: 271–84.

13 Zigmond A and Snaith P (1983) The Hospital Anxiety and Depression Scale (HAD). *Acta Psychiatr Scand.* **67**: 361–70.

14 Lindesay J (1991) Phobic disorders in the elderly. *Br J Psychiatry.* **159**: 531–41.

15 Oyebode F (2008) *Sims' Symptoms in the Mind: An Introduction to Descriptive Psychopathology* (4e). Saunders, London.

16 Forstl H, Burns A, Levy R and Cairns N (1994) Neuropathological correlates of psychotic phenomena in confirmed Alzheimer's disease. *Br J Psychiatry.* **165**: 53–9.

17 Hodkinson HM (1972) Evaluation of a mental test score for assessment of mental impairment in the elderly. *Age Ageing.* **1**: 233–8.

18 Blessed G, Tomlinson BE and Roth M (1968) The association between quantitative measures of dementia and senile change in the grey matter of elderly people. *Br J Psychiatry.* **144**: 797–811.

19 Kay DW, Black SE, Blessed G and Sahgal A (1992) The prevalence of dementia in a general practice sample: upward revision of reported rate after follow-up and reassessment. *Int J Geriatr Psychiatry.* **5**: 179–86.

20 Holmes J and Gilbody S (1996) Differences in use of abbreviated mental test score by geriatricians and psychiatrists. *BMJ.* **313**: 465.

21 Molloy DW, Alemayehll E and Roberts CR (1991) Reliability of a standardized mini-mental state examination compared with the traditional mini-mental state examination. *Am J Psychiatry.* **148**: 102–5.

22 Greifenhagen A, Kurz A, Wiseman M, Haupt M and Zimmer R (1994) Cognitive assessment in Alzheimer's disease: what does the CAMCOG assess? *Int J Geriatr Psychiatry.* **9**: 743–50.

23 Curran S and Wattis J (1997) Measuring the effects of anti-dementia drugs in patients with Alzheimer's disease. *Hum Psychopharmacol.* **12**: 347–59.

24 Christensen H and Jorm AJ (1992) The effect of premorbid intelligence on the mini-mental state and IQCODE. *Int J Geriatr Psychiatry.* **7**: 159–60.

25 Shulman KI, Gold DP, Cohen CA and Zucchero CA (1993) Clock-drawing and dementia in the community: a longitudinal study. *Int J Geriatr Psychiatry.* **8**: 487–96.

26 Ronnberg L and Ericsson K (1994) Reliability and validity of the hierarchic dementia scale. *Int Psychogeriatrics.* **6**: 87–94.

27 David AS, Fleminger S, Kopelman MD, Lovestone S and Mellors JDC (2009) *Lishman's Organic Psychiatry.* Wiley-Blackwell, Chichester.

28 Moore V and Wyke MA (1984) Drawing disability in patients with senile dementia. *Psychol Med.* **14**: 97–105.

29 Woods R and Clare L (2008) *Handbook of the Clinical Psychology of Ageing.* Wiley, Chichester.

30 Holden UP and Woods RT (1995) *Positive Approaches to Dementia Care.* Churchill Livingstone, Edinburgh.

31 Golding E (1989) *The Middlesex Elderly Assessment of Mental State.* Available from www.pearsonassessments.com.

32 Wilson B, Cockburn J and Baddeley A (1985) *The Rivermead Behavioural Memory Test.* Thames Valley Test Company, Bury St Edmunds.

33 Woods RT (ed.) (1999) *Psychological Problems of Ageing: Assessment, Treatment and Care.* Wiley, Chichester.

34 Philp I (1994) *Assessing Elderly People in Hospital and Community Care.* Farrand Press, London.

35 National Institute for Health and Clinical Excellence (NICE) (2006 and 2011) *CG42 Dementia: Supporting People with Dementia and their Carers in Health and Social Care.* http://nice.org.uk/dementia-cg42/guidance#diagnosis-and-assessment-of-dementia (accessed March 2012).

36 Capildeo R, Court C and Rose FC (1976) Social network diagram. *BMJ.* **1**: 143–4.

37 Department of Health (1990) *Joint Health/Social Services Circular: Health and Social Services Development – 'Caring for People', the Care Programme Approach for People with a Mental Illness Referred to the Specialist Psychiatric Services.* Department of Health Publications Unit, London.

38 Burns T (1997) Case management, care management and care programming. *Br J Psychiatry.* **170**: 393–5.

39 Charlwood P, Mason, A, Goldacre M, Cleary R and Eilkinson E (1999) *Health Outcome Indicators: Severe Mental Illness. Report of a Working Group to the Department of Health.* National Centre for Health Outcomes Development, Oxford.

40 Stein GS (1999) Usefulness of the Health of the Nation Outcome Scales. *Br J Psychiatry.* **174**: 375–7.

41 Wattis JP, Butler A, Martin C and Sumner T (1994) Outcome of admission to an acute psychiatric facility for older people: a pluralistic evaluation. *Int J Geriatr Psychiatry.* **9**: 835–40.

3

General principles of treatment

INTRODUCTION

Before patients can be effectively treated it is important that they have had a detailed medical, psychological and social assessment so that the most appropriate treatment can be initiated. This has been described in Chapter 2. Establishing the facts is an important aspect of assessment, but there is another aspect of assessment and treatment that can be characterised as 'personal' or 'relational'. It is difficult to characterise but it pervades good practice. It signifies accepting patients and carers as individuals who have their own values. This helps to develop a relationship of trust in which shared decision making can work effectively. This facilitates the more technical aspects of assessment and treatment. The assessment of the patient is important not only to enable an accurate diagnosis to be made, but also because it is during this period that the doctor begins to develop a relationship with the patient. If this relationship is not developed, and if the patient does not trust the doctor or other healthcare professional, it is likely that it will be more difficult to engage them in treatment. Diagnosis can be especially difficult in older people who are coping with age-related changes in somatic and cognitive functions, physical illness, the effects of (often numerous) drugs, and losses (including loss of health, mobility, income, family, friends, partners and independence, to name but a few). A quote from Menninger et al[1] is particularly relevant to older people: 'There are no psychiatric disorders, only psychiatric patients'. Older people with mental health problems may be considerably more difficult to compartmentalise into specific psychiatric categories compared with younger people. In addition, treatment of the individual patient often requires working with the whole family, especially in the case of patients with moderate to severe dementia. It also requires that we inform patients and involve them (and sometimes their carers) in decisions about how to manage their problems.

CARE PATHWAYS

Care pathways present a way of considering the overall management of patients. The National Institute for Clinical Excellence (NICE) has produced a series of care pathways that link NICE guidance, including evidence-based guidance and technology appraisals (http://pathways.nice.org.uk/). The pathways include several in the mental health field, of which the following are relevant to old age psychiatry:
- dementia
- depression
- generalised anxiety disorder
- panic disorder
- post-traumatic stress disorder
- self-harm
- alcohol-use disorders.

These pathways generally produce a stepped or staged approach to the management of disorders, depending on severity, chronicity, complexity, risk and response (or failure of response) to treatment. The early steps are generally in primary care, and for many conditions involve self-help, guided self-help and low-intensity psychological interventions. Higher-intensity psychological interventions and simple pharmacological interventions often come next, and more complex or risky cases (including dementia at the diagnostic stage) are often recommended for referral to specialist services. Although the details of the care pathways only apply to the English NHS, the principles have universal validity and readers can adapt them to their local circumstances or use parallel local guidance.

Another initiative in the English part of the UK is Improving Access to Psychological Therapies (IAPT: www.iapt.nhs.uk/iapt/). A useful practice guide on their website discusses the problems of access to psychological therapies for older people and some initiatives to overcome the barriers (http://iapt.nmhdu. org.uk/silo/files/older-people-positive-practice-guide.pdf). However, it remains likely that access to psychological therapies for older people lags behind that for younger adults in many areas.

When discussing individual conditions in later chapters we have used the broad outlines provided by the NICE pathways, although we have concentrated on the more complex cases that are likely to find their way to secondary mental health services for older people.

DEVELOPMENT AND PSYCHOSOCIAL INTERVENTIONS IN OLD AGE

The concepts of 'old age' and 'normal ageing' have been discussed in Chapter 1. This section is concerned with development in old age, particularly in relation to psychological approaches to treatment. Most people have a rough plan for their life from an early stage. This will include events such as leaving school, getting a job, building a career, going to university, getting married and having children, to name but a few. Mid-life is typically a time for reconsidering one's aims and goals in life and, if not successfully negotiated, this may lead to a 'mid-life crisis'. As was discussed in Chapter 1, Erikson has produced a useful model of the psychosocial stages that individuals pass through from infancy to old age (for a summary of this, *see* Table 1.1).

At each stage there is a 'conflict' that has to be 'resolved' either positively or negatively before the individual is able to proceed to the next stage. In old age this conflict is between 'ego-integrity' and 'despair', as individuals struggle to come to terms with the limits of their existence and their achievements, and the loss of a future. Erikson's model is based on psychoanalytic theory, and implies that personal growth is achieved through the successful resolution of psychosocial conflicts which are brought about by maturational processes and external conditions. This model suggests that psychosocial development continues through to old age, and it emphasises that this process is an active and dynamic one.

People experience many changes as they grow older. It is surprising how well most older people cope with these changes, which can include normal changes in bodily appearance (e.g. loss of hair, loss of skin tone, wrinkles, greying of the hair and loss of physique) as well as changes to health (e.g. arthritis, heart disease and dementia, to name just a few). Loss of mobility may be particularly crippling for older people, and this, combined with changes in sensory function, particularly vision and hearing, can rapidly result in isolation. In addition, older people experience a wide range of other losses, including relationships and roles. These include children moving away, loss of friends and partners due to death, and role changes such as retirement. To compound the situation, older people have a reduced economic base and may have to give up their home and everything that this entails in order to go into a nursing or residential home. There they may be further de-skilled to the extent that virtually everything is done for them. They may also be treated like children and find their choices restricted by staff. Despite this, many older people adapt well but, not surprisingly, others may experience difficulties. Older people in these circumstances may feel that they have lost 'control' of their lives, and this can lead to depression, which often goes unrecognised and untreated.

An important and inescapable aspect of old age is that of death. Old age requires people to face death. In late adulthood, individuals have to come to terms with the meaning of their existence and decide for themselves whether their life has been worthwhile. It is during this time that the conflict between 'integrity' and 'despair' has to be resolved, and if old age is to be successful, this conflict has to be resolved in favour of 'integrity'. If this conflict is successfully resolved, the traditional quality attributed to old age, namely wisdom, will emerge. Fear of death seems to become less common as people age.[2] This is partly due to the fact that older people have often experienced a number of frightening or stressful events in life, which to some extent prepare them for the final experience, namely death. However, different individuals may react to the prospect of death in different ways.[3] These include denial, depression and despair, anger, attempts to bargain and control, and acceptance and hope. Older people have as much capacity to enjoy life as younger individuals, and the great majority of older people do so. For those people who find the challenges of old age too much, psychological input can provide a means to enable them to enjoy and reach their full potential during their remaining few years of life.

PSYCHOLOGICAL THERAPY

A simple way of conceptualising psychological therapy is to think of the interdependence between behaviour (actions), cognitions (beliefs and attitudes) and feelings or emotions in a given situation. Psychological therapy aims to change one or more of these elements, thus leaving the person better able to cope. These three aspects of self (behaviour, cognitions and emotions) have some theoretical basis in psychological therapy, including behaviour therapies, cognitive therapies and the psychodynamic therapies. In addition to these three core schools of therapy, there are additional techniques which can be particularly useful, including family therapy, which could theoretically be based on any of the three broad therapeutic models, and which also takes into account systems theory. Age is no longer viewed as a contraindication for psychological therapy, but there are many practical difficulties in accessing psychological therapies for older people, and the majority of psychotherapeutic work is still done with younger patients. However, if one returns to the model proposed by Erikson, it is clear that development continues into old age and conflicts still have to be resolved. It is also clear from therapists who have worked successfully with older people that it is quite possible to use the full range of psychotherapeutic models in a conventional way, although modified by knowledge of the ageing process and the difficulties associated with older patients. Moreover, studies have shown that the full range of therapies has been successful in older people, including psychodynamic approaches,[4] behaviour therapy,[5] cognitive behaviour therapies,[6] counselling[7] and family therapy.[8] There are also a number of therapies that have been specifically developed for use in older people with dementia, including reality orientation, reminiscence therapy and validation therapy. These are described in more detail in Chapter 4.

In general, with the exception of reality orientation, reminiscence therapy and validation therapy, patients should be cognitively well preserved if they are to get the most out of psychological therapy. The problem should not be entirely defined by family members. The patient must also accept that there is a problem and be willing to accept the role of psychological factors in the development and maintenance of their problems. Patients who 'normalise' (deny that there is a problem) or 'somatise' (blame physical illness for everything) are difficult to help.

A therapeutic relationship must be established with the patient at an early stage. The patient must have clear, realistic expectations, and the therapist should show respect for the patient, refrain from exploitation or abuse, and accept the patient as a valued individual regardless of his or her behaviour, thoughts or feelings. The therapist should clearly demonstrate a willingness to listen and understand, and convey genuineness, warmth and empathy. Some therapists may become 'an active advocate for the patient', justifying this because of the patient's physical infirmity and illness. Others avoid this approach at all costs, suggesting that to act on behalf of the patient outside therapy is to take on a role that is inappropriate between two adults. A common-sense approach is needed, and either approach may be suitable given a particular therapist's training and the individual circumstances. One may have to be more flexible than with younger patients, and this is particularly the case with regard to settings and attendance. Reduced mobility and frailty often mean that home visits or other strategies to increase accessibility are required, and frequent poor physical health may mean that appointments have to be cancelled. One needs to be conscious of these limitations and adopt a pragmatic and practical approach to treatment. However, although the therapist may engage in treatment in the patient's own home, and this may be convenient for the patient, it may give rise to difficulties and the setting may inhibit therapy, partly due to lack of privacy.

The overall process of therapy usually involves a number of stages, regardless of the approach adopted by the therapist. After an initial assessment, a therapy contract is drawn up between the patient and the therapist, following which the patient enters a period of therapy. At the end of this process there should be a follow-up assessment, and the patient may then be discharged, or a new therapy contract might need to be negotiated if there has been no progress or if new problems have arisen. Compared with younger adults, much greater flexibility may be needed in the contract described above.

In older people a number of factors are known to enhance the therapeutic contract. These include the following:
➤ flexible session length
➤ flexibility of session location
➤ time-limited contract
➤ explicit, concrete and realistic goals
➤ awareness of real social and physical limitations
➤ an active rather than passive therapist

➤ an awareness of ageism in the therapist
➤ an awareness of medication effects in the elderly.

The implications of the developmental model proposed by Erikson for psychological therapy with older people are clear. Conflicts and issues specific to age can be recognised as normal. Each individual will bring to their current situation a set of beliefs, attitudes and resources that have been accumulated through previous years, and it is these which affect how resilient the older person will be in the face of change.

General issues

Ageing brings with it changes in a number of domains, including attitudes, health, self-image, relationships, status, generational changes, sexual functioning and an awareness of time and mortality. These general themes all appear regularly in clinical work with older people as they come to terms with the realities of retirement or illness. Much of the therapeutic work with older people involves their coming to terms with losses of various types.

A detailed discussion of each of the various psychological approaches is beyond the scope of this book. The reader is referred to more specialised texts for a discussion of psychological approaches.[6–8] A discussion of validation therapy, reminiscence therapy and reality orientation can be found in Chapter 4. Two of the most commonly used approaches with older people are group therapy (particularly in a day hospital setting) and family therapy (which can be extremely useful for dealing with distressed and sometimes dysfunctional families).

Family therapy

The well-being of the older person is affected by those around them. Many older people live either with a partner or with other relatives, and even those who live alone often have some contact with relatives who are within easy travelling distance. For many older people, an understanding of the family context may be the key to finding the most appropriate psychological approach. Increasingly, family therapy is being viewed as a valuable and effective method for families in which there are difficulties in adapting to transitions due to ageing.[8] The focus of assessment is the family system and the interactions of the family members. The involvement of other members of the family in perpetuating or alleviating the distressed or disturbing behaviour of the elderly referred person is emphasised.

Most family members are caring and attempt to help the referred person, even though these family members may appear difficult, intransigent or occasionally openly destructive. In general, they have attempted to solve problems that have arisen from a change in life circumstances in one or more other family members. However, if these attempts are faulty the initial problems can be exacerbated.

The initial contact between therapist and family, and the way in which this is organised, are both important to success. Copies of the appointment letter are sent to all invited members of the family individually, including the referred patient. Normally at least two professionals work together. This is partly because large amounts of information will be supplied by a variety of different family members, and it would be very difficult for one therapist to follow this effectively. If both sexes are represented on the co-therapists' team, they may obtain more information from the family. In initial interview sessions with the whole family present, therapists are interested not only in what is being said and how it is being said, but also in the non-verbal communication within the family. When using family therapy techniques, we need to consider the impact of transitions for the family members concerned, and the impact of these on others. Sometimes the needs of one family member may conflict with the responsibilities of others.

Behavioural therapy

There are many possible factors that contribute to a person's behaviour, including environmental and internal factors. Sometimes individuals may behave in ways that are troubling or dangerous to themselves or others, and such individuals are commonly referred to services for older people. The patient may or may not be suffering from dementia. Troubling behaviours include aggression, inappropriate sexual activities, dangerous behaviours, rejection of care or control, and stereotyped or repetitive behaviour. A behavioural assessment will involve observation and analysis of behaviour (*see* Chapter 2). These approaches are often quantitative in nature. In addition, the aim of assessment may be to clarify a sequence of events in order to identify the triggers and consequences of a particular behaviour. The function of the behaviour for the patient and others can then be better understood. This may be summarised as the *ABC approach*, with A denoting antecedents, B denoting behaviour and C denoting consequences. The procedure may be as follows.

A baseline measurement of the behaviour is taken (*see* Chapter 2). This is easiest with discrete symptoms or easily defined behaviour. A careful analysis of the behaviour will often facilitate the development of an appropriate treatment strategy. For more detailed information the reader is referred to more specialist works.[9] However, it is unlikely that such a 'mechanistic' approach would be successful in isolation. In clinical practice it is important to develop a good relationship with the patient, to regard them as a valued individual and to be flexible in one's approach. To achieve success with older people who have psychological difficulties it might be (and frequently is) necessary to use several psychological approaches in a variety of settings.

Cognitive behaviour therapy (CBT)

This approach is founded on the understanding that how we think affects how we feel and act, and vice versa. Faulty ('unrealistic') thoughts can reinforce depressed mood and increase disability in other disorders, including schizophrenia. CBT has been widely researched, mostly in working-age adults, and forms one of a group of interventions labelled psychosocial interventions (PSI). Generally these interventions are under-researched and under-funded in old age services, but there are moves to make them more readily available to older people. CBT is generally short term and concentrates on helping the client to identify unrealistic thoughts, stop them and replace them with more realistic thoughts. Often there is also a behavioural component – for example, with graded re-engagement in activities from which the client had withdrawn.

For further details of CBT, readers are referred to standard texts[6] and self-help manuals.[10-12] CBT needs to be adapted for use with some older individuals to take into account a slower pace of change. Group cognitive therapy with old people can work successfully, and theoretical aspects of CBT with older people are beginning to be explored.

PHARMACOLOGICAL TREATMENTS

In the same way that it has proved difficult to classify mental disorders, it has also proved difficult to classify psychotropic drugs, and a number of different classifications exist based on chemical structures, mechanisms of action, or the main effects on brain function. The classification is complicated by the fact that many drugs overlap and do not fit neatly into discrete categories. In general, the broad categories include *antidepressants, mood stabilisers, anxiolytics, hypnotics, antipsychotics* and *antidementia drugs*. Subclassification is usually on the basis of chemical structures (e.g. tricyclic antidepressants), pharmacokinetic properties (e.g. short- and long-acting benzodiazepines) and specific properties (e.g. sedation). There is considerable overlap and this classification, although useful, is very broad and has a number of limitations. The problem of classification is well illustrated by antidementia drugs. These have a number of different names (e.g. nootropics and cognitive enhancers), and individual drugs often have several important effects on the CNS. Furthermore, the drugs in this category have different detailed mechanisms of action, making classification very difficult. It is also interesting to note that most psychotropic drugs were first developed in the 1950s or later, making the field of psychopharmacology relatively new compared with many other branches of psychiatry and pharmacology. For a more detailed consideration of psychopharmacology in old age the reader is referred to *Practical Old Age Psychopharmacology: a Multiprofessional Approach.*[13]

A detailed assessment of the patient is important for a number of reasons.

➤ First, it enables an accurate diagnosis to be made, and this has implications for both the treatment and the prognosis of the specific condition under consideration.

➤ Secondly, it is the beginning of the process of developing a trusting relationship with the patient that will be crucial for providing a sound basis for treating the patient and maintaining compliance.

➤ Thirdly, the assessment of the patient's past and current medical problems will indicate which drugs to avoid, and will highlight potential drug interactions.

➤ Finally, a knowledge of the patient's past psychiatric history might point to the most appropriate treatments.

Informing the patient

The *Drug and Therapeutics Bulletin*[14] has recommended that patients should be given the following information about their medication, and over 30 years later this advice remains highly relevant:

➤ the name of the medicine

➤ the aim of the treatment (relief of symptoms, cure, prevention of relapse, or prophylaxis)

➤ how the patient will know if the drug is or is not working

➤ when and how to take it

➤ what to do if a dose is missed

➤ how long to take it for

➤ side-effects

➤ effects on performance (e.g. driving ability)

➤ interactions with other drugs.

Beginning treatment

Lader and Herrington[15] have wisely suggested that 'unless there is intense distress there is no need to proceed with haste'. There are a number of important reasons for delaying treatment for a short time.

➤ The additional time enables a more detailed assessment to be conducted which will make the eventual treatment more informed.

➤ Psychotropic drugs can be harmful, and older people are often very sensitive to their side-effects, so they should not be given unnecessarily.

➤ For a number of conditions the initial management may best be by means of psychological therapies or social intervention.

➤ Some patients improve after the initial assessment/admission, making the use of psychotropic drugs unnecessary. For example, in general practice, patients with minor disorders often improve after simple discussion, and drugs may reinforce the patient's view that they have a 'serious illness'.[16]

➤ Admission to hospital may be associated with a significant improvement in symptoms.[17] However, this is not always sustained.

➤ Other reasons include the increased risk of drug interactions and the financial implications.

Older people should be on as few drugs as possible. However, if a decision is made to prescribe, choosing the most appropriate medication can be a complex process. Response to previous treatments is sometimes helpful but not always a reliable guide.[15] There is also variation in the response depending both on the illness and on comorbid clinical factors, such as personality factors.[18] Age itself is an important determinant of the response to treatment, due to reduced drug clearance, increased side-effects, a reduction in receptor density and increased risk of interactions with other drugs. Physical illness can also impair the response to treatment through a variety of mechanisms. Reduced diet can also have an impact through changes in the proportion of body fat, reduced plasma protein levels, reductions in amino acid and vitamin levels (with consequences for enzyme function),[19] and changes in receptor density.[20]

In general, it is better to know about a few drugs in detail so that one becomes familiar with their doses, side-effects and interactions with other drugs. Confusion and costs will also be reduced if the generic name is used wherever possible. Complex drug regimes should be avoided and, in general, it is not necessary to use two or more drugs from the same class of drugs (e.g. two or more antipsychotic drugs). Drugs should be commenced cautiously, and they should also be stopped cautiously and over a few days or weeks, particularly if the patient is on high doses and/or has been taking the drug for an extended period of time. This will depend in part on the individual patient, the drug in question, the dose and the duration of treatment. A range of factors have to be considered before prescribing drugs for older people. One of the questions that should always be considered is the advantage of prescribing nothing.[15]

Consent is also an important issue. In order to consent to treatment, the patient should have a broad understanding of the treatment, including its risks and benefits, the consequences of not taking the treatment, and the alternatives currently available, with their risks and benefits. Patients with serious psychiatric disorder who lack the capacity to give consent should normally be treated under the Mental Health Act (1983, 2007, accessed through www.legislation. gov.uk/). Patients with dementia who lack the capacity to give consent should normally be treated within the framework of the Mental Capacity Act (2005, also accessed through www.legislation.gov.uk/). Patients with dementia who are refusing treatment should be treated under the Mental Health Act (2007).

The Mental Capacity Act (2005) formalises the area assessing whether the patient is mentally capable of making decisions. The Mental Health Act (2007) describes the circumstances when a patient can be treated against their wishes.

The general principles relating to consent are as follows:
➤ Consent must be obtained before an examination or treatment.
➤ Consent must be voluntary (i.e. the person must not be put under any undue influence).
➤ It is assumed that the person has capacity unless this can be demonstrated not to be the case.
➤ Competent adults have the right to refuse treatment.
➤ People need sufficient time to make a decision, and they can change their mind.
➤ To be capacitous the person should understand the purpose and nature of the treatment, should understand the benefits, risks and alternatives, should be able to retain and weigh up the pros and cons of the treatment, and be able to communicate their decision.
➤ No one can give consent on behalf of an incompetent adult.

Patients who lack capacity (i.e. are incompetent) can still receive medication if it is in their best interests. A number of factors should be considered, including:
➤ the patient's own wishes and values, including advance decisions
➤ clinical judgement
➤ the likelihood of improvement
➤ the views of relatives, carers and significant others
➤ knowledge about the patient's religious, cultural and other relevant information that might have an impact on the patient's wishes.

More information on the Mental Capacity Act (2005), the Code of Practice (2005) and the Mental Health Act (2007). See Chapter 10 for more details of relevant legislation and the following websites:
➤ Mental Health Act 2007
   www.legislation.gov.uk/ukpga/2007/12/c (accessed 10.05.12)
➤ Mental Capacity Act 2005
   www.legislation.gov.uk/ukpga/2005/9/co (accessed 10.05.12)
➤ Mental Capacity Act Code of Practice
   www.legislation.gov.uk/ukpga/2005/9/pdfs (accessed 10.05.12).

Assessing response to treatment

Evaluation of the patient's response to treatment is intricately linked with assessment and initiation of treatment. The response should be evaluated fairly frequently after commencing treatment, but there are no universally accepted guidelines, and practice depends in part upon clinical judgement. It is usual for contact with the patient to be maintained for as long as they remain on psychoactive drugs, unless specified otherwise in local 'shared care guidelines' between primary and secondary care. In any event there should be clear discussion with the GP and the team if formal contact comes to an end. It is also important to determine the aim of treatment (e.g. relief of acute symptoms, prevention of relapse, or prophylaxis).

Psychoactive drugs

A wide range of drugs can be used in older people with mental illness, and a detailed knowledge of these is necessary to ensure that drugs are safely and appropriately used. It is also important to monitor side-effects, and some of these may not be obviously related to the prescribed medication (e.g. there is an increased risk of falls with psychotropic drugs in older people, but this may be wrongly diagnosed as being due to an underlying medical condition). Antidementia agents, antidepressants, antipsychotics and anxiolytics are described in detail in Chapters 4, 5, 6 and 7, respectively. Hypnotics are a frequently neglected group of drugs. As sleep disturbance is common in many disorders, the use of hypnotic drugs is described in greater detail in this chapter. Before considering the use of these drugs, underlying medical conditions such as paroxysmal nocturnal dyspnoea and severe depression should be ruled out.

Hypnotic drugs – 'sleeping tablets'

Despite recent progress in the use of non-benzodiazepines, clinicians continue to remain reluctant to prescribe hypnotics. Insomnia affects less than 10% of the population, and in approximately half of the cases it is associated with another psychiatric diagnosis (e.g. depressive disorder). Sleep problems can be due to a variety of health problems (e.g. moving or restless legs) or to alerting medication or poor sleep habits. Where insomnia is associated with another disorder or cause, this should usually be dealt with first. If distressing insomnia persists despite good sleep habits, treatment should be considered. If the problem is related to short-term stress, treatment for 3–7 days with one of the 'Z' drugs (see below) may be appropriate. Cognitive behavioural therapy for insomnia (CBTi) is now the first-line treatment for more prolonged insomnia, and slow-release melatonin is also recommended.

➤ Patients should have a full history and physical examination as well as laboratory investigation as appropriate.

➤ It is also useful to ask the patient to keep a sleep diary, and to ask the partner to corroborate the patient's account (there is often little correlation between subjective experience of sleep and objective measures such as the sleep polygraph).

➤ Sleep can also be promoted by improving the sleep environment (e.g. comfortable bed, low level of noise, comfortable temperature) and adopting habits that do not interfere with sleep (e.g. avoiding caffeine, exercise and large meals before sleep). These simple measures (known as sleep hygiene) are often very effective in promoting sleep without the need to use drugs. A useful patient information sheet produced by the Royal College of Psychiatrists, *Sleeping Well*, is available at rcpsych.ac.uk/mentalhealthinfoforall/pro (accessed 10.5.12).

Box 3.1   Drugs associated with insomnia

➤ Decongestants
➤ Caffeine
➤ Nicotine
➤ Alcohol
➤ Aminophylline
➤ Beta-blockers
➤ Corticosteroids
➤ Calcium-channel blockers
➤ Diuretics
➤ CNS stimulants

Hypnotics with long half-lives should be avoided (e.g. diazepam), and hypnotics should normally only be prescribed for short periods e.g. 2–4 weeks (i.e. benzodiazapine and 'Z' drugs). NICE (2004) has concluded that there is a 'lack of compelling' evidence to distinguish between the 'Z' drugs (zaleplon, zolpidem and zopiclone) or the shorter-acting benzodiazepine hypnotics, and that the drug with the lowest cost should be prescribed. However, in older people, benzodiazepines may increase the risk of falls and cause confusion. In our opinion, the 'Z' drugs are more appropriate in older people as a first-line treatment after non-pharmacological interventions have been tried. Benzodiazepines that can be used include nitrazepam, temazepam, flurazepam, loprazolam and lormetazepam.

For a full summary of the NICE guidance on insomnia, visit the following guideline:

Guidance on the use of zaleplon, zolpidem and zopiclone for the short-term management of insomnia, NICE (2004) Technology Appraisal 77 www.nice.org.uk/nicemedia/pdf/TA077fullg (accessed 10.5.12).

For an excellent and detailed review of the assessment, diagnosis and treatment of insomnia, visit the following guideline:

British Association for Psychopharmacology consensus statement on evidence-based treatment of insomnia, parainsomnias and circadian rhythm disorders (2010) at www.bap.org.ui/pdfs/BAP_Sleep_Guidelines (last accessed on 10.5.12).

This consensus statement also reviews the use of other drugs such as antidepressants in the management of insomnia.

Box 3.2 Potential side-effects of hypnotics

➤ Residual sedative effect (falls!)
➤ Rebound insomnia
➤ Physical dependence
➤ Tolerance
➤ Drug interactions (especially CNS depressants)
➤ Memory impairment
➤ Respiratory depression

Currently there are no hypnotics which are entirely free from side-effects, and they should all be used with caution and only after careful evaluation and alternative measures (where appropriate).

Sedative drugs, particularly benzodiazepines, are also commonly used in medically ill patients, and are particularly useful in the intensive care unit (ICU) environment because of their anxiolytic, sedative, hypnotic and memory-dulling properties. Although these drugs have high therapeutic to toxic ratios, they can nevertheless be associated with serious complications, including airway obstruction, respiratory depression, hypotension and pain at injection sites. Benzodiazepines are metabolised by hepatic microsomal enzymes, either via oxidation (e.g. diazepam) or via glucuronide conjugation (e.g. lorazepam). Drug oxidation is particularly susceptible to the effects of a number of drugs. Cimetidine in particular prolongs the half-life and thus increases the sedative effects. Another important interaction is between erythromycin and midazolam. Erythromycin significantly decreases the metabolism of midazolam.

The term 'sedative' is much used but difficult to define. How much sedation should be used? The clinician needs a precise definition of what constitutes sedation and how to measure it. This is particularly important if the patient may have to drive a car and/or operate potentially dangerous machinery either at home or in the workplace. Sedation in conscious patients is termed *conscious sedation* and has been defined as 'a minimally depressed level of consciousness that retains the patient's ability to maintain a patent airway independently and continuously and respond to physical stimulation and/or verbal command'. This may be an adequate definition for patients being treated in emergency departments, but would be inappropriate, say, for an elderly demented patient requiring 'sedation' for behavioural disturbance on a medical ward.

The definition of sedation is not absolute, and it will vary depending on the patient's age and clinical circumstances.

CONCLUSION

The full range of therapeutic approaches can be used with older people. The general principles of treatment are the same, but there may be a need to make minor modifications and the therapist may need to be more flexible. All psychological therapy is underpinned by good relationships. Family therapy techniques and behaviour therapy are particularly useful. In addition, there is a range of therapeutic approaches that have been specifically developed for use with older people, including reminiscence therapy and validation therapy. Flexibility on the part of the therapist is extremely important and, as with younger patients, a careful assessment is required prior to commencing treatment. Therapists need appropriate training and supervision, particularly when dealing with sometimes extremely difficult families. It is important to emphasise that psychological approaches will not solve all of the problems that older people encounter in later life, and goals need to be clearly defined and realistic.

REFERENCES

1 Menninger K, Ellensberger H, Pruyser P and Mayman M (1958) The unitary concept of mental illness. *Bull Menn Clin.* **22**: 4–12.
2 Bengston VL, Cuellar JB and Ragan PK (1997) Stratum contrasts and similarities in attitudes towards death. *J Gerontol.* **32**: 76–88.
3 Kübler-Ross E (1969) *On Death and Dying.* Macmillan, New York.
4 Colthart NEC (1991) The analysis of an elderly patient. *Int J Psychoanal.* **72**: 209–19.
5 Barraclough C and Fleming I (1986) *Goal Planning with Elderly People.* Manchester University Press, Manchester.
6 Laidlaw K, Thompson LW, Gallagher-Thompson D and Dick-Siskin L (2003) *Cognitive Behaviour Therapy with Older People.* Wiley-Blackwell, Chichester.
7 Scrutton S (1999) *Counselling Older People* (2e). Hodder Arnold, London.
8 Peluso PR, Watts RE and Parsons M (2012) *Changing Aging, Changing Family Therapy: Practising with 21st Century Realities (Family Therapy and Counselling).* Routledge, London.
9 Zarit SH (1997) Behavioural and environmental treatment in dementia. In: C Holmes and R Howard (eds) *Advances in Old Age Psychiatry* (2e). Wrightson Biomedical Publishing, Petersfield.
10 Williams C (2012) *Overcoming Anxiety, Stress and Panic: a Five Areas Approach* (2e). Hodder Arnold, London.
11 Williams C (2012) *Overcoming Depression and Low Mood: a Five Areas Approach* (3e). Hodder Arnold, London.
12 Williams C (2011) *Overcoming Functional Neurological Symptoms: a Five Areas Approach.* Hodder Arnold, London.

13 Curran S and Bullock R (eds) (2005) *Practical Old Age Psychopharmacology: a Multiprofessional Approach.* Radcliffe Publishing, Oxford.

14 Drug and Therapeutics Bulletin (1981) What should we tell patients about their medicines? *Drug Ther Bull.* **19**: 73–4.

15 Lader M and Herrington R (1990) *Biological Treatments in Psychiatry.* Oxford Medical Publications, Oxford.

16 Thomas KB (1978) The consultation and the therapeutic illusion. *BMJ.* 1:1327–8.

17 Lieberman PB and Strauss JS (1986) Brief psychiatric hospitalisation: what are its effects? *Am J Psychiatry.* **143**: 1557–62.

18 Young MA, Keller MB, Lavori PW *et al* (1987) Lack of stability of the RDC endogenous subtype in consecutive episodes of major depression. *J Affect Disord.* **12**: 139–43.

19 Williams RT (1978) Nutrients in drug detoxification reactions. In: JN Hathcock and J Coon (eds) *Nutrition and Drug Interactions.* Academic Press, New York.

20 Goodwin GM, Fraser S, Stump K, Fairburn CG, Elliott JM and Cowen PJ (1987) Dieting and weight loss in volunteers increases the number of α_2-adrenoceptors and 5-HT receptors on blood platelets without effects on ^{3}H-imipramine binding. *J Affect Disord.* **12**: 267–74.

4

Confusion: delirium and dementia

INTRODUCTION

The confused patient does not usually ask for help – indeed, sometimes it can be very difficult to get them to accept help. The general practitioner, social services or others are usually called in by worried relatives or neighbours. The confusion might also be noticed when the patient is admitted to hospital for another reason, or when a sudden bereavement unmasks confusion that was previously managed by the deceased partner.

Helping the confused person is a difficult and complex task. It can sometimes take a long time even to gain entry to the patient's home. Patients may deny that they have a problem and refuse all offers of help, including assessment. Full physical, psychological and social assessments are required, and this can usually only be achieved by the multidisciplinary team working together in an integrated way. Confused, frail, elderly patients may be living on a 'knife-edge', and there may be concerns not only about mental health but also about physical health, nutrition, safety (e.g. falls, wandering, leaving the gas turned on, etc.) and exploitation by others. Such people can be very vulnerable, especially if they live alone. If they live with a carer, or are cared for by family members, there is nearly always considerable family stress. The family also needs help. The whole issue is complicated when patients, and occasionally relatives, refuse to accept help, and the Mental Health Act (1983) may sometimes have to be used. When the patient lacks capacity, various aspects of the Mental Capacity Act (2005) may also have to be invoked (see Chapter 10, pp. 269–283). However, there is a danger of overstating the difficulties, and most confused patients will respond positively to skilled intervention.

ANALYSING THE PROBLEM

Figure 4.1 presents an interactive model of confusion which stresses that factors in the brain, the internal environment, the special senses and the external

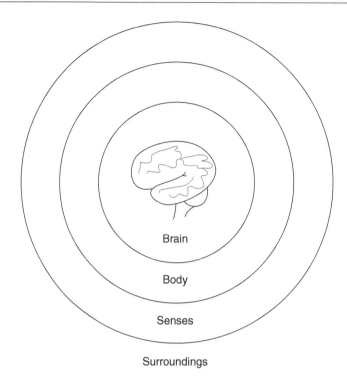

Brain

Body

Senses

Surroundings

Figure 4.1 An interactive model of confusion.

environment may all interact to cause confusion. In any one patient the contribution of environmental and personal factors will be unique and, even where there is irreversible brain damage, treating the sufferer as a human being, as well as attention to such factors as constipation, a malfunctioning hearing-aid and environmental design, may produce marked improvement. Disturbances in the internal environment are largely involved in delirium, whereas brain-intrinsic factors are more important in the dementias. These factors will be considered individually in the remainder of this chapter. Referring back to this figure will help to remind the reader of the need to analyse the problems facing confused people in each of the 'layers'. Management plans based on this kind of analysis will recognise the importance of paying attention to the environment and communication, as well as general health and any specific brain damage.

DELIRIUM

Introduction

The term *delirium* (ICD-10, F05)[1] describes a syndrome in which there is disturbance of consciousness, impaired attention/concentration, and associated problems with memory, behaviour and the sleep–wake cycle. In addition, perceptual distortions (illusions) and hallucinations (usually visual) are frequently present. The term *acute confusional state* is used to describe the same syndrome. Old people, especially if they have cognitive impairment, are particularly vulnerable to delirium.

Epidemiology

The prevalence of delirium in the community is unknown. In medical inpatients it is sometimes not recognised and sometimes confused with dementia.[2] Around 10–22% of elderly medical admissions have delirium. However, if patients are carefully assessed and delirium is specifically looked for, the prevalence rises to 33%. Following surgery in older people, the prevalence of delirium is 5–10%, and this figure rises to 40% in those who need intensive care.[3]

Clinical description

The hallmark of delirium is sudden onset. The patient's behaviour is often erratic and bizarre, and this may precipitate referral. The patient's level of awareness of the environment is diminished and it fluctuates, often being worse at night. The patient may look perplexed and fearful and their speech may be incoherent. Perceptual misinterpretations (illusions) and hallucinations (especially visual) are very common. Attention and concentration are reduced and memory is impaired. Depending on the underlying cause and other factors, the patient may be hyperactive or hypoactive, the latter being more difficult to diagnose.

Case History 4.1

Mrs C is a 77-year-old woman with arthritis and mild heart failure who was admitted to a nursing home following the death of her husband. It was also thought that she might have mild cognitive impairment. She developed low mood and was seen by her GP, who prescribed a tricyclic antidepressant (amitriptyline, 75 mg at night) to treat her low mood and help her to sleep. Shortly after commencing treatment she became increasingly distressed and confused. Her memory and attention/ concentration became impaired, and she became very agitated and frightened and appeared to be responding to visual hallucinations. Staff found it increasingly difficult to manage her. After 5 days a psychiatrist saw her in the nursing home. The amitriptyline was stopped. The patient then made a quick and full recovery from the delirium, which was related to the anticholinergic side-effects of the amitriptyline.

The time course of delirium is variable depending on the underlying cause, ranging from a few hours or days (e.g. with an acute infection) to weeks or months (e.g. with chronic metabolic disorders such as chronic liver disease)[3,4] (*see* Figure 4.2 and Case History 4.1).

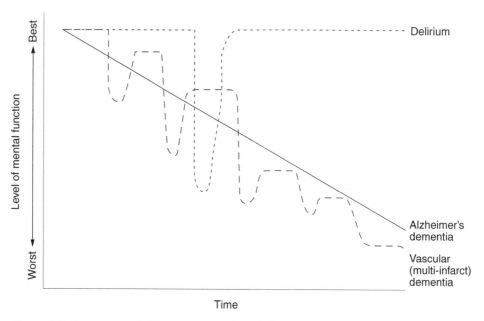

Figure 4.2 Time course of different causes of confusion.

Detection

The Confusion Assessment Method (CAM) of Inouye *et al*[5] has been widely used in research, and has been validated in Europe as a screening tool for delirium.[6] It is a simple algorithm with four questions (*see* Box 4.1). The diagnosis of delirium requires the presence of features 1 and 2 and either 3 or 4.

These features reflect the diagnostic criteria in the *American Diagnostic and Statistical Manual* versions III-R and IV. This test has only moderate sensitivity and specificity, but if the questions were asked about every acutely ill older person they would undoubtedly lead to a higher rate of diagnosis of this often hidden condition.

Aetiology

Heart failure and infections, especially chest and urinary tract infections, are probably the commonest causes of delirium in older people. Prescribed drugs, especially those with anticholinergic side-effects (e.g. the older antipsychotic and antidepressant drugs), may cause memory impairment and delirium.

Other drugs reported to be associated with delirium include benzodiazepines and steroids. In addition, the side-effects of some older antipsychotic drugs (extrapyramidal side-effects) are sometimes managed by using anticholinergic drugs (e.g. procyclidine), with the result that the acute confusional state may be worsened. Some of the common causes of delirium are summarised in Box 4.2. Thiamine deficiency is classically associated with alcoholism and it causes a delirium called Wernicke's encephalopathy, characterised by confusion, ataxia and double vision due to paralysis of the eye muscles. This may be followed by permanent loss of short-term memory and confabulation (Korsakoff's psychosis), and constitutes a medical emergency that requires immediate treatment with parenteral thiamine.

Box 4.1   The Confusion Assessment Method*

1   *Acute onset and fluctuating course*
    This feature is assessed by asking an informant 'Is there evidence of sudden change from the patient's previous mental state?' and 'Did the abnormal behaviour tend to fluctuate (come and go, increase and decrease) through the day?'

2   *Inattention*
    Also usually assessed by asking an informant. 'Did the patient have difficulty focusing attention, were they easily distractible or did they have difficulty keeping track of the conversation or what was happening?'

3   *Disorganised thinking*
    'Was the patient's thinking disorganised, was their conversation rambling or incoherent, or was there unpredictable switching from subject to subject?'

4   *Altered level of consciousness*
    This feature is shown by any answer other than 'alert' to the question 'Overall, how would you rate this patient's level of consciousness?' (alert [normal], vigilant [hyperalert], lethargic [drowsy, easily aroused], stuporose [hard to arouse] or comatose [unarousable]).

---

*Modified from Inouye *et al.*[5]

Management

Patients must have a thorough medical and psychiatric history taken as well as a thorough physical examination, and additional investigations may need to be undertaken in order to identify the underlying cause. Care must be taken to avoid diagnosing 'dementia' unless all of the criteria for dementia are present (see below). Unless the cause of the delirium is obvious and not serious, it will be necessary to admit the patient under the care of a physician in order to identify and treat the underlying physical illness. Treatment of the underlying cause is the mainstay of therapy. However, admission to hospital may increase the confusion because of disorientation. Good nursing care is essential at this time, and management may be supplemented by the use of an antipsychotic drug. This should be chosen with care (*see* Chapter 6). An antipsychotic with low anticholinergic side-effects (e.g. risperidone, haloperidol) is preferable. A small dose should be given initially and any increases should be gradual, bearing in mind the extended half-life of some of these medications. The drug should be given only until the delirium resolves, and it should then be gradually withdrawn. If there is underlying dementia, antipsychotics should be avoided when possible and only used for short periods if essential. Prescriptions should differentiate between oral and parenteral administration because of increased potency per unit dose when given intramuscularly (IM), and should state the maximum cumulative dose in any 24-hour period. The use of antipsychotic drugs is discussed further in Chapter 6.

Box 4.2   Causes of delirium

Severe infection	*Dehydration*
Chest	*Drugs/toxins*
Urinary tract	Carbon monoxide
	Alcohol
	Anticholinergic drugs
Metabolic causes	Benzodiazepines
Diabetes	Digoxin
Thyroid dysfunction	Barbiturates
Vitamin B$_{12}$ deficiency	Some antibiotics
Thiamine deficiency	Antihistamines
	Tricyclic antidepressants
Intracranial lesions	Antipsychotic drugs
	ACE inhibitors
Systems failure	Diuretics
Cardiac	Non-steroidal anti-inflammatory drugs
Renal	Steroids
Hepatic	Calcium-channel blockers
Respiratory	

Prognosis

There is usually a physical cause for the delirium, and if this can be identified the prognosis for recovery of the mental state in the short to medium term is good. In addition, because the physical treatment of the underlying condition is now very much better than in the past, only about 10% of the patients admitted to hospital with delirium now die before 6 months have elapsed, although around one-third will die in the following 2 years, and the prognosis is usually worse for prolonged delirium.

DEMENTIA

Introduction

Since 1900, the percentage of elderly people in the population has increased dramatically. For example, at the turn of the last century, approximately 4% of the population were aged 65 years or over. Today the proportion is about four times higher, and it is still rising. Dementia is now recognised as a leading cause of death in developed countries. Its prevalence is likely to increase as the numbers of old and very old people increase, and this has important medical, social and economic implications.

Symptoms and signs of dementia were described by Greek and Roman physicians. The concept of old age as a cause of dementia was popularised by Galen in the second century. However, there was little progress in our understanding of Alzheimer's disease until 1906, when Alois Alzheimer presented a paper at a scientific meeting. His presentation concerned a 51-year-old woman whose symptoms consisted of memory loss, disorientation, depression and hallucinations. After 5 years she had profound dementia, and she subsequently died. At post-mortem, marked cerebral atrophy was noted. Using a new silver-staining technique, Alzheimer demonstrated for the first time neurofibrillary tangles and neuritic plaques in the brain. Despite the importance of this finding, it provoked little discussion. However, as a result of further work by Alzheimer and others, Kraepelin decided to name the condition 'Alzheimer's disease'. Since then there has been an exponential increase in research, with advances in diagnosis and a much greater awareness of aetiology. However, the condition continues to cause enormous morbidity and mortality, the causes remain speculative, and there is currently no successful treatment for this devastating illness, although the new generation of antidementia drugs have an important contribution to make in some cases.

Epidemiology

Alzheimer's disease is by far the most common form of dementia in late life, accounting for around 75% of diagnoses either alone or in combination with vascular dementia. Vascular dementia (mostly multi-infarct dementia, MID) is probably the second most common form, with Lewy body dementia (LBD) a close third. Other rarer causes of dementia (fronto-temporal dementia, Pick's disease, etc.), and conditions which can cause 'chronic brain syndrome', such as thyroid deficiency, account for less than 10% overall. The relative prevalence of different causes may have to be revised further in the light of emerging evidence and the complexities of overlapping pathology, pathogenesis and biochemistry.

Prevalence of dementia

Alzheimer's Disease International estimates that there are currently 30 million people with dementia in the world.[7] There is invariably a preponderance of females in any demented population, although this partly reflects the greater number of elderly women in the general population. The prevalence of dementia increases with age[7] (*see* Table 4.1). It is now generally believed that the prevalence of dementia increases more or less exponentially with increasing age, with a widening gap between men and women over the age of 85 years.

Table 4.1 Age-specific prevalence of dementia in Western Europe[7]

Age range (years)	Prevalence (%)
60–64	0.9
65–69	1.5
70–74	3.6
75–79	6.0
80–84	12.2
85–89	24.8

The prevalence of Alzheimer's disease approximately doubles for every 4.5 years of lifespan beyond 60 years of age. This exponential rise continues until the age of 90 years. Thereafter it is difficult to estimate the prevalence because of the small numbers of cases involved.

Incidence of dementia

The incidence refers to the number of new cases occurring in a given population during a specified time period, and it is generally regarded as a more useful indicator than prevalence. This is partly because differences in prevalence rates could be due either to differences in the number of new cases or to differences in survival rates. Despite this, there have been comparatively few studies of incidence. In order to yield reliable data, studies either need to be very large or conducted over many years. This is because incidence rates are so low. The few data that are available suggest that the incidence of dementia, like the prevalence, increases exponentially between 60 and 90 years of age. At age 65 years the incidence is 350 in 100 000, rising to 3400 in 100 000 at age 85 years. The incidence of dementia levels off in the very old, but the precise reason for this is unknown. The incidence of dementia in men and women has also been examined, but the results are inconsistent.

Clinical description of dementia

Numerous definitions of dementia have been suggested. Roth[8] proposed that it is 'an acquired global impairment of intellect, memory and personality'. Definitions of this type are useful for the purpose of communication, but are of less value in clinical research. More recently, definitions have been included in standardised diagnostic criteria, the *Diagnostic and Statistical Manual of the American Psychiatric Association, DSM-IV,*[9] and the *International Classification of Diseases, ICD-10* (*see* Box 4.3).[1]

Box 4.3   ICD-10 diagnostic criteria for dementia

The primary requirement for the diagnosis is evidence of a decline in both memory and thinking which is sufficient to impair personal activities of daily living. The impairment of memory typically affects the registration, storage and retrieval of new information, but previously learned and familiar information may also be lost, particularly in the later stages. Dementia is more than impaired memory. There is also impairment of thinking and of reasoning capacity, and a reduction in the flow of ideas. The processing of incoming information is impaired, in that the individual finds it increasingly difficult to attend to more than one stimulus at a time (e.g. taking part in a conversation with several people), and to shift the focus of attention from one topic to another. If dementia is the sole diagnosis, evidence of clear consciousness is required. However, a double diagnosis of delirium superimposed on dementia is common. The above symptoms and impairments should have been evident *for at least 6 months* for a confident clinical diagnosis of dementia to be made.

Different types of dementia

The specific cause of dementia must then be determined. Such distinctions are achieved by interviewing the patient and carer, conducting a physical examination, undertaking a number of laboratory investigations to exclude the secondary causes of dementia, and performing special investigations (e.g. computed tomography (CT), magnetic resonance imaging (MRI), single positron emission spectography (SPECT) scan) to identify various pathologies that might cause dementia. Historically, dementias were grouped by age of onset into 'presenile' (early onset) and senile dementias. A more useful division is according to pathogenesis. *Neurodegenerative* dementias include Alzheimer's disease and the fronto-temporal dementias, of which the best known is Pick's disease. At the subcortical level, Huntingdon's disease and parkinsonism with dementia also come into this broad category. The *vascular dementias* include (most commonly) multi-infarct dementias but also strategic infarct dementia, hypertensive encephalopathy (Binswanger's disease) and hypoxic dementia. *Secondary dementias* may be due to endocrine disorder, vitamin deficiencies and infective causes, including HIV.[10] The attempt to divide dementias into distinct classes by localisation of pathology, underlying causes or other criteria is always confounded by overlap between different categories and the not infrequent presence of more than one pathological process. The final stage involves confirmation of the diagnosis by recourse to histopathology, but this rarely happens except in research settings.

Detection

Detection of early dementia has improved markedly since the introduction of cholinesterase inhibitors. It seems that relatives especially are more motivated to bring dementia to the attention of doctors following publicity surrounding the launch of these medications. Nevertheless, the Alzheimer's Society[11] reports that 68% of their respondents with dementia had to wait over a year between noticing their symptoms and getting a diagnosis, and 8% had to wait 5 years or longer. Worse still, it reports that only 43% of people with dementia have been formally identified in the UK. Memory clinics and other services for the delivery of the medications have developed rapidly.[11] The National Dementia Strategy[12] has, as a second objective, 'good quality early diagnosis and intervention for all'. Any suggestion of memory impairment should lead to a formal assessment of memory (*see* Chapter 2) and further investigations as indicated.

Assessment

Patients with a suspected diagnosis of dementia should have a full assessment, including the following:

➤ full history (including a history from an informant)
➤ cognitive and mental state examination
➤ physical examination and other appropriate investigation
➤ a review of medication to identify and minimise the use of drugs, including over-the-counter products that may adversely affect cognitive function.[13]

In addition, it is vitally important to obtain information from nursing staff (often the community psychiatric nurse), the patient's social worker, general practitioner and occupational therapist, as well as other professionals involved with the patient (including those working in the voluntary sector). This enables a clear picture to emerge with regard to the patient's difficulties and areas of risk, and it allows a package of care to be put together that is tailored to the needs of the individual patient and their carers. A fuller discussion of early detection can be found in *Practical Management of Dementia*.[14]

Primary degenerative dementias

Alzheimer's disease (F00)

In ICD-10,[1] Alzheimer's disease (AD) is divided into 'Dementia in AD with early onset' (F00.0) and 'Dementia in AD with late onset' (F00.1). These categories include the definition of dementia discussed above (*see* Box 4.3). For 'Dementia in AD with late onset', onset is after the age of 65 years. AD has an insidious onset with a gradual decline in the mental performance. Memory difficulties, especially with regard to new memories, are usually the first symptoms to be noticed. Memory problems may be attributed to 'old age' or 'absent-mindedness'. The onset is so gradual that even a close relative living with the patient may find it difficult to put a date on the time when the patient was last well. In the early stages, previous personality may strongly influence the presentation. Patients with a tendency to be suspicious of others or to deny their own limitations may upset carers by accusing them of stealing misplaced items. Others may react to these early changes by becoming extremely dependent on relatives, especially if family patterns of behaviour encourage this. Mood disturbance is not a diagnostic feature of AD, although it can be present in 15–30% of patients with early AD. It may also be common in more advanced AD. Here it may not be reported by the patient, but may be inferred from behavioural changes and response to treatment with antidepressants. The patient usually lacks insight, and as the disease progresses their behaviour may become more erratic. Disorientation with regard to time, place and person will also increase, usually in that order. The combination of disorientation in time and place and topographical disorientation may cause the patient to wander, resulting in considerable distress for the family, risk to the patient, and the involvement of neighbours, other individuals and the police, who may have to bring the patient home. Patients may get up in the early hours believing that it is time to go to work or get the children ready for school. Hallucinations (usually visual) are fairly common, but are not usually evident except through the description of carers (e.g. 'he spends a lot of time picking up imaginary food from the floor'). As the disease progresses, the patient will become unable to recognise their relatives, who often find this very upsetting. The patient may then become distressed, as they may believe that their partner or son or daughter is an intruder. In addition, the patient may fail to recognise him- or herself, and this can also cause considerable distress. Carers often find that removing mirrors solves the problem. Other difficulties with moderate to severe impairment include apraxia, which presents with difficulties in dressing and washing and other tasks involving visuo-spatial skills. Dysphasia (inability to express oneself in words or to understand words) can lead to severe frustration when combined with all of the other impairments and confusion. Incontinence (both urinary and faecal) usually develops late in the disease, and for many carers is the 'final straw'. Eventually the point is reached when the patient is unable to do anything for him- or herself, including the following:

➤ dressing
➤ personal hygiene
➤ domestic tasks
➤ toileting
➤ feeding.

The burden of looking after patients with AD is immense, and carers and families become physically and emotionally exhausted. Family feuds are not uncommon, often because of arguments about residential care. At this time families need support from the multidisciplinary team (*see* Case History 4.2).

Case History 4.2

Mr M is an 82-year-old retired miner who lives with his wife and one of his three sons. He has had a gradual deterioration of memory for the past 4 years. He is now unable to do anything for himself and needs help with all of his activities of daily living. He is disorientated with regard to time, place and person, and spends much of the day pacing up and down the house. He is sleeping poorly and has been urinating and defaecating in inappropriate places. His wife is physically exhausted. He now believes that his son is having an affair with his wife, and he has become verbally and physically aggressive towards his son, whom he regards as an intruder.

Diagnosis. The diagnosis of AD (*see* Box 4.4) is a multistage process. Initially the patient is interviewed, symptoms and signs identified, and the degree of illness severity determined. If the patient has early or a mild degree of cognitive impairment, it is then important to distinguish the changes of normal ageing from dementia. Once the symptoms and severity have been established, the course of the illness must be defined. If the symptoms are of relatively recent origin, the cognitive impairment may be due to delirium.

Box 4.4   ICD-10 diagnostic criteria for dementia in Alzheimer's disease

The following features are essential for a definite diagnosis:
1   presence of a dementia as described above (*see* Box 4.3)
2   insidious onset with slow deterioration. Although the onset usually seems to be difficult to pinpoint in time, realisation by others that the defects exist may occur suddenly. An apparent plateau in the progression may occur
3   absence of clinical evidence, or findings from special investigations, to suggest that the mental state may be due to other systemic or brain diseases which can induce a dementia (e.g. hypothyroidism, hypercalcaemia, vitamin B_{12} deficiency, niacin deficiency, neurosyphilis, normal-pressure hydrocephalus or subdural haematoma)
4   absence of a sudden, apoplectic onset, or of neurological signs of focal damage such as hemiparesis, sensory loss, visual field defects, and poor coordination occurring early in the illness (although these phenomena may be superimposed later).

There is now increasing sophistication in the diagnosis of different types of dementia, and an international working group has recently proposed a diagnostic framework that gives a higher degree of certainty for clinical diagnosis of Alzheimer's disease and enables (currently only for research purposes) the identification of a prodromal stage.[14,15]

Box 4.5   Diagnostic criteria for Alzheimer's disease[15]

Probable AD: A plus one or more of the supportive features B, C or D

Core diagnostic criteria
A   Presence of an early and significant episodic memory impairment that includes the following features:
➤   gradual progressive change in memory function reported by the patient or informant over more than 6 months
➤   objective evidence of significantly impaired episodic memory on testing. This generally consists of memory performance that

does not improve significantly with cueing or recognition testing and after effective encoding of information has been previously controlled

➤ the episodic memory impairment can be isolated or associated with other cognitive changes at the onset of AD or as AD advances.

Supportive features

B   Presence of MTL atrophy:

Volume loss of hippocampal, entorhinal cortex or amygdala evidenced on MRI with:

➤ qualitative ratings using visual scoring (referenced to well-characterised population with age norms) or quantitative volumetry of regions of interest (referenced to well-characterised populations with age norms).

C   Abnormal CSF biomarkers:

➤ decreased Aβ 1–42 and/or increased total tau and/or increased phosphor-tau

➤ other well-validated markers to be discovered in the future.

D   Specific pattern in functional neuroimaging with PET:

➤ reduced glucose metabolism in bilateral temporal parietal regions

➤ other well-validated ligands, including those that will emerge, such as PiB or FDDNP.

Exclusion criteria

History:

➤ sudden onset

➤ early occurrence of the following symptoms: gait disturbances, seizures, behavioural changes.

Clinical features:

➤ focal neurological features, including hemiparesis, sensory loss and visual field deficits

➤ early extrapyramidal signs.

Other medical conditions severe enough to account for memory and related symptoms:

➤ non-AD dementia

➤ major depression

➤ cerebrovascular disease

➤ toxic and metabolic abnormalities, all of which may require specific investigation

> ➤ MRI FLAIR or T2 signal abnormalities in the MTL that are consistent with infectious or vascular insults.
>
> AD, Alzheimer's disease; MTL, medial temporal lobe; CSF, cerebrospinal fluid; PET, photon emission tomography; PiB, Pittsburgh compound B; FDDNP, 2-(1-{6-[2-[F18]fluoroethyl) (methyl) amino]-2-naphthyl}ethylidene) malononitrile; MRI FLAIR, magnetic resonance imaging fluid attenuation inversion recovery.

*Box 4.5 lists the proposed diagnostic criteria for probable Alzheimer's disease. The NICE guidance[13] referred to above does *not* recommend CSF examination in the routine investigation of dementia. It does recommend the use of standardised cognitive testing. It also recommends the use of standardised diagnostic criteria for the differential diagnosis of Alzheimer's disease, vascular and other types of dementia. It supports the use of structural imaging to exclude other cerebral pathologies and to help to establish the subtype diagnosis. For a more detailed discussion of the types of neuroimaging available, the reader is referred to the guidance[13] and to *Practical Management of Dementia*.[14]

Fronto-temporal dementia. This is a primary degenerative dementia with both clinical and neuropathological features that distinguish it from AD. It generally occurs in those under 65 years of age, and Elfgren *et al*[16] have reported that it accounts for approximately 10% of all cases of dementia. In fronto-temporal dementia, the neuropathological changes are non-specific and include neuronal loss, gliosis and microvacuolation. The clinical features include a slowly progressive dementia, with early personality change, frontal lobe signs including disinhibition, and subsequently dementia.[16] As a group, these dementias are not specifically mentioned in ICD-10[1] or other contemporary international classifications, but they are becoming increasingly recognised. NICE recommends the use of the Lund–Manchester criteria for the diagnosis of fronto-temporal dementia. Useful discriminators of this type of dementia include:
> ➤ loss of personal awareness
> ➤ hyperorality
> ➤ stereotyped and perseverative behaviour
> ➤ progressive reduction of speech
> ➤ preserved spatial orientation
> ➤ MRI and SPECT imaging can help to confirm the diagnosis.[13]

Dementia in Pick's disease (F02.0). Pick's disease is classified as a fronto-temporal lobe dementia. It accounts for approximately 2% of all cases of dementia. It differs from other fronto-temporal dementias in its characteristic neuropathological lesions, which are known as Pick's bodies.[17] This form of dementia usually commences between the ages of 50 and 60 years, is slowly progressive, and is characterised by early changes in personality and social functioning. Such changes are followed by impairment of memory, intellect and language functions, together with apathy or euphoria and extrapyramidal phenomena. There is selective atrophy of the frontal and temporal lobes, but neuritic plaques and neurofibrillary tangles are not seen in excess of those observed in normal ageing. Diagnosis depends on establishing first the presence of dementia and then the predominance of frontal lobe features.

Dementia in Creutzfeldt–Jacob disease (CJD) (F02.1). This is a progressive dementia with extensive neurological signs due to specific neuropathological changes termed spongiform encephalopathy. This condition is thought to be due to a transmissible agent termed a prion. The onset of the condition is usually in middle to late life. The clinical course is rapid, leading to death within 1 to 2 years. The diagnosis should be suspected in all cases of dementia that progress rapidly in the presence of multiple neurological symptoms and signs. Occasionally the neurological symptoms and signs may precede the onset of dementia. The diagnosis is usually based on three main criteria, namely a rapidly progressive and devastating dementia, pyramidal and extrapyramidal signs with myoclonus, and characteristic triphasic waves on the electroencephalogram. Following the bovine spongiform encephalopathy (BSE) epidemic, a number of cases of new-variant CJD have been reported and, because of the long 'incubation periods' involved, it is uncertain whether there may be an epidemic in humans, although as time passes this seems less likely. CSF examination should be used to clarify the diagnosis if CJD or other forms of rapidly progressive dementia are suspected.[13]

Dementia in Huntington's disease (F02.2). This disorder is transmitted by a single autosomal dominant gene with almost 100% penetrance. This means that if the gene is identified when the patient is well, it is certain that symptoms will develop. These usually emerge in the third and fourth decades, and the incidence in men and women is probably equal. In a proportion of cases the early symptoms include depression, anxiety and paranoid illness, and personality change may be prominent. The condition is slowly progressive over 10–15 years. The triad of choreiform movement disorder, dementia and a family history of Huntington's chorea is highly suggestive of the diagnosis, but cases may occasionally occur without a family history. The choreiform movements typically involve the face, hands and shoulders, and usually precede the dementia. The dementia involves predominantly the frontal lobes in the early stages, with relative preservation of memory until later in the course of the illness.

Dementia in Parkinson's disease (F02.3). This is dementia that occurs in the course of established Parkinson's disease. Although there is some overlap with AD, the dementia that occurs in Parkinson's disease is classified as a subcortical dementia, the main features of which are slowing of thought processes (bradyphrenia), apathy and an inability to manipulate acquired knowledge.

Histologically, the dementia appears to be due to the presence of diffuse Lewy body formation.[17]

Lewy body dementia (LBD). More recently, there has been increasing interest in this condition, which is characterised by episodic confusion, prominent visual hallucinations, cognitive impairment and gradual deterioration. Parkinsonian-type symptoms are often present, including tremor, rigidity and bradykinesia. There appears to be a profound cholinergic deficit in Lewy body dementia, and it has been suggested that this form of dementia may be particularly likely to respond to treatment strategies that enhance cholinergic neurotransmitters. Patients with this form of dementia should not be given antipsychotic medication. SPECT can help to confirm the diagnosis.[13,14]

Vascular dementias (F01)

Vascular dementias are distinguished from AD by their history of onset, clinical features and subsequent course (*see* Figure 4.2). Typically there is a history of transient ischaemic attacks, fleeting pareses and visual loss. The dementia may follow a succession of acute cerebrovascular accidents or, less commonly, a single stroke. Diagnosis is based on the presence of dementia and uneven impairment of cognitive function, and focal neurological signs may be present. The patient may have considerable insight, and personality may be relatively well preserved. An abrupt onset or stepwise deterioration is often observed. Associated features include hypertension, carotid bruits, emotional lability and transient clouding of consciousness. A number of subtypes have been described in ICD-10.

Vascular dementia of acute onset (F01.0). Dementia develops rapidly after a succession of strokes from cerebrovascular thrombosis, embolism or haemorrhage.

Multi-infarct dementia (F01.1). This is more gradual in onset, and follows a number of minor ischaemic episodes which produce multiple infarcts in the cerebral cortex.

Subcortical vascular dementia (F01.2). Here there is ischaemic destruction in the white matter of the cerebral hemispheres, and the cerebral cortex is usually well preserved. The term 'Binswanger's encephalopathy' is sometimes used. There is usually a history of severe hypertension, acute strokes and an accumulation of focal neurological signs.

Differentiation of Alzheimer's disease from vascular dementia

The Ischaemic Score[18,19] is based on 13 clinical features, each of which is scored as 0, 1 or 2. The maximum score on some items is 1 (e.g. 'nocturnal confusion'), whereas on the remaining items the highest score is 2 (e.g. 'history of strokes').

The maximum possible score after all items have been rated is 18. A score of 7 or more is indicative of vascular dementia, whereas a score of 4 or less is suggestive of AD (*see* Table 4.3).

The Ischaemic Score is a widely used but not very reliable instrument for distinguishing AD from vascular dementia. The classification of dementia is becoming increasingly complex. AD is only one of several neurodegenerative dementias, and there are several forms of vascular dementia. This scale must therefore be used and interpreted with caution.

Table 4.3 Components of the Ischaemic Score[18]

Abrupt onset	2
Stepwise deterioration	1
Fluctuating course	2
Nocturnal confusion	1
Relative preservation of personality	1
Depression	1
Somatic complaints	1
Emotional incontinence	1
History of hypertension	1
History of strokes	2
Associated atherosclerosis	1
Focal neurological symptoms	2
Focal neurological signs	2
Total	18

Risk factors for vascular dementia

The risk factors for vascular dementia are summarised in Box 4.6.

Box 4.6   Risk factors for vascular dementia

Increased risk
➤ Male sex
➤ Increasing age
➤ Hypertension
➤ Diabetes mellitus
➤ Previous stroke
➤ Cardiovascular disease
➤ High levels of low-density lipoproteins

Possible increased risk
➤ Smoking
➤ Alcohol misuse
➤ Poor education
➤ 'Blue-collar' occupations
➤ Psychological stress in early life
➤ Previous exposure to pesticides, fertilisers, etc.

Reproduced from Richman and Wilson[10] with permission

Other causes of dementia

Vitamin B$_{12}$ deficiency. This is usually, but not always, associated with a megaloblastic anaemia. The patient's mental state may be indistinguishable from AD, but an admixture of apparently depressive symptoms with marked slowing and apathy can sometimes provide a clue. Patients with AD may also have lower than normal vitamin B$_{12}$ levels, and this may be one reason why the response to vitamin B$_{12}$ injections is sometimes poor. When there is a response, it is often (but not always) slow and incomplete.

Folic acid deficiency. Low serum folate levels are often an incidental finding in demented patients, and are only rarely of aetiological significance. Red cell folate level is a better indicator of deficiency, as it is less affected by short-term dietary intake. Treatment with folic acid, which is cheap and may produce some benefit, is justified until the diet can be improved.

Thyroid deficiency. Coarsening of the hair, a puffy facial appearance, pretibial myxoedema and a deep voice may be noted, but are not always present. The changes of hypothyroidism are sometimes so insidious that they are mistaken for normal ageing, and when mental changes supervene they are attributed to AD. Hypothyroid patients often complain of the cold and put extra garments on when those around them are quite warm enough. Marked slowing and apathy are again characteristic, but treatment with gradually increasing doses of thyroxine often partially and occasionally fully restores mental function.

Subdural haematoma. Chronic subdural haematoma is notoriously difficult to diagnose before death. The clinical picture may be of dementia or delirium. A high index of suspicion is essential, and if there is a history of head injury or if the level of consciousness is varying markedly, an expert opinion and structural scan are justified.

Other space-occupying lesions. Unexplained mental symptoms are sometimes due to intracranial growths. If these are malignant, they are often 'aggressive' and inoperable. Slow-growing, benign meningiomas can mimic mental illness, and a parasagittal meningioma can produce a picture very similar to that of normal-pressure hydrocephalus.

Normal-pressure hydrocephalus. This is characterised by the triad of confusion, abnormal gait and incontinence, more severe than would be expected in an early dementia. Patients presenting with this triad should be referred early for specialist assessment, as an operation can sometimes reverse the disability. There is still a lack of clarity surrounding the diagnosis and treatment of this condition.[20]

Alcoholic dementia. When alcohol is consumed to excess, approximately 10% of cases develop dementia.[21] Age is a major risk factor for alcoholic dementia. Disinhibition and impaired judgement are more common early in this form of dementia than in AD. Its progress may be arrested by abstention from alcohol. It may also be an accelerating factor in the deterioration due to multi-infarct dementia (MID) or AD, and may act as a risk factor for MID through the mechanism of hypertension. A history of excessive alcohol intake may be difficult to elicit, but hard-drinking friends or relatives, unexplained macrocytic anaemia or abnormal liver function tests may provide a clue.

Neurosyphilis. This is now a rare cause of dementia in old age, but should not be discounted, especially if there is a relevant past history or if the clinical picture is atypical. Serological tests can confirm or exclude the diagnosis.

HIV (F02.4). Dementia in human immunodeficiency virus (HIV) disease, also known as AIDS–dementia complex, is a rare condition but is not unheard of in older people. It presents with complaints of forgetfulness, slowness and poor concentration, or sometimes atypically with affective or psychotic symptoms. Progress of the disease is usually relatively rapid (of the order of weeks or months), leading to global dementia, mutism and death.[22]

Depressive pseudodementia. This is not an ICD-10 diagnostic term, but it is widely used and serves as a useful reminder that some severely depressed patients, especially those with severe psychomotor retardation or agitation, may appear to be suffering from dementia. A history of relatively rapid onset, with loss of interest rather than loss of memory as the first symptom, and a positive personal or family history of affective illness, are useful pointers. Sleep deprivation may be useful for distinguishing between the two conditions in cases where there is diagnostic doubt. Sleep deprivation improves cognitive function in those with an affective disorder, and worsens it in those with a dementing illness.

Cortical and subcortical dementia

A clinical distinction has been made between cortical and subcortical dementia. AD is the classic cortical dementia, with marked aphasia, amnesia and impaired judgement. The subcortical dementias include the toxic and metabolic dementias, and are characterised by forgetfulness, marked psychomotor slowing, apathetic or depressed mood, and often by abnormal posture, muscle tone and movements. MID often produces a mixed picture. The terms 'cortical' and 'subcortical' are anatomically misleading, due to the complicated interactions of systems within the brain. Nevertheless, they are clinically relevant, especially as so-called subcortical features can provide an important clinical clue to an early and potentially treatable dementia.

Measuring the severity of dementia

At the beginning of 1982, two scales were published to assess severity, and they are still in use, namely the Global Deterioration Scale (GDS)[23] and the Clinical Dementia Rating (CDR).[24] The GDS has tended to be more widely used in a clinical context, and the CDR has been more often used in epidemiological research. The GDS has seven categories: no, very mild, mild, moderate, moderately severe, severe and very severe cognitive decline. The CDR is divided into five categories: healthy, and questionable, mild, moderate and severe dementia. However, there are a large number of instruments for measuring symptoms in confused patients. For a more detailed discussion, with information about individual instruments, the reader is referred to a helpful book devoted to rating scales,[25] and some of these scales are considered below and in Chapter 2.

Behavioural disturbance

BEHAVE-AD. This was designed specifically to assess behavioural symptoms in patients with AD, but it is also useful in patients with dementia generally. There are 26 questions in total, one of which is a global rating. Areas covered include delusional ideas, hallucinations, disturbed activity, aggressiveness, sleep, and mood disturbance and anxiety symptoms.[26]

Activities of daily living

Bristol Activities of Daily Living Scale. This is a 20-question instrument with a maximum score of 60 (equivalent to very severe). It covers areas such as eating, dressing, personal hygiene, toileting, mobility, orientation, communication and domestic tasks.[27]

Staging instruments

Functional Assessment Staging (FAST). This is used for the assessment of functional change (staging) in ageing and dementia. Staging ranges from 1 (no difficulties) to 7f (unable to hold head up).[28]

Delirium

Delirium Rating Scale (DRS). This is a 10-item instrument for assessing delirium, with a maximum score of 32 (very severe).[29] The CAM[5] is also useful, particularly as a screening instrument.

Potentially reversible causes of dementia

A smaller number of patients have a potentially reversible dementia, and there are many potential causes[14] (*see* Table 4.4). The proportion of dementia patients with a potentially reversible cause ranges from 8%

Table 4.4 Some causes of reversible dementia

Intracranial causes	Subdural haematoma
	Tumour
	Abscess
Central nervous system infection	Syphilis
	Tuberculosis
	Fungal infections
Endocrine causes	Hyper/hypothyroidism
	Hyper/hypoparathyroidism
	Hyper/hypoadrenalism
Collagen diseases	Systemic lupus erythematosus
	Temporal arteritis
Metabolic diseases	Liver disease
	Renal disease
	Wilson's disease
	Pernicious anaemia
	Folate deficiency
Toxic causes	Alcohol
	Heavy metals and aluminium
Psychiatric causes	Depression/mania
	Schizophrenia
	Conversion disorder
	Ganser syndrome
Miscellaneous causes	Communicating hydrocephalus
	Epilepsy
	Parkinson's disease
	Remote effect of various cancers
	Cardiac insufficiency
	Respiratory insufficiency

to 40%. The prevalence will depend on a number of factors, including the population studied and the definition of 'reversible'. For example, geriatric inpatients may have a higher prevalence of hypothyroidism than community-based patients, and this may result in a higher prevalence of hypothyroidism in demented patients on medical wards compared with those at home. In addition, the presence of a 'reversible cause' does not mean that the dementia is necessarily due to that potential cause or even that it can be reversed in any individual case. It is crucial that patients with dementia have a full assessment and that any potentially treatable cause of dementia is identified and corrected. Generally the earlier such problems are identified and treated, the better the prognosis.

The aetiology of Alzheimer's disease

The precise aetiology of AD is poorly understood. The most favoured current understanding is based on the idea that the initiating event in Alzheimer's disease is related to abnormal processing of β-amyloid (Aβ) peptide. Understanding the process is important because such an understanding may have implications for both prevention and treatment. The relationship between cause and effect may be difficult to establish, particularly with regard to neurotransmitter deficits and the characteristic neuropathological changes that are seen in AD. The most important risk factor for AD is old age. Other risk factors include Down's syndrome, head trauma, a family history of Alzheimer's disease, and obesity in middle age. Many other factors have been suggested, but the evidence for these is very limited. Possible causative factors can be considered under the following headings:

➤ genetic factors
➤ toxic exposure
➤ infectious agents
➤ free radicals
➤ ageing/environmental interaction
➤ neurochemical changes
➤ neuropathological changes.

Genetic factors

Genetics is perhaps one of the most interesting and promising areas of research in terms of the aetiology of AD. Neuritic plaques, the neuropathological hallmark of AD, are extracellular aggregates 50–200 mm in diameter (see below).

Hardy and Higgins[30] have proposed the 'amyloid cascade hypothesis', in which they suggest that Aβ is directly or indirectly neurotoxic and this leads to the development of neuritic plaques and neurofibrillary tangles, with subsequent neuronal cell death. Aβ is derived from another larger protein called amyloid precursor protein (APP). The normal function of APP is unknown, although it may be important for maintaining the integrity of synapses. Interestingly, it has been known for some time that patients with Down's syndrome (trisomy 21) who live into their fifties also develop neuropathological features of AD. In addition, the gene for APP has been localised on chromosome 21.[31] It appears that approximately 25% of early-onset familial AD may be due to mutations of the APP gene on chromosome 21. Another gene on chromosome 14 is thought to be responsible for the remaining 75% of familial early cases of AD. However, early cases account for only a small percentage of all cases of AD. There have been some important developments in the genetics of late-onset AD. Three alleles (ε2, ε3 and ε4) code for apolipoprotein E (ApoE), and these alleles are located on chromosome 19. ApoE is a major component of very-low-density lipoproteins (VLDLs), whose normal function includes removing excess cholesterol from the blood and transporting it to the liver for metabolism. The alleles occur with different frequencies, and in normal individuals, ε4 is the least common. However, in late-onset AD, ε4 is the most common. The ε4 allele is associated through an as yet uncertain mechanism with increased accumulation of Aβ in the brain. Based on a review of 42 studies,[32] the lifetime risk of AD in individuals who are homozygous for ε4 is approximately 91%.

Hypoxia

Hypoxia associated with chronic obstructive pulmonary disease and cardiovascular disease such as stroke or even persistent or repeated cardiac arrhythmia can increase the incidence of Alzheimer's disease. The mechanism for this appears to involve increased expression of APP and increased formation of Aβ with dysregulation of calcium channels in the neuronal membrane.[33]

Toxic exposure

The substance which has received most attention is aluminium, and there is evidence both for and against (mostly against) this hypothesis. Aluminosilicates are present in the cores of the neuritic plaques which are one of the 'hallmarks' of AD.[34] Neuritic plaques are found throughout the hippocampus and neocortex, and their presence has been correlated with the severity of dementia. However, there is still some debate as to whether these abnormalities are primary or secondary. Aluminium salts directly applied to the brain produce neurofibrillary tangles in rabbits and cats. However, these abnormalities are not identical to the neurofibrillary tangles seen in AD. There have also been studies of human subjects exposed to high levels of aluminium. For example, renal dialysis patients develop high levels of serum aluminium, but at post-mortem the associated neuropathology is also quite distinct from AD. Other toxic substances have also been implicated, but the evidence is limited and inconclusive. However, when alcohol is drunk to excess, approximately 10%

of individuals develop dementia.[20] The pathological changes are different to those found in AD. However, the conditions may overlap.

Infectious agents

A number of neurological conditions similar to AD are caused by a transmissible agent. These include kuru, Creutzfeldt–Jakob disease (CJD) and Gerstmann–Straussler syndrome.[35] These diseases are due to prions which, until relatively recently, were unknown infectious agents. Prions have a long incubation period with none of the inflammatory responses that are seen with viral infections. This raised the possibility that AD might also be caused by a transmissible agent, but this now seems unlikely.

The free radical hypothesis

Free radicals are atoms or molecules with one or more unpaired electrons, and they are particularly likely to arise in chemical reactions involving oxygen. When oxygen is reduced, free radicals may be formed, including the superoxide and hydroxyl radicals. These interact with other molecules to produce new free radicals and thus set in motion a 'chain reaction'. Such substances are particularly toxic to biological molecules (e.g. DNA and proteins), and the body uses a number of natural defences to deal with them, including enzymes (e.g. superoxide dismutase) and antioxidants (e.g. vitamin E). Free radicals may be responsible for both ageing and AD, which may be due to the progressive accumulation of irreversible damage caused by free radicals.

Ageing and environmental interaction

Certain environmental events (e.g. trauma, exposure to toxins or infectious agents) may cause neuronal loss, but this loss is not of sufficient severity to produce clinical symptoms. However, later in life when the effects of cortical loss due to ageing are superimposed, clinical manifestations of dementia may arise. This is thought to be the case with regard to a number of neurological conditions, including Guam parkinsonism–dementia complex, Parkinson's disease and post-poliomyelitis syndrome. Environmental exposure may magnify the Alzheimer-type changes that are seen in normal ageing. If AD is an exaggeration of the normal ageing process, these hypotheses fit together well. Unfortunately, the notion that AD is an exaggeration of the normal ageing process is very controversial, with evidence on both sides.

Neurochemical changes

The four classic neurotransmitters, namely acetylcholine, dopamine, noradrenaline and serotonin, have been examined in both elderly subjects and patients with AD.[36]

Acetylcholine. This neurotransmitter is found predominantly in the cerebral cortex, caudate nucleus and parts of the limbic system. The presence of this neurotransmitter may be indirectly assessed by the presence of either the synthetic enzyme choline acetyltransferase (CAT) or the metabolic enzyme acetylcholinesterase (AChE). Using such methods, it has been shown that there is an age-dependent decrease in CAT. CAT concentrations show a larger decrease in patients with AD, and this decline in cholinergic activity is said to be a key factor in the aetiology of AD.

Dopamine. This neurotransmitter shows a decrease in levels with age (e.g. in the nigrostriatal system). In addition, there is a reduction in the number of dopamine D2-receptors with increasing age. The situation in patients with AD has been little studied, and few data are currently available.

Noradrenaline. In the cerebellum and locus caeruleus, noradrenaline levels decrease with increasing age, but there does not appear to be a similar reduction in levels in the cortex. The concentration of monoamine oxidase B (MAO-B), which metabolises noradrenaline, increases with age, and there is a significant increase in MAO-B levels in patients with AD compared with age-matched controls.

Serotonin. Levels of this neurotransmitter may decrease with increasing age. The cell bodies are located in the raphe nuclei of the brainstem and have both ascending and descending projections. Although some studies have suggested that there are no age-dependent changes in 5-HT receptors, other workers have shown that ageing is associated with an increase in 5-HT1 receptors and a decrease in 5-HT2 receptors. The situation in patients with AD is less clearly defined.

Neuropathological changes

It may be difficult to make a clear distinction between the normal ageing process and the pathological features of early AD.[36] Some of the changes that are seen in the normal ageing brain include decreased brain weight, decreased brain volume, dendritic loss, widening of sulci and ventricles, neuritic plaques, neurofibrillary tangles, and deposits of lipofuscin, aluminium, copper, iron and melanin.[36] These changes are also the primary neuropathological features seen in AD. During the first 50 years in normal elderly individuals, grey matter is lost at a greater rate than white matter, but during the second 50 years, white matter is lost at a greater rate. The loss in patients with AD is similar but greater (i.e. there is a quantitative difference rather than a qualitative one). The neuritic plaque is initially composed of a few amyloid fibres intermingled with degenerating neurons. This is replaced by a central core of amyloid surrounded by amyloid fibres and degenerating neurites. Finally, the amyloid plaque is surrounded by astrocytes. Neurofibrillary tangles are lesions within the cytoplasm of the perikaryon of medium and large pyramidal cells of the neo- and paleocortex. They occur less frequently in the subcortical nuclei. Under the electron microscope they can be seen as paired helical filaments, but precisely how they impair cortical function is not known. Some authors have identified an association between cholinergic neurons and neuritic plaques, and this has been proposed in support of the cholinergic hypothesis of AD.

Management: the memory service

NICE guidance[13] now gives detailed advice on all aspects of the diagnosis and management of dementia. Increasingly this is done by a specialist memory service or clinic.

Typically the memory service will be run by mental health services for older people. The first point of contact for concerned relatives will usually (in the UK) be the primary care team. They will often make an initial assessment including standard investigations agreed under a 'shared care protocol' with the local memory service. If there appear to be significant memory problems, the patient will be referred to the memory service. These are increasingly nurse-led and adopt a person-centred approach. They gather further information from the patient and family with a view to aiding an accurate diagnosis and formulating a care plan. This care plan may involve medication for Alzheimer's disease (see below), psychological approaches to support the patient and carers, and social measures. The assessment will also take into account any concurrent physical illness and treatment and any sensory problems, and seek to ensure their optimal management.

Neuroimaging investigations will be undertaken in keeping with NICE guidance,[13] and the patient will usually be seen by a psychiatrist who will make a formal diagnosis and explain the issues to the patient and carers. Giving the diagnosis is a sensitive matter, and services usually do this with great care and forethought. Often the patient and carers will be supported at the point of diagnosis by a member of the memory services team, who will provide ongoing support and initial monitoring of the effects of any treatment with anticholinesterase or similar medication, as well as overseeing the effectiveness of other parts of the care plan. In many areas the Alzheimer's Society is taking an increasing role in supporting patients and carers, working in close collaboration with memory services.

Psychological management

The patient and their family will require considerable support to discuss the implications of the diagnosis. This may require several meetings and may be done in the patient's home, depending on their circumstances, by a member of the memory team. The worker will be able to direct the patient and carer to relevant information about the condition, and discuss the long-term prognosis and natural history. This will help the patient and carer to think about future needs and how best the service will be able to help them. If the Alzheimer's Society is not an integral part of the service, patients and carers can be put in contact with www.alzheimer.org.uk. Patients and carers usually benefit from the opportunity to discuss in greater depth their anxieties about the condition and its implications. The occupational therapist or clinical psychologist may also be able to help in more specialised areas, such as simple techniques to help with orientation and 'risk' behaviours. For example, a large board in the kitchen could display the day of the week and the date *(reality orientation)*, and large-print sheets on the door and cooker could remind the patient to 'lock the door' and 'light the gas'. These can be adapted to individual patients' needs.

According to NICE guidance,[13] people with mild to moderate dementia should be given the opportunity to participate in a structured group cognitive stimulation programme. A Memory Services National Accreditation Programme run by the College Centre for Quality Improvement (CCQI) at the Royal College of Psychiatrists (www.rcpsych.ac.uk) provides a process for developing and accrediting services. Support is crucial for both patient and carer, and will continue to be needed for an extended period of time. The management of the patient will also change as the illness progresses.

Social aspects of management

A number of social aspects of management need to be considered. First, it is important to undertake an assessment of the patient in their own home. This may be done by the memory service nurse or by the occupational therapist when one is available. This assessment will focus on a number of aspects, including the ability of the patient to undertake routine tasks such as dressing, toileting, personal hygiene (e.g. bathing), making a hot drink and a simple meal, managing their finances and undertaking tasks outside the home (e.g. shopping). It is also important to undertake a risk assessment. This will include an assessment of 'personal' risk (e.g. suicidal ideas, common in the early stages of Alzheimer's disease, violent behaviour and falls due to medication) and 'environmental' risk. The latter will include a detailed examination of the patient's environment. Areas that require closer examination might include use of gas cookers and fires, use of electrical appliances, risk of leaving doors unlocked, risk of eating defrosted/rotten food, and risk due to steep stairs or loose carpets that might increase the likelihood of trips or falls. Once a risk assessment has been completed, it is important to implement risk management (i.e. each identified area of risk needs to be reduced to a minimum). It will not be possible to remove all risk completely. Reducing the risk to a minimum has to be balanced against the needs and wishes of the patient and their carers.

During the early stages of the condition, the patient and carer may need to seek advice from a social worker, solicitor or voluntary agencies about managing their assets. They should consider the need to make a will (if one has not already been made) and also issues relating to Power of Attorney and Lasting Power of Attorney. If appropriate, the psychiatrist can undertake an appropriate assessment of the patient's capacity to sign such agreements.

A range of services can usually be provided for patients and their carers depending on their individual needs and wishes, including the following:

➤ home care (help with cleaning, shopping, collecting pension, etc.)
➤ meals on wheels
➤ laundry service
➤ help with personal hygiene
➤ help with getting up and going to bed
➤ night service (to let the carer get some sleep)
➤ day care (to give the carer some respite and provide stimulation for the patient)
➤ respite care (a period away from home to give the carer a break)
➤ luncheon clubs
➤ day trips.

The availability of these services from local authorities varies greatly for financial and organisational reasons. Voluntary groups such as the Alzheimer's Society are taking an increasing role in organising and providing them.

Medical aspects of management

There are now four antidementia drugs available for the treatment of mild to moderate Alzheimer's disease. The first three – donepezil, rivastigmine and galantamine – are all cholinesterase inhibitors that prevent the breakdown of acetylcholine, the principal neurotransmitter thought to be depleted in Alzheimer's disease and associated with memory formation. Galantamine also modulates nicotinic-receptor function. The fourth drug, memantine, which acts on glutamate pathways, is a useful alternative in patients with moderate Alzheimer's disease who are intolerant of or have a contraindication to cholinesterase inhibitors. It is also recommended for people with severe Alzheimer's disease, and evidence is emerging that cholinesterase inhibitors may help this group, too, although this is outside current NICE guidance. The criteria for using antidementia drugs in England and Wales are summarised in the National Institute for Health and Clinical Excellence (NICE) guidelines.[13]

For the patient to be eligible for a cholinesterase inhibitor drug, the following criteria must be met.

➤ The patient must have mild to moderate Alzheimer's disease.
➤ The drug must be prescribed by a specialist (an old age psychiatrist, geriatrician or neurologist).
➤ The patient must be carefully monitored after commencing treatment. This is usually achieved by using one measure of cognitive function and one measure of activities of daily living (see above).
➤ The initial assessment should normally be at 2 to 4 months. If there is no improvement after 3 months, the drug should be discontinued.

In general terms, approximately 30–50% of patients will derive some benefit from treatment, but data on longer-term treatment are relatively scarce. If these drugs are used, individual outcome must be assessed systematically, usually in a memory clinic. An assessment (cognitive assessment and measure of activities of daily living) should be undertaken prior to commencing treatment and then at week 4 and week 12. After 3 months, information from clinical observations, input from other healthcare professionals and social services, the results from rating instruments and information from the patient and carer will all need to be pooled and a decision made about whether there has been any clinical benefit. If there has been improvement, the antidementia drug should be continued and re-evaluated every 3 months. If there has been no improvement, the drug should be stopped. However, as the illness progresses it may be increasingly difficult to determine whether there has been any improvement. Since the condition gradually deteriorates, a situation where there has been no change or where the decline was less severe than one would predict could be interpreted as 'improvement'. The use of other medications (e.g. antidepressants, antipsychotics) is described below. The currently available drugs are being increasingly used, but a wide range of drugs has been tried or suggested as treatments for Alzheimer's disease (*see* Table 4.5), highlighting the complexity of this rapidly growing area.

Treatment of non-cognitive features of dementia

Mood disorders

When patients present with a cluster of symptoms suggestive of a depressive illness, antidepressants may be indicated, although environmental manipulation and psychological approaches should also be considered. The side-effect profile and individual preference of the clinician normally govern the choice of drug. The anticholinergic effects of the tricyclics may further impair cognitive function and should be avoided. Selective serotonin reuptake inhibitors (SSRIs) seem to be well tolerated at standard doses in older people, and are preferable in patients with cardiac problems or for

Table 4.5 Current and possible future pharmacological treatments for patients with Alzheimer's disease

Current treatments	Examples
Cholinesterase inhibitors	Donepezil
	Rivastigmine
	Galantamine
NMDA antagonist	Memantine

Future treatments/augmentation strategies

Folate (increased synthesis of acetylcholine plus additional neurochemical benefits)

Selegiline (improves dopamine functioning plus antioxidant and neuroprotection)

Vitamin E (antioxidant, and may help to reduce disease progression)

Lithium (can block the hyperphosphorylation of tau in animal models; studies are in progress)

Disease-modifying agents (a number of vaccines and drugs are in development that act on amyloid processing)

β-amyloid antagonists (these drugs bind to β amyloid and may prevent the assembly of amyloid plaques; they are in development)

Gamma secretase inhibitors (these inhibit the enzyme gamma secretase, thus reducing the formation of A-beta-42 formation, which is important in the formation of amyloid plaques; in development)

Beta secretase inhibitors (also work by preventing beta amyloid formation; in development)

whom the anticholinergic effects of the tricyclics make them inadvisable. Some clinicians would make an SSRI their first choice of antidepressant regardless of the patient's age. The atypical antidepressants (e.g. trazodone), the newer selective reversible monoamine oxidase inhibitors (e.g. moclobemide), and drugs that act on both noradrenergic and serotonin receptors (e.g. venlafaxine, duloxetine) also have a role in the treatment of depression in patients with dementia. There is also emerging evidence of benefit with agomelatine, a $5HT_{2A}$ antagonist and melatonin agonist. As well as having antidepressant activity, it also improves sleep. However, research remains very limited in this area, as recently demonstrated in a systematic review and meta-analysis of seven randomised controlled trials of antidepressants in patients with dementia.[37] Evidence for effectiveness was 'inconclusive', and larger studies were noted to be needed. In more severe dementia, depression may be manifested by behavioural problems such as agitation, wandering or unwillingness to be left alone. In such cases a trial of antidepressant therapy may be justified. If the patient is unable to report a change in mood, then target behaviours must be identified and monitored to ascertain the effectiveness of the treatment.

Psychotic symptoms

Psychotic symptoms, including delusions and hallucinations, are common in dementia, and if they are distressing or result in behavioural disturbances it may be appropriate to treat them pharmacologically. It is not yet clear how far cholinesterase inhibitors and memantine work in this group, but it may be worth a trial of treatment. Antipsychotic medication carries an appreciable mortality and should be avoided if possible. If antipsychotic drugs have to be used, the newer atypical antipsychotics such as risperidone, olanzapine and quetiapine may be used cautiously for short periods. There is currently a national 'call to action' to reduce the use of antipsychotics in people with dementia, in recognition of the risks associated with these drugs. This has been organised by the NHS Institute of Innovation and Improvement and the Dementia Action Alliance. Further information is available at www.institute. nhs.uk/dementia c2a (accessed 13/5/12). Occasionally benzodiazepines may be useful, but they should not be used routinely or long term.

Behavioural disorders

Antipsychotics should not generally be prescribed for agitation and aggression, regardless of the cause of the symptom, and their use should not replace assessment of the cause of the behaviour, which may often be physical or environmental. Most studies have shown antipsychotics to be more effective than placebo in the treatment of symptoms of agitation, overactivity and restlessness. However, recent concern about the safety of antipsychotics in people with dementia has led to a situation where they can only be recommended when the disturbance is otherwise unmanageable, and then only for short periods at low doses. Generally the newer antipsychotics are to be preferred, but none are without risk. The drug dosage should be reduced or the drug stopped completely if side-effects are bothersome. Aggression and irritability can also be helped by SSRIs or trazodone in some patients. These effects on aggression, irritability and inner drive are often seen much earlier than would be expected from an antidepressant effect, and it is likely that antidepressant drugs have specific effects in addition to their antidepressant actions. Trazodone also seems to be of benefit in a minority of patients without depression, in stopping apparently purposeless shouting, but more research is needed to confirm these findings, which are generally based on clinical observation and small trials.

Non-pharmacological treatments

Specific psychological treatments for some of the symptoms of dementia have been developed, and it is argued that both patients and their families derive benefit from them, but few of the treatments are easily evaluated, although the evidence for structured group cognitive stimulation has been accepted by NICE.[13] The management of patients with dementia must always involve supporting patients and relatives, allowing them an opportunity to express their feelings, and maintaining patients' self-esteem by emphasising their skills rather than focusing on their failures.

Memory training

At present most patients with dementia are referred to specialist services when their illness is too severe to benefit from memory training. However, for the normal elderly and for those with mild memory impairment the maxim 'use it or lose it' is relevant. Techniques to aid memory (e.g. by making visual associations or using prompts) have been shown to be helpful. Such techniques are often intuitively used by patients and their families, and the increase in the number of memory clinics seeing patients with mild impairment should lead to increased formal teaching of such techniques, including structured group cognitive stimulation.

Behaviour modification

Behaviour modification is another technique which is often used by carers in an intuitive way, but which can also be used as a formal therapy. The therapy depends on operant conditioning techniques whereby the desired behaviour is positively reinforced (e.g. by spending time in an enjoyable activity with the patient) and undesirable behaviours are negatively reinforced – that is, the reward is withdrawn (e.g. by ignoring the patient's behaviour). Behaviour modification can be useful for a range of undesirable behaviours, including aggression, screaming and some types of incontinence.

The basis of the technique is the ABC of behaviour, where A is the antecedent, B is the behaviour itself and C is the consequences of the behaviour. Carers are first asked to give a detailed description of the undesired behaviour, including environmental factors such as the time of day and the activities of others. Charting the behaviour can allow its cause to be determined, which could be a physical symptom (e.g. constipation, or pain on moving) or environmental (e.g. the noise and arousal of other patients at mealtimes diverting the carer's attention away from the patient). Attempts can then be made to modify the antecedents. Even if the cause of the behaviour cannot be removed, the behaviour can still be modified by operant conditioning.

A valuable part of the therapy is the support and advice that are given to the carer in a non-judgemental way, and the hope that improvements can be made in the quality of the lives of both the patient and their carers. Psychological and psychotherapeutic techniques underpin the management of patients with dementia and severe behavioural problems who are cared for on continuing care wards.

Reality orientation

Disorientation with regard to time and place is an early symptom of dementia, and two main forms of reality orientation (RO) have been described.[38] In the first type, known as informal reality orientation or 24-hour reorientation, all opportunities are taken to orientate the patient with regard to time and place. The orientation boards that are found in most institutions are examples of this type of reorientation technique.

In formal structured reality orientation sessions, a small number of patients undergo a programme of discussion, exploring topics of interest, which allows reorientation to take place. Exponents of formal reality orientation emphasise that formal RO sessions are intended as a supplement rather than an alternative to 24-hour RO. It is essential in both types of RO that the staff or carers do not agree with the patient if they are clearly wrong. RO has been criticised as a 'dehumanising' behaviour modification technique that is solely preoccupied with targeting symptom management, but its supporters argue that this reflects the way in which the technique is used in unskilled hands, rather than its original aim.

Research designed to evaluate the effectiveness of RO has clearly demonstrated an improvement in verbal orientation,[38] but attempts to demonstrate lasting improvement in orientation have been disappointing, with patients failing to generalise from their experiences in the groups. RO techniques have been shown to have a positive effect on staff and carers both in increasing staff satisfaction, and in increasing staff knowledge of individual patients and thus improving the quality of interactions between them.

Validation therapy

Validation therapy is a more patient-centred therapy, which aims to validate the patient's past and present experiences and feelings. It was designed for use in elderly patients with dementia, and it emphasises the need to interact in 'whatever reality they are in, in order to ease distress and restore self-worth'.[39] Thus, for example, if a patient became anxious about the need to collect her children from school, the therapist would start by sharing the anxiety associated with these thoughts and then gradually move the patient through that phase of her life to the present day. As with reality orientation, these techniques can either be used formally in groups or can be incorporated into round-the-clock care for the patient.

Validation therapy is very widely used in institutions, but the evidence that it is useful is anecdotal. Evaluations have failed to produce convincing evidence of its effectiveness, either on patients or on staff morale, largely because of problems with the design of the studies.

Reminiscence therapy

Reminiscence therapy is widely used. It has its roots in psychodynamic theory and ideas about the process of life review in later life where past experiences are reviewed and past conflicts can be examined again and reintegrated. Most often groups of patients meet with a therapist. Photographs of past times, music or other sensory experiences such as smells are used as triggers to memory, and then the therapist aims to facilitate discussion. Specifically designed packages of audio-visual material have been produced for use in reminiscence therapy. According to King,[40] meeting in groups provides the opportunity for socialisation and social reintegration, resolution of old conflicts through life review, identification of current concerns and struggles, recognition of oneself as a survivor, and appreciation of one's own achievements and those of others.

Much of the published work on reminiscence therapy is anecdotal, and many of the studies have not included a control group. Reminiscence therapy groups are reported as often being enjoyed by both staff and patients, increasing staff's knowledge of their patients, and increasing the quality of interactions between patients and staff. It is not clear to what extent these positive benefits are non-specific or related to the reminiscence therapy. No lasting effects on memory have been reported in controlled trials.

Expressive therapies

Other techniques are used with patients with dementia, not only to provide interest and occupation, but also to reduce anxiety and aid self-expression, often by non-verbal means. Art, music and techniques involving physical contact (e.g. hand massage and aromatherapy employing specific oils) are used. The Snoezlen technique was developed for use with severely demented patients with the aim of providing sensory input through a range of senses.

Research studies have not demonstrated the efficacy of these treatments compared with spending the equivalent amount of time with patients. However, techniques such as dementia care mapping, in which the quality of interactions as well as the time spent with patients are documented, show that in most institutions little time is devoted to attending to patients' social or psychological rather than physical needs, and hence any moves to promote quality interactions between staff and patients should be encouraged.

Enriched opportunities programme

This highly structured approach to improving the quality of life of people with dementia in residential or nursing care combines a variety of approaches. In one study its implementation increased well-being, diversity of activity and positive staff interactions, with a significant reduction in depression.[41] The reader is referred to the original paper, available through www.alzheimers.org.uk, for further details.

Communication with people with dementia

Communication is a key skill for all health workers. The ability to communicate with people with dementia needs to be developed in training. The starting point is a belief that we can communicate effectively with most – if not all – people, however confused they may be. Good communication involves much more than verbal communication. It includes how we dress, our facial expression, our body language and our tone of voice. Patients, especially if they have been through the disorientating process of illness and admission to hospital, perhaps compounded by sensory impairment, will be glad to see a nurse or doctor who is willing to spend time helping them to make sense of the situation in which they find themselves. Communication includes respectful listening as well as asking questions and imparting information. If there are specific sensory deficits, they should be corrected as far as possible. If there are specific verbal deficits (e.g. various forms of aphasia), speech should be simple and well articulated, in order to facilitate easy answers. A speech therapist may be able to help in particularly difficult cases.

In addition, the Royal College of Psychiatrists has produced a variety of information leaflets for patients and carers, and this is available by following the links on the College website (www.rcpsych.ac.uk/).

Prognosis

This has usually been studied in terms of length of survival, but quality of life of patients and carers is also important and much more amenable to intervention. The demented patient who lives in a sympathetic enabling environment, whose physical health and sensory abilities are optimised and whose carers use the available knowledge about dementia and are well supported will fare better. In general, patients with Alzheimer's disease steadily deteriorate over a period of 2–5 years, and death is often due to pneumonia or some other physical illness. The time course is usually longer with multi-infarct dementia, especially if the underlying cardiovascular risk factors are reduced or well controlled (e.g. stopping smoking, well-controlled hypertension). Overall, dementia, particularly in the very old, is associated with a higher mortality and shortened life.[42]

CONCLUSION

Dementia is common, and its prevalence rises with increasing age. Delirium is also common in older people. Figure 4.3 summarises some of the important factors in distinguishing between the different causes of confusion in old age. Confusion has many different causes, including physical illness, making a detailed physical assessment essential. The two commonest types of dementia are Alzheimer's disease and multi-infarct dementia. There are now treatments

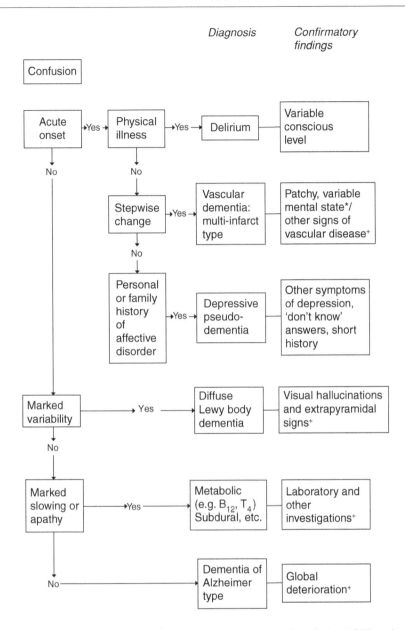

Figure 4.3 Flow chart for diagnosis of some important causes of confusion. *Diffuse Lewy body disease also produces marked variability, often with visual hallucinations and/or extrapyramidal symptoms. [+]In all cases neuroimaging may support the diagnosis.

available that might aid the management of Alzheimer's disease, and simple measures such as the control of hypertension and use of aspirin can help to prevent further deterioration in patients with vascular dementia. Patients and carers are often in a very distressed state. Good interpersonal skills are vital to reduce distress and to communicate clearly. Good teamworking skills are also essential because patients and carers may require the full back-up of the multidisciplinary team to ensure that they receive the support which they need. The management of patients with dementia and support for their families can be extremely challenging but also very rewarding.

REFERENCES

1 World Health Organization (1992) *The ICD-10 Classification of Mental and Behavioural Disorders*. World Health Organization, Geneva.
2 Bowler C, Boyle A, Branford M *et al* (1994) Detection of psychiatric disorders in elderly medical inpatients. *Age Ageing*. 23: 307–11.
3 O'Keeffe ST (1999) Delirium in the elderly. *Age Ageing*. 28: 5–8.
4 O'Keeffe ST and Lavan JN (1999) Clinical significance of delirium subtypes in older people. *Age Ageing*. 28: 115–19.
5 Inouye SK, van Dyck CH, Alessi CA *et al* (1990) Clarifying confusion: the Confusion Assessment Method. A new method for the detection of delirium. *Ann Int Med.* 113: 942–8.
6 Laurila JV, Pitkala KH, Strandberg TE and Tilvis RS (2002) Confusion Assessment Method in the diagnostics of delirium among aged hospital patients: would it serve better in screening than as a diagnostic instrument? *Int J Geriatr Psychiatry.* 17: 1112–19.
7 Alzheimer's Disease International (2008) *The Prevalence of Dementia Worldwide.* www.alz.co.uk/adi/pdf/prevalence.pdf
8 Roth M (1955) The natural history of mental disorder in old age. *J Ment Sci.* 101: 281–301.
9 American Psychiatric Association (1994) *Diagnostic and Statistical Manual of Mental Disorders* (4e). American Psychiatric Association, Washington, DC.
10 Richman AV and Wilson KCM (2012) Diagnosis and classification. In S Curran and J Wattis (eds) *Practical Management of Dementia* (2e). Radcliffe Publishing, London.
11 Alzheimer's Society (2012) *Dementia 2012.* www.Alzheimers.org.uk/dementia2012 (accessed 29 March 2012).
12 Department of Health (2009) *Living Well with Dementia: a National Dementia Strategy.* Available at https://www.gov.uk/government/publications/living-well-with-dementia-a-national-dementia-strategy (accessed 26 November 2012).
13 National Institute for Health and Clinical Excellence (2006/2011) *CG42: Dementia: Supporting People with Dementia and their Carers in Health and Social Care.* http://publications.nice.org.uk/dementia-cg42.
14 Krüger S, Bertoni MA and Curran S (2011) Early detection of dementia. In S Curran and J Wattis (eds) *Practical Management of Dementia* (2e). Radcliffe Publishing, London.

15 Dubois B, Feldman H and Schletens P (2007) A new concept and new criteria for Alzheimer's disease. *Eur Neuro Dis*, Issue 2.

16 Elfgren C, Brun A, Gustafson L *et al* (1994) Neuropsychological tests as discriminators between dementia of Alzheimer type and frontotemporal dementia. *Int J Geriatr Psychiatry.* **9**: 635–42.

17 Godwin-Austen RB (1994) Dementia and Parkinson's disease. In: JRM Copeland, MT Abou-Saleh and DG Blazer (eds) *Principles and Practice of Geriatric Psychiatry.* John Wiley & Sons, Chichester.

18 Hachinski V (1978) Differentiation of Alzheimer's disease from multi-infarct dementia. In: R Katzman, RD Terry and KL Bick (eds) *Alzheimer's Disease: Senile Dementia and Related Disorders.* Raven Press, New York.

19 Loeb C and Godolfo C (1983) Diagnostic evaluation of degenerative and vascular dementia. *Stroke.* **14**: 399–401.

20 Mulley G (2011) The role of the physician for the elderly: the assessment, diagnosis and treatment of people with dementia. In S Curran and J Wattis (eds) *Practical Management of Dementia* (2e). Radcliffe Publishing, London.

21 Joyce EM (2011) Alcohol and other toxic dementias. In: JRM Copeland, MT Abou-Saleh, C Katona and A Kumar (eds) *Principles and Practice of Geriatric Psychiatry* (3e). John Wiley & Sons, Chichester.

22 Esiri M and Morris JH (1997) *The Neuropathology of Dementia.* Cambridge University Press, Cambridge.

23 Reisberg B, Ferris SH, de Leon M *et al* (1982) The Global Deterioration Scale for assessment of primary degenerative dementia. *Am J Psychiatry.* **139**:1136–9.

24 Hughes CP, Berg L, Danziger WL, Coben LA and Martin RL (1982) A new clinical scale for the staging of dementia. *Br J Psychiatry.* **140**: 566–72.

25 Burns A, Lawlor B and Craig S (2004) *Assessment Scales in Old Age Psychiatry* (2e). Informa Healthcare, London.

26 Reisberg B, Borenstein J, Salob SP, Ferris SH, Franssen E and Georgotas A (1987) Behavioural symptoms in Alzheimer's disease: phenomenology and treatment. *J Clin Psychiatry.* **48 (Suppl. 5):** 9–15.

27 Bucks RS, Ashworth DL, Wilcock GK and Siegfried K (1996) Assessment of activities of daily living in dementia; development of the Bristol Activities of Daily Living Scale. *Age Ageing.* **25**: 113–20.

28 Reisberg B (1988) Functional Assessment Staging (FAST). *Psychopharmacol Bull.* **24**: 653–9.

29 Trzepacz PT, Baker RW and Greenhouse J (1988) A symptom rating scale for delirium. *Psychiatr Res.* **23**: 89–97.

30 Hardy JA and Higgins GA (1992) Alzheimer's disease: the amyloid cascade hypothesis. *Science.* **256**: 184–5.

31 Goldgaber D, Lerman MI, McBride OW, Saffiotti U and Gajdusek DC (1987) Characterisation and chromosomal localisation of a cDNA encoding brain amyloid of Alzheimer's disease. *Science.* **235**: 877–80.

32 McLoughlin DM and Lovestone S (1994) Alzheimer's disease: recent advances in molecular pathology and genetics. *Int J Geriatr Psychiatry.* **9**: 431–44.

33 Peers C, Boyle JP, Scragg JL and Pearson MA (2007) Probing the mechanisms linking hypoxia with Alzheimer's disease: a key role for Ca^{2+} channels? *J Qual Res Dementia.* **4**: 3–6.

34 Edwardson JA, Klinowski J and Oakley AE (1986) Aluminosilicates and the ageing brain: implications for the pathogenesis of Alzheimer's disease. In: *Silicon Biochemistry.* Ciba Foundation Symposium 121. John Wiley & Sons, Chichester.

35 Harrison PJ and Roberts GW (1991) 'Life, Jim, but not as we know it?' Transmissible dementias and the prion protein. *Br J Psychiatry.* **158:** 457–70.

36 Stahl SM (2008) Dementia and its treatment. In: *Essential Psychopharmacology* (3e). Cambridge University Press, Cambridge. pp. 899–942.

37 Nelson JC and Devanand DP (2011) A systematic review and meta-analysis of placebo-controlled antidepressant studies in people with depression and dementia. *J Am Geriatr Soc.* **59:** 577–85.

38 Bleathman C and Morton I (1994) Psychological treatments. In: A Burns and R Levy (eds) *Dementia.* Chapman & Hall, London.

39 Morton I and Bleathman C (1991) The effectiveness of validation therapy in dementia – a pilot study. *Int J Geriatr Psychiatry.* **6:** 327–30.

40 King K (1982) Reminiscing psychotherapy with ageing people. *J Psychosoc Nurs Ment Health Serv.* **20:** 21–5.

41 Brooker D and Woolley R (2008) Development and evaluation of a multi-level activity-based model of care. *J Qual Res Dementia.* **5:** 9–18.

42 Aguero-Torres H, Fratiglioni L and Gou Z (2000) Dementia in advanced age led to higher mortality rates and shortened life. *Evid Based Ment Health.* **3:** 57.

FURTHER READING

➤ Curran S and Wattis JP (eds) (2011) *Practical Management of Dementia: a Multidisciplinary Approach* (2e). Radcliffe Publishing, London.

5

Mood disorders

DEPRESSION

The feeling of 'depression' is something that most people have experienced. However, someone with a depressive illness has an experience that is both qualitatively and quantitatively different, often with psychological, social and physical consequences. Depressive illness is often pervasive and affects all aspects of the individual's life. Unfortunately, the term 'depression' is used to describe both the everyday experience and the more serious pervasive form of depression. For this reason, people often find it difficult to accept that those with a depressive illness are unable to 'shake themselves out of it'. There is also the feeling that depression is an 'understandable' consequence of the many losses that old people may experience. These include loss of health, relationships, home, independence, income, and many others. Depressive illness in old age is common and is frequently undiagnosed or else pushed aside as being 'understandable'. Severe depressive illness is a serious condition associated with a high mortality and morbidity if left untreated. It is important to recognise depression in old age and to make a full assessment since, with adequate treatment, patients can make a full recovery.

Epidemiology

Depression in old age is common. Its prevalence will depend to some extent on the diagnostic criteria used, and in general the stricter the diagnostic criteria, the lower the prevalence. The prevalence of depressive symptoms far exceeds that of depressive illness.[1] One early study undertaken in Newcastle[2] found a prevalence of approximately 10% in community-based subjects, but after more careful assessment only 1.3% of these individuals met the criteria for a depressive illness. Copeland *et al*,[3] using AGECAT (a diagnostic algorithm based on the Geriatric Mental State (GMS) Examination), found a prevalence of 11.3% for 'diagnostic syndrome cases' in Liverpool, with 3% having 'depressive psychosis'. Prevalence rates are also influenced by a number of different factors, including the proportion of very elderly patients, and some of the studies have included relatively small numbers of subjects. Similar rates for depression were found among both younger and older old people.[4] Although depressive symptoms are very common in old age, the evidence that depressive illness is significantly more or less prevalent among older people than among younger individuals is poor. Community-based samples suggest a prevalence of approximately 6–7% for less severe depressive syndromes and 2–4% for more severe depressive illness (or 'major depression'). The prevalence of depression in older people in other settings may be considerably higher. For example, the prevalence in hospitalised elderly patients rises to 12–45%.[5] In addition, as many as 40% of patients in residential homes may have depression. Despite the high prevalence of depression, many patients are not diagnosed, and if they are diagnosed, treatment may not be offered or may be inadequate. It is therefore important to ensure that older patients with depression receive a full assessment and have access to the full range of treatments that are available for younger people with depression.

Clinical description

Symptoms of depression include low mood, anhedonia (inability to experience pleasure), sleep disturbance, poor appetite, weight loss, hopelessness, fatigue and suicidal ideas[6] (see below). The diagnosis of depression may be more difficult in older people than in younger patients. For example, older people with depression are more likely to have somatic complaints and hypochondriacal worries,[7] and patients presenting with these symptoms may be more likely to be diagnosed as suffering from physical illness. Similarly, older people with depression are more likely to display agitation,[8] which may be attributed to anxiety rather than to depression. Other areas which may cause diagnostic confusion include paranoid ideas and depressive pseudodementia, with symptoms being attributed to paranoid illness and dementia, respectively. The overlap of symptoms caused by depression and physical illness is particularly important. Many of the features associated with physical illness (e.g. insomnia, weight loss, fatigue and poor appetite) are also seen in depression, making diagnosis more difficult. Clues to the emergence of a depressive illness include the presence of new symptoms (e.g. early-morning wakening in the setting of sleep disturbance), and the presence of fatigue, even at rest. In addition, older people are more likely to dismiss their feelings of depression because it is 'understandable'.[9] Impaired vision and hearing are additional barriers in the elderly. It is therefore essential to obtain a careful history from the patient (and informant). It is particularly important to ask carefully about anhedonia, which is a core feature of depression. However, even anhedonia may not be a reliable indicator of depression in physical illness.[10] Depressive thoughts should also be examined, including reduced self-esteem, guilt, worthlessness and suicidal ideas.[1] A full physical examination, including appropriate investigations, should form an integral part of the assessment in more severe cases, or in less severe cases that fail to respond to appropriate treatment. A family history and personal history of depression are also important, and evidence of recent major life events should be sought. A US consensus meeting in 1992 found that depression in older people was under-recognised, associated with a suicide rate that was twice that among younger people, and was strongly associated with physical illness.[11]

Screening for depression

A number of instruments can be used to screen for depression. Unfortunately, many of these have been developed in younger people and rely heavily on physical symptoms, making them unsuitable for elderly depressed patients. The Geriatric Depression Scale (GDS) overcomes some of these difficulties. It assesses mainly cognitive aspects of depression rather than physical symptoms, and it has a simple 'yes/no' format. Although it contains 30 questions, it can be administered relatively quickly, with a score of 11 or higher being suggestive of depression.[12] As well as screening for depression, this instrument can also be used to monitor the patient's response to treatment, and there is now good evidence for its use as a screening instrument for depression.[13] Shorter forms are available (e.g. GDS-15), which trade some loss of sensitivity and/ or specificity for brevity.[14] There are a number of other instruments which do not rely on an evaluation of physical symptoms, and the Hospital Anxiety and Depression Rating Scale is widely used.[15] This instrument does not perform well as a screening instrument in general medical inpatients,[16] but it does appear to be particularly useful as a self-rated outcome measure in depressed older people.[17]

In areas where prevalence is high, for example in those with chronic physical illness, those who are isolated, and those in general hospital and residential care, screening is particularly likely to yield useful results. When a screening programme is undertaken, there should be a clear plan to treat detected cases.

A STAGED APPROACH TO THE RECOGNITION AND MANAGEMENT OF DEPRESSION

The National Institute for Health and Clinical Excellence (NICE) provides useful interactive guidance on the evidence-based detection and management of depression in adults of all ages (http://pathways.nice.org.uk and click through). The following is an abbreviated version of the NICE guidance with some suggested modifications for older people. Readers are advised to review the full NICE guidance online. This suggests a pathway with the following steps:

1. recognition, assessment and initial management of depression
2. persistent subthreshold depressive symptoms or mild-moderate depression
3. persistent subthreshold depressive symptoms or mild-moderate depression with inadequate response to initial interventions and moderate and severe depression
4. complex and severe depression.

Recognition, assessment and initial management of depression

Health workers are advised to be aware of the possibility of depression, especially in those with a previous history or those with chronic physical illness and functional impairment (which includes many older people). To these we would add, specifically for older people, the issue of being particularly alert to the presence of depression in those who are socially isolated, living in residential care, in general hospital care, caring for relatives with dementia or who have recently been bereaved or subject to other major life events. NICE suggests the following two simple screening questions:

During the last month have you often been:
➤ feeling down, depressed or hopeless?
➤ having little interest or pleasure in doing things?

In addition, where there are chronic physical health problems, further questions are suggested to improve the accuracy of diagnosis:

During the last month, have you often been bothered by:
➤ feelings of worthlessness?
➤ poor concentration?
➤ thoughts of death?

If the patient answers 'yes' to either of the first two questions then a practitioner 'who is competent in mental health assessment' should, it is suggested, make a further assessment of the patient's mental state and associated functional, interpersonal and social difficulties, using appropriate validated measures for symptoms, functions and/or disability. The assessment should take account of the degree of associated functional impairment or disability and the duration of the episode. The history of the depression and any comorbid disorders, any past history of mood elevation, response to previous treatments, the quality of relationships and living conditions and social isolation should also be considered. In the presence of learning disability or acquired cognitive impairment, it may be appropriate at this stage to consult relevant specialist services. Management for people with learning disability or dementia should, as far as possible, follow the same lines as for everyone else, with modifications depending on the patient's comorbid condition.

Most importantly, a person with depression should always be asked about suicidal ideation and intent, and issues of self-neglect should also be explored for older people (see below). People who present a considerable immediate risk to themselves or others should be referred urgently to specialist services. Patients and relatives/carers should also be advised of the possibility of increased agitation, anxiety and suicidal ideation early in treatment, and the need to seek urgent help if these problems occur. They should also be advised to watch out for mood changes, negativity, hopelessness and suicidal ideation, particularly at times of stress. These issues are especially important for people who are socially isolated, who may require more intensive treatment and support to manage risk effectively. Whoever provides initial management should ensure adequate monitoring of progress with particular attention to the issues mentioned above. In the presence of risk of suicide, increased support and referral to specialist mental health services should be considered. In the view of the authors it is especially important to involve specialist mental health services for older people at an early stage because of the frequent complexity and higher suicide risks in this group.

Persistent subthreshold depressive symptoms or mild to moderate depression

Here NICE recommends low-intensity psychosocial interventions or group-based CBT. Guided self-help, including written materials and supported by a trained practitioner, can be supplemented by structured group-based activities suitable to the individual's needs and taking into account any chronic physical health problems. Computerised cognitive behavioural therapy can also be part of this package. In the author's opinion, older people may have difficulty in accessing the activities provided by 'age-blind' services, and services need to be designed which take into account the special problems with mobility, motivation and group work that some older people may experience.

Antidepressants are not recommended routinely at this stage, but should be considered where there is a past history of moderate or severe depression, where subthreshold symptoms have been present for at least 2 years at initial presentation, or where subthreshold or mild depression persists after other interventions. The presence of chronic physical illness may also be an indication for the earlier than usual use of antidepressants, but also requires consideration as to whether the physical condition is receiving optimal treatment, the possible depressogenic side-effects of some drugs, and the risks of interactions with any prescribed antidepressant.

Persistent subthreshold depressive symptoms or mild to moderate depression with inadequate response to initial interventions, and moderate and severe depression

High-intensity psychological treatments and/or antidepressant treatment should be considered at this level. For details the reader is referred to the NICE guidance. Briefly, the high-intensity treatments include individual CBT and various other approaches. The issue of choice of antidepressant is dealt with later in this chapter, although generic SSRI prescribing is generally the first line. If there is a failure to respond to this treatment, NICE has several further suggestions, but the authors would suggest that, for older people, this is probably the place to consider referral to a specialist mental health team for the elderly (members of which may well already have been involved in some of the treatments suggested above).

Complex and severe depression

For people with severe depression, or with moderate depression and complex problems, consider referral to specialist mental health services for a programme of coordinated multiprofessional care.

The rest of this chapter is written from the point of view of how the specialist services would deal with such a referral.

Making the diagnosis

As mentioned above, it is important to include the following:
➤ a full history
➤ an appropriate physical examination
➤ any laboratory or other investigations deemed to be necessary, depending on the clinical picture.

As much information as possible about the clinical problem should be obtained from as many other sources as possible, including the following:
➤ the patient's partner and/or family
➤ the patient's general practitioner
➤ other professionals involved in the patient's care.

The history should look for evidence of change and details about any previous history of depression and/or a family history of depression. A full drug history should be obtained, since drugs are a common cause of depression in old age (see below). Other important components of the history include a social assessment and a history of life events. At this stage it is useful to compare the information collected from the patient with the diagnostic criteria listed in the *International Classification of Diseases (ICD-10)*.[6]

There are a number of different types of depression included in the *ICD-10*,[6] and these are listed below with a brief summary of each type. These categories represent clinically recognised syndromes. However, in practice they may often overlap. If there are persistent depressive symptoms sufficient to interfere with everyday life, intervention is justified whatever the exact diagnostic label. In older people, a low threshold for diagnosis leading to a trial of interventions may be the best way of confirming the diagnosis.[18]

F32 Depressive episode

In typical depressive episodes, the affected individual usually experiences the following:
➤ depressed mood*
➤ loss of interest and enjoyment*
➤ reduced energy*
➤ increased fatiguability
➤ diminished activity
➤ reduced concentration and attention
➤ reduced self-esteem and self-confidence
➤ ideas of guilt and unworthiness (even in a mild type of episode)
➤ bleak and pessimistic views of the future
➤ ideas or acts of self-harm or suicide
➤ disturbed sleep
➤ diminished appetite.

Somatic symptoms such as headache, abdominal discomfort, constipation and other 'aches and pains' may or may not be present in mild, moderate and severe types. In a moderate depressive episode, at least two of the three most typical symptoms (denoted by an asterisk in the above list) should be present, plus at least three (and preferably four) of the other symptoms. Several symptoms are likely to be present to a marked degree. The minimum duration of the whole episode is approximately 2 weeks. In patients with a severe depressive episode, all three of the typical symptoms noted for mild and moderate depressive episodes (marked with an asterisk) should be present, plus at least five other symptoms, some of which should be of severe intensity. However, if important symptoms such as agitation or retardation are marked, the patient may be unwilling or unable to describe many of their symptoms in detail. Patients may or may not have psychotic symptoms. Delusions usually involve ideas of sin, poverty or imminent disasters, responsibility for which may be assumed by the patient. Auditory or olfactory hallucinations are usually of defamatory or accusatory voices, or of rotting filth or decomposing flesh. Severe psychomotor retardation may progress to stupor. During a severe depressive episode it is very unlikely that the patient would be able to continue with normal social activities, occupational work or domestic activities. It may help to use a simplified flow chart to facilitate the diagnosis of depression based on *ICD-10*[6] diagnostic criteria (see Figure 5.1).

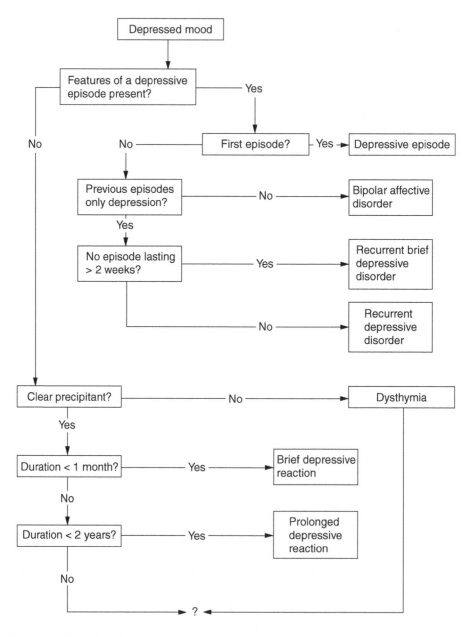

Figure 5.1 Flow chart for the diagnosis of a patient with depressed mood according to simplified *ICD-10* criteria.

F33 Recurrent depressive disorder

This disorder is characterised by repeated episodes of depression as described for mild, moderate and severe depressive episodes (see above). The age of onset, severity, duration and frequency of the episodes of depression are all highly variable. In general, the first episode occurs later than in bipolar affective disorder (see pp. 143–147), with a mean age of onset in the fifth decade. Individual episodes last for between 3 and 12 months (median duration about 6 months), but recur less frequently than in bipolar disorder. Recovery is usually complete between episodes. The disorder may be mild, moderate or severe. For diagnosis, the criteria for depressive episode should be met. In addition, at least two episodes should have lasted for a minimum of 2 weeks and be separated by several months without significant mood disturbance. Somatic symptoms may or may not be present.

F34 Persistent mood (affective) disorders

These are persistent and usually fluctuating disorders of mood in which individual episodes are rarely, if ever, sufficiently severe to warrant being described as hypomanic or even mild depressive episodes.

F34.1 Dysthymia

This is a chronic depression of mood that does not currently fulfil the criteria for recurrent depressive disorder, although the criteria for mild depressive episode may have been fulfilled in the past, particularly at the onset of the disorder. The balance between individual phases of mild depression and intervening periods of comparative normality is very variable.

Aetiology

The aetiology of depression in older people is complex. Biological factors include the following:
➤ the normal ageing process
➤ neurodegenerative changes
➤ alterations in neurotransmitters (especially noradrenaline and serotonin)
➤ genetic predisposition
➤ physical illness
➤ drug-related factors.

Drugs associated with depression include psychotropics (e.g. benzodiazepines, buspirone), anticonvulsants (e.g. carbamazepine, clobazam, phenobarbital), anti-parkinsonian drugs (e.g. anticholinergics, levodopa), cardiovascular drugs (e.g. beta-blockers, clonidine, enalapril, methyldopa), gastrointestinal drugs (e.g. cimetidine, ranitidine), non-steroidal anti-inflammatory drugs (NSAIDs), respiratory drugs (e.g. aminophylline, theophylline) and steroids.[19]

Social factors are also important in the elderly, and include reduced social networks, loneliness, bereavement and poverty.[20]

Finally, psychological factors play an important role. Personality dysfunction is more likely to be associated with 'mild' depression than with severe/psychotic depression, especially in those prone to anxiety. Life events are particularly relevant as precipitating factors, and acute physical illnesses are important in this regard. Murphy[21] found that among older people with depression, just under 50% have experienced a severe life event, compared with 23% in the control group. However, older people experience a wide range of 'life events', especially losses, including the following:

➤ loss of health
➤ loss of youth
➤ loss of home
➤ loss of income
➤ loss of family
➤ loss of partner
➤ loss of children.

It is surprising (and encouraging) that the prevalence of depression is not higher in older people. The development of depression in an older person will depend on a number of factors working together. This will often be a combination of a physical illness, previous life experiences, the presence of vulnerability factors and premorbid personality. In most cases, depression in older people will have several causes, making a detailed medical, psychological and social assessment essential. Physical illness is particularly important as a cause of depression in old age (see Case History 5.1).

Physical illness and depression may occur concomitantly, and the overlap of symptoms may lead to diagnostic difficulties. Physical illness/disease may predispose to, precipitate or perpetuate depression, and some of the specific illnesses known to be associated with depression in later life are listed in Table 5.1.

A number of different aspects of physical illness can act as vulnerability factors for depression, including the following:

➤ pain
➤ disability
➤ poor diet
➤ reduced physical activity.

Alternatively, patients with depression may only complain of physical symptoms (somatisation), especially pain for which no physical evidence can be found (see Case History 5.2).

It is also important to consider the patient's response to physical illness. Although physical illness will mean different things to different patients, it will usually be interpreted as a threat, a loss or a restriction. The way in which a patient responds to their illness will also have a bearing on the prognosis.

Case History 5.1

Mrs B was a 68-year-old woman with a long history of chronic renal failure who was awaiting a kidney transplant. She complained of low mood, low energy, disturbed sleep and weight loss, and for the previous 3 months she had begun to think that life was not worth living. She had been taking paroxetine, 20 mg, for approximately 3 months with no clinical benefit. On examination she was noted to be very pale, and routine laboratory investigations revealed that she had a very low haemoglobin level. Anaemia is a well-recognised cause of feelings of depression, and after treatment with several transfusions (packed red cells), Mrs B made a full recovery from her depressive illness.

Table 5.1 Physical illnesses associated with depression

Endocrine disorders	Hypothyroidism
	Hyperparathyroidism
	Addison's disease
	Cushing's syndrome
Metabolic disorders	Hypercalcaemia
	Iron vitamin B_{12}/folate deficiency
Neurological disorders	Cerebrovascular accident
	Parkinson's disease
	Intracranial tumours
	Epilepsy
	Multiple sclerosis
Cardiovascular	Myocardial infarction
Orthopaedic	Hip fracture
Chronic pain	Various causes
Alcohol dependence	
Infections	Post influenza
	Infectious mononucleosis
	Hepatitis
Sensory deficits	Impairments of vision and hearing

There may be a subgroup of resistant depression with late onset in which vascular factors have a more significant aetiological role, but this is not undisputed. 'Vascular depression' has little practical value as a concept, since it does not affect the approach to management (although it may provide a post hoc rationalisation for treatment resistance).

Case History 5.2

Mrs R was a 71-year-old woman who had been an inpatient on a general medical ward for several months with severe and disabling lower abdominal pain. She denied having any symptoms of depression with the exception of onset insomnia (difficulty getting to sleep), and extensive investigations, including a laparotomy, revealed no physical abnormality. After a psychiatric assessment she was transferred to a psychiatric ward and commenced on trazodone, 50 mg at night. This was gradually increased to 300 mg/day. Her distress and preoccupation with her pain gradually lessened, and after 4 months she had fully recovered from her pain and distress. She was never able to accept that her illness had a psychological origin, but she was willing to continue taking the antidepressant and was able to resume a normal life.

Factors that will influence the patient's response to physical illness include how independent they remain, the degree to which the illness is felt to be within the patient's sphere of influence (locus of control), and how active or passive the patient is with regard to problem solving. Physical illness is associated with higher morbidity and mortality in older people with depression,[21] although other factors are important, including severity of depression, duration of illness, social class and severity of life events in the year following the initial episode. Because of the complex and diverse range of factors that can cause depression in older people, it is essential to ensure that the aetiological factors (including psychological, biological and social factors) are thoroughly evaluated and taken into account in the management plan. The relationship between physical illness and psychiatric morbidity is explored more fully in Chapter 9.

Usually a range of factors contribute to the aetiology of depression, and these are summarised in Figure 5.2.

Treatment of depression

As discussed in the NICE guidance referred to earlier, depression can be treated using a range of different approaches, from 'general support', problem solving

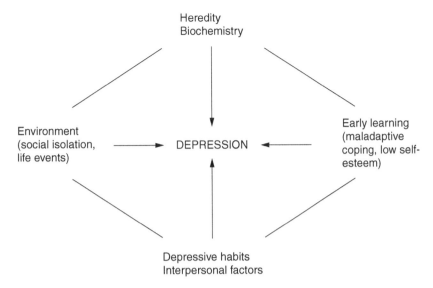

Figure 5.2 Factors that are implicated in causing and maintaining depression.

and formal psychological techniques (including individual and group CBT) to pharmacotherapy and electroconvulsive therapy (ECT). Two useful information leaflets for patients and carers have been published by the Royal College of Psychiatrists, namely *Depression in Older Adults* and *Bereavement* (follow the links on www.rcpsych.ac.uk/). Depression in later life is frequently not treated at all, or under-treated. In addition, benzodiazepines are commonly given inappropriately to treat symptoms of depression (e.g. anxiety).[22] Appropriate and effective treatment is important, particularly in cases where other illnesses or disability complicate the picture. The treatment of depression should include treatment of any underlying physical illness, whether it is directly or indirectly related to the depression.

Psychological treatments
The main psychological approaches to treatment are cognitive behaviour therapy (CBT) and interpersonal therapy (IPT). Both are effective in mild to moderate depression and for severe depression, too, provided that the patient is accessible to treatment. Psychological treatments can be delivered as a guided self-help package, in a group setting or in a more intensive one-to-one format. In moderate to severe depression they are often used in combination with pharmacotherapy and appear to work synergistically. Those delivering these therapies need appropriate training and supervision. For a fuller description of these approaches and how they are delivered in practice, the reader is referred to *Practical Management of Affective Disorders in Older People*.[23]

Pharmacological treatments

Factors that should be taken into consideration when prescribing an antidepressant include the following:

➤ concomitant physical illness

➤ previous response to treatment

➤ patient preference

➤ the clinical experience of the clinician

➤ the presence of bipolar disorder, for which a different pharmacological approach is needed.

Whichever drug is chosen, the patient should be given an adequate therapeutic dose (within *British National Formulary (BNF)* limits) for an adequate period of time. In one study, Waern *et al*[24] found that in 75 elderly suicides, a large proportion of patients were taking antidepressants but the doses were sub-therapeutic (*see* Case History 5.3).

Case History 5.3

Mrs P was a 77-year-old woman referred to the outpatient clinic with a 2-year history of moderately severe depression. She was taking imipramine, 50 mg at night. She noted that this helped her to sleep and she denied having any significant side-effects, but it had not helped her underlying depression. She was very reluctant to stop her imipramine, so this was gradually increased over several weeks to 150 mg daily. She had no significant side-effects, and within 8 weeks she had made a good recovery.

In addition, the response to drug treatment may take up to 12 weeks in older people with depression,[11] which is much longer than in younger patients. Once recovery is evident, treatment should be continued at full dose for at least 6 months, and where risk of relapse is high for up to 2 years, possibly indefinitely.[25] However, relatively few studies have been conducted specifically in older people with depression. In recurrent depressive disorder, lifelong maintenance therapy may be indicated. In general, most of the available antidepressants appear to have efficacy for the treatment of major depression, and most antidepressants 'work' by interacting with serotonergic and/or noradrenergic systems to varying degrees, and their different mechanisms of action largely explain their different side-effect profiles. Side-effects may be more serious with the older antidepressants (tricyclic antidepressants or TCAs and monoamine oxidase inhibitors or MAOIs) than with the newer drugs, and they include sedation, anticholinergic effects (blurred vision, confusion, urinary retention, exacerbation of glaucoma), cardiotoxicity and a greater propensity to induce convulsions. However, lofepramine (a tricyclic) is generally well tolerated in older people with depression, and has considerably fewer side-effects and lower toxicity in overdose than amitriptyline or imipramine. The relatively newer drugs, such as selective serotonin reuptake inhibitors (SSRIs) (e.g. fluvoxamine, sertraline, fluoxetine, paroxetine, citalopram and escitalopram), serotonin and noradrenaline reuptake inhibitors (SNRIs) (e.g. venlafaxine and duloxetine) and noradrenaline and serotonin-specific antidepressants (NaSSAs) (e.g. mirtazapine) are better tolerated, have fewer side-effects, are safer in overdose and are less likely to cause convulsions compared with tricyclic antidepressants.[25] There is also emerging evidence for agomelatine in older people, which partly works by enhancing melatonin functioning. Resistant cases of depression may respond to lithium augmentation (the addition of lithium) and various other strategies, but these should only be used in consultation with local psychiatric services. ECT is also a safe and effective treatment for depression in the elderly, especially severe depression with psychotic features and psychomotor retardation, but caution should be exercised when prescribing antidepressants with ECT, as these may be associated with increased duration of seizures.[26] ECT is normally only given by specialist psychiatric services. Recently, transcranial magnetic stimulation[26] has shown promise as an effective alternative to ECT, although experience with this new treatment is still limited to research settings in the UK.

CHOICE OF ANTIDEPRESSANTS

Antidepressants should be chosen according to the needs of individual patients. Unless there are special factors, most evidence and guidance suggests the choice of SSRI antidepressants or other newer antidepressants.[23] Side-effects, previous efficacy and cost should all be taken into account, and generic forms of the SSRIs probably represent the best starting point for most patients. The summary information below is not complete, and prescribers should consult relevant guidance (e.g. the *British National Formulary*, *BNF*) before using these drugs.

Selective serotonin reuptake inhibitors (SSRIs)

These drugs are widely used in the treatment of depression, and have advantages over TCAs and MAOIs. In particular they are associated with the following:

➤ less sedation
➤ less postural hypotension
➤ fewer anticholinergic side-effects (and therefore less confusion, memory impairment and cardiac problems)
➤ less serious consequences in overdose
➤ fewer seizures.

SSRIs have been shown to be effective in the treatment of depression, as well as for anxiety and eating disorders. These drugs do not bind to any specific neuroreceptor, but rather they produce a pharmacological effect by blocking serotonin reuptake from the synaptic cleft into the presynaptic neuron, thereby increasing the concentrations of serotonin that are available to act on one or more of the post-synaptic serotonin receptors. They have the advantage that the therapeutic dose for depression is generally more straightforward than is the case with TCAs or MAOIs, and this tends to improve compliance. The starting and therapeutic doses are usually, but not always, the same. Liquid preparations are also available for fluoxetine and paroxetine, and escitalopram is available as drops (*see* Case History 5.4). This has a number of advantages for patients who may have difficulty in swallowing.

Case History 5.4

Mr A was a 68-year-old man who had a history of depression of at least 5 years' duration. He had been tried on at least nine different antidepressants, all for relatively short durations and frequently at sub-therapeutic doses. In all cases sensitivity to side-effects had been the reason for either stopping the drug early or not giving a therapeutic dose. We commenced him on citalopram drops (5 mg) for 1 week followed by 10 mg for 1 week and only increasing to 20 mg (therapeutic dose) in week 3. He was able to tolerate this regime, and after approximately 6 weeks he had improved sufficiently to start planning a holiday. Six months later he had made a full recovery and he had no problems with drug tolerability.

These drugs have highly variable half-lives, which may influence the choice of drug, depending on individual clinical circumstances. The long half-life of fluoxetine may or may not be a clinical problem. For example, it makes withdrawing the drug less problematic, and there are likely to be fewer difficulties if the patient misses one or two doses. However, if it is necessary to have a wash-out period before commencing another drug (e.g. an MAOI), this may have to be up to 5 weeks. Overall, the SSRIs are associated with less troublesome side-effects than are TCAs or MAOIs. The commonest side-effects include dizziness, dry mouth, sweating, anxiety/agitation, drowsiness, nausea and diarrhoea. These tend to be worse during the early phase of treatment and subside after a couple of weeks or so. Sometimes it is found that giving patients a smaller dose initially helps them to adjust to the medication and many of these side-effects can be prevented. Abnormal movements may also occasionally be associated with SSRIs, but these are usually transient and subside once the drug has been discontinued. If a patient is taking an MAOI, there should be a 2-week wash-out period before commencing an SSRI. If the patient is on an SSRI, the wash-out period should be five times the half-life of the SSRI before the MAOI is commenced, because of the risk of causing a serotonin syndrome (i.e. confusion, restlessness, myoclonus, hyper-reflexia, shivering, tremor, and sometimes coma and death). The cost of SSRIs is higher than that of TCAs, but generic forms of several SSRIs are now available, bringing the costs down considerably. In addition, the side-effects of TCAs may require treatment (e.g. constipation), which adds to the cost of treatment with TCAs. The SSRIs are also considerably safer in overdose and are a better option for many older people.

Serotonin and noradrenaline reuptake inhibitors (SNRIs)

The principal antidepressants in this group are venlafaxine and duloxetine. The main side-effects include nausea, dizziness, dry mouth, insomnia, nervousness, headache and constipation, and these tend to be dose dependent. SNRIs are relatively safe in overdose and have a low propensity to induce seizures compared with tricyclic antidepressants.

Venlafaxine and duloxetine are both dual reuptake inhibitors of both serotonin and noradrenaline. In particular, a number of studies have shown duloxetine to be effective and to have good safety and tolerability in older people with depression.

In 2006 the Committee on Safety of Medicines updated its advice on the use of venlafaxine. It is not recommended as a first-line treatment. Because the risk of toxicity is higher than that associated with SSRIs it should be prescribed in limited amounts (no more than 2 weeks at a time) where suicide risk is appreciable, and it should be used with caution in patients with cardiac disease. Higher doses (over 300 mg) should only be initiated by appropriate specialists (the full guidance can be found at www.mhra.gov.uk).

Noradrenergic and specific serotoninergic antidepressants (NaSSAs)

Mirtazapine belongs to this new class of antidepressant. It is a selective presynaptic α_2-adrenoreceptor antagonist that increases the synaptic availability of noradrenaline. It also blocks 5-HT_2 and 5-HT_3 receptors and thus enhances the transmission of 5-HT_1 receptors, which have been associated with anxiolytic properties. It is completely absorbed after administration and has an elimination half-life of approximately 43 hours. It is therefore given once daily, typically 15 mg at night. It has been shown to be more effective than a placebo, trazodone and amitriptyline. Side-effects include dry mouth, drowsiness, increased appetite and weight gain, but these are significantly less than with TCAs. The reported incidence of seizures is very low, and this figure is not significantly different to that for placebo. The available data suggest that mirtazapine is safe in overdose.

Table 5.2 provides a summary of the different antidepressants.

Table 5.2 Antidepressants, available preparations and indications

Drug	Available types	Indications	Comments
Amitriptyline	Tablets	Depressive illness	Initially 30–75 mg daily, increasing to 150–200 mg daily
Clomipramine	Capsules Tablets Slow release	Depressive illness Phobias OCD	Initially 10 mg, gradually increasing to 30–75 mg daily
Dosulepin	Capsules	Depressive illness	Initially 50–75 mg daily, increasing gradually to 150 mg daily
Imipramine	Tablets	Depressive illness	Initially 10 mg, increasing gradually to 30–50 mg daily
Lofepramine	Tablets	Depressive illness	70–210 mg daily
Nortriptyline	Tablets	Depressive illness	30–50 mg daily
Mianserin	Tablets	Depressive illness	Initially 30 mg daily, increasing to a maximum of 90 mg daily. Check FBC every 4 weeks during first 3 months of treatment
Trazodone	Capsules Tablets	Depressive illness	Initially 100 mg daily, increasing to 300 mg
Phenelzine	Tablets	Depressive illness	Initially 15 mg three times a day, increasing to four times a day after 2 weeks if necessary. Usual maintenance dose is 15 mg on alternate days
Isocarboxazid	Tablets	Depressive illness	5–10 mg daily
Tranylcypromine	Tablets	Depressive illness	10 mg twice a day increasing to 30 mg daily Maintenance dose is 10 mg daily
Moclobemide	Tablets	Depressive illness Social phobia	Initially 300 mg daily, increasing to a maximum of 600 mg daily
Citalopram	Tablets Drops	Depressive illness Panic disorder	20–40 mg daily
Escitalopram	Tablets Drops	Depressive illness Panic disorder Social phobia GAD	Initially 5 mg, increasing to 10–20 mg daily

Drug	Available types	Indications	Comments
Fluoxetine	Capsules Liquid	Depressive illness Bulimia nervosa OCD	20–40 mg daily
Paroxetine	Tablets Liquid	Depressive illness OCD Panic disorder Social phobia PTSD GAD	20–40 mg daily
Sertraline	Tablets	Depressive illness OCD PTSD	Initially 50 mg, increasing to 200 mg. Usual maintenance dose is 50 mg
Flupenthixol	Tablets	Depressive illness Psychoses	**Initially 500 mcg daily, increasing to 2 mg in divided doses**
Venlafaxine	Tablets Modified release (MR)	Depressive illness GAD	Initially 75 mg daily, maximum 375 mg daily. MR: maximum 225 mg daily
Duloxetine	Capsules	Depressive illness	60 mg daily
Mirtazapine	Tablets Orodispersible	Depressive illness	Initially 15 mg daily, increasing to 45 mg daily
Agomelatine	Tablets	Depressive illness	Initially 25 mg every night, increasing to 50 mg every night after 2 weeks

PTSD, post traumatic stress disorder; GAD, generalised anxiety disorder; OCD, obsessive compulsive disorder; FBC, full blood count.

Recent developments

Agomelatine, a melatonin MT1/MT2 agonist and serotonin 5-HT2c antagonist, is the most recent antidepressant. As well as treating depression it also improves sleep onset and sleep quality. The usual starting dose is 25 mg every night, increasing to 50 mg every night after 2 weeks. There is emerging evidence of benefit in older people, but further research is needed. Side-effects include GI disturbance, headache, blurred vision and very rarely hepatitis, but in clinical practice the drug appears to be well tolerated and can be a useful addition in patients with treatment-resistant depression, especially if sleep disturbance is a prominent feature.

Selective noradrenaline reuptake inhibitors (NARIs)

Selective noradrenaline reuptake inhibitors (NARIs) specifically target the reuptake of noradrenaline. At the time of writing, reboxetine, the only member of this class, is not licensed for the treatment of depression in older people in the UK.

Serotonin antagonist/reuptake inhibitors (SARIs)

Several antidepressants have the ability to block serotonin 2A and 2C receptors as well as serotonin reuptake, the prototype drug being trazodone. Trazodone is an effective antidepressant, and subtherapeutic doses (e.g. 50 mg) are frequently used in the management of insomnia in older people. However, trazodone should be used with caution as it has a number of side-effects, including sedation, postural hypotension and the serotonin syndrome, if used with other drugs with predominantly serotonergic mechanisms (e.g. SSRIs).

Tricyclic antidepressants

The efficacy of tricyclic antidepressants in the treatment of depression is well established. They have also been found to be helpful in the treatment of depression with psychotic features, dysthymia, recurrent depression and depression occurring in other medical settings (e.g. schizophrenia). They work principally, after a delay of 2 to 3 weeks, through down-regulation of α_1 and 5-HT$_2$ receptors. There is a wide range of drugs with variable half-lives (e.g. amitriptyline has a half-life of 9–46 hours and imipramine has a half-life of 6–28 hours). For this reason, tricyclics may have to be given more than once per day, depending on the response of individual patients. The side-effects are also quite extensive, and in general these drugs are less acceptable to older patients. Side-effects include anticholinergic effects such as blurred vision, urinary retention, constipation and dry mouth. TCAs can also impair memory, which may be a serious problem for older patients with early dementia. Care also needs to be taken with patients who have compromised cardiovascular function. Cardiovascular problems include orthostatic hypertension and an increased risk of cardiac arrhythmias. There is also a risk of heart block, and careful ECG monitoring may be needed. Tricyclic antidepressants may also occasionally cause increases in liver enzymes or delirium, probably through anticholinergic mechanisms, especially in the elderly (*see* Case History 5.5).

Many TCAs are very sedating, and this may be associated with falls. They are also potentially fatal in overdose. Usually the starting dose is small, and this is gradually increased until a therapeutic response has been achieved. In addition, TCAs may be more likely than more modern antidepressants to provoke mania in susceptible patients.

Monoamine oxidase inhibitors (MAOIs)

These are also a well-established group of drugs. Although they are effective as a treatment for depression, the database is smaller than for tricyclic antidepressants, and they are rarely used in modern practice, certainly not

---

Case History 5.5

Mrs C was a 79-year-old woman who had recently been admitted to a residential home. She had been finding it increasingly difficult to manage at home and she had no close relatives. Although initially she had been excited about the prospect of moving into a home and making new friends, approximately two months after the move she started to feel low in mood, and this gradually became worse over the following weeks. The staff felt that she was depressed. She was seen by her GP and commenced on amitriptyline, 50 mg at night. Within a few hours of commencing the amitriptyline she became very agitated, verbally aggressive and was experiencing visual hallucinations. She was reviewed by the psychiatric team, the amitriptyline was stopped and the symptoms of delirium subsided. We were able to manage her reaction to being admitted to the residential home through the community psychiatric nurse, with a very positive result. This involved giving Mrs C an opportunity to discuss her anxieties and worries, and providing her with a clear explanation of the reaction she had to amitriptyline.

---

as a first-line treatment. They should be reserved for use under specialist supervision, and are now more often used as one option for the management of treatment-resistant depression. MAOIs (e.g. phenelzine, tranylcypromine) act by inhibiting monoamine oxidase, an enzyme responsible for the breakdown of noradrenaline and serotonin. Usually the drug dosage has to be gradually increased, and typically the drug is given twice daily. If the patient is switched to another antidepressant, a wash-out period of at least 2 weeks is advisable because of the risk of severe hypertension. A wash-out of 2 weeks should also be observed before ECT. Side-effects of MAOIs are well documented, and include hypomania, hypertensive crisis, convulsions, syncope, disorientation, oedema, rash, weight gain, urinary retention and drowsiness. Because of the risk of a hypertensive crisis, patients have to observe a strict diet, and should avoid foods rich in tyramine (e.g. cheeses, certain alcoholic beverages, yeast products, game). For these reasons, these drugs are particularly unattractive for older people with depression. However, moclobemide (see below), a relatively new and selective MAOI, does not require such dietary restrictions.

Reversible inhibitors of monoamine oxidase A (RIMAs)

Moclobemide, a reversible inhibitor of monoamine oxidase A (RIMA), is only indicated for major depression. It causes less potentiation of the pressor effects of tyramine, but patients should still avoid eating large amounts of tyramine-rich food. Although the risk of interactions with other drugs is less than with MAOIs, sympathomimetics (e.g. ephedrine) should still be avoided. In addition, moclobemide should not be given with another antidepressant. Because of its short half-life, no treatment-free period is required after it has been stopped. However, it should not be started until other antidepressants have been removed from the body (five times the half-life). It has a number of side-effects, including sleep disturbance, dizziness, nausea, headache, agitation and confusional state. The usual dose is 300 mg daily in divided doses after food. This twice-daily administration is a slight disadvantage, and no liquid preparation is available. Moclobemide is safe in overdose and has a very low propensity to cause seizures.

Lithium

Lithium is usually administered as a salt. It is found in natural spring and spa water, and was first recommended for 'mania' in the second century AD by Soranus of Ephesus.

In the 1940s, John Cade, an Australian, gave lithium to guinea pigs and found that they became lethargic. This was followed by an open trial in 1949, when lithium was found to be helpful in manic patients. Unfortunately, it has a very narrow therapeutic range. If too much lithium is present it is associated with side-effects, and if insufficient drug is present there are usually no therapeutic benefits. Lithium levels as well as renal and thyroid function must be carefully monitored. Lithium is rapidly absorbed and its levels peak after only 2–3 hours. It is not protein bound or metabolised in the body (i.e. it is excreted unchanged). Its mechanism of action is poorly understood, but it increases the activity of the enzyme $Na^+/K^+ATPase$ (intracellular Na^+ levels are therefore decreased). After acute doses there is an increase in brain 5-HT, but after chronic administration there is down-regulation of 5-HT receptor sites.

The initial starting dose is usually 400 mg/day in older people. It takes approximately 5 days to reach steady state, so the first lithium level is usually measured after 1 week of treatment. Once stabilised, the lithium level should be checked every 3 months, and thyroid function tests and urea and electrolytes every 6 months. This is usually done at a lithium clinic. An excellent review on lithium has been published.[28] Factors associated with good and poor responses to lithium are summarised in Box 5.1. Lithium is clinically indicated in a number of conditions, including the following:

➤ mania
➤ bipolar affective disorder (either two episodes each lasting at least
   1 month over a 2-year period, or three episodes over a 5-year period)
➤ schizoaffective disorder

➤ lithium augmentation (to augment the effects of other antidepressants in patients with treatment-resistant depression).

Lithium should only normally be prescribed by a specialist after careful assessment and with planned and assertive follow-up.

Box 5.1   Factors associated with good and poor responses to lithium

Factors associated with a good response to lithium
➤ Good compliance
➤ Good previous response
➤ Bipolar affective disorder/endogenous-type depression
➤ Family history of bipolar affective disorder

Factors associated with a poor response to lithium
➤ Rapid cycling
➤ Paranoid features
➤ Substance abuse
➤ Poor social circumstances

Side-effects are commonly observed with lithium, and are sometimes very serious or even fatal. It is therefore essential that patients who are taking lithium are carefully monitored for side-effects and their lithium levels are checked regularly (at least every 3 months in patients who are stabilised on lithium). Common side-effects (which are usually dose related and increase with increasing age) include memory impairment, thirst, polyuria, tremor, drowsiness and weight gain. In addition, lithium levels may become very high, and the patient will then become toxic. If the patient is taking a standard dose of lithium, this toxicity could be due to a number of factors, including dehydration, decreased clearance or drug interactions (e.g. thiazide diuretics).

Clinical symptoms include the following:
➤ vomiting
➤ cognitive impairment
➤ diarrhoea
➤ lassitude
➤ coarse tremor
➤ restlessness
➤ dysarthria
➤ agitation
➤ ataxia
➤ seizures and coma (which can lead to death).

It is important that these symptoms are recognised early and that appropriate management or treatment is initiated quickly. The mainstay of treatment includes the following:

➤ stopping lithium
➤ supportive measures
➤ anti-epileptics if indicated
➤ regular measurement of lithium levels and clinical monitoring
➤ increased fluid intake (if kidney function is normal)
➤ isotonic saline infusion
➤ haemodialysis if lithium levels are very high.

There are also a number of important drug interactions. These are summarised in Table 5.3.

Table 5.3 Drug interactions with lithium

Drug	Comments
Diuretics	Thiazide diuretics decrease the renal clearance of lithium and can cause toxicity
Neuroleptics	Concern has been expressed about a possible toxic interaction between lithium and haloperidol, even at therapeutic levels. Overall, the evidence does not support this, but caution is recommended
Non-steroidal anti-inflammatory drugs	These drugs tend to reduce lithium clearance and thus increase plasma levels of lithium
Anticonvulsants	Lithium and carbamazepine may interact to cause a neurotoxic interaction even when both drugs are within their respective therapeutic ranges

The use of antipsychotics in severe (psychotic) depression

When depression has marked psychotic features, augmentation of antidepressant treatment with a suitable antipsychotic (e.g. olanzapine) may be helpful.

Electroconvulsive therapy

Electroconvulsive therapy (ECT) has been used in psychiatry for over 50 years, but despite good evidence for its safety and efficacy, it still arouses controversy. Most older people who are treated with ECT have a severe depressive illness, particularly one with psychotic symptoms and/or psychomotor retardation. However, psychotic symptoms are regarded as the main indication by old age psychiatrists.[26] ECT is also useful in a number of other conditions, including schizoaffective disorder and, very occasionally, depressive illness with dementia, particularly if pharmacological treatment has been unsuccessful. It might be particularly useful in patients with the following conditions:

➤ depressive illness which has failed to respond to antidepressant drugs
➤ depressive illness where previous episodes responded to ECT but not to antidepressant drugs
➤ depressive illness with psychotic symptoms
➤ depressive illness with severe agitation
➤ depressive illness with high suicidal risk
➤ patients with depressive stupor.

Prior to commencing ECT, the patient should receive a full explanation of the procedure and should generally provide their written informed consent. Occasionally patients who have severe mental illness are unable to give informed consent, and it may be necessary to give ECT compulsorily under the Mental Health Act (1987). This will require a second opinion from an independent psychiatrist appointed by the Care Quality Commission. The Mental Health Act Commission was replaced by the Care Quality Commission (www.cqc.org.uk) in April 2009. The CQC checks hospitals in England to ensure that government standards are being met, including those relating to the Mental Health Act (2007). These reviews are undertaken by Mental Health Act Commissioners.

It is also important to ensure that the patient has had a full physical examination and routine laboratory assessments undertaken, and in most cases an ECG and chest X-ray should be taken. If there are any concerns about the patient's physical health, these should be discussed with the anaesthetist *before* the final decision is made to proceed with treatment. Patients will normally require between six and eight treatments, but this figure can vary depending on the response to treatment by each individual patient.

The choice of electrode placement will to some extent be governed by the need of the individual patient. Bilateral electrode placement is preferable for patients whose concurrent medical conditions make it advisable to minimise the number of general anaesthetics. It might also be preferable in patients who are suicidal, as it tends to be more quickly effective than unilateral ECT. Unilateral electrode placement is indicated for patients with pre-existing cognitive impairment, in order to minimise cognitive side-effects during treatment.[26]

ECT itself is a safe treatment, and most of the serious adverse events are associated with the anaesthetic. ECT is a low-risk procedure with a mortality of approximately two deaths per 100 000 treatments. This is very similar to the mortality rate for anaesthesia for minor surgical procedures. Immediately after treatment, patients may experience a number of side-effects, including the following:
➤ headaches
➤ muscular aches
➤ drowsiness

➤ weakness
➤ nausea
➤ anorexia.

These side-effects are usually only mild and respond to symptomatic treatments. In addition, ECT can affect memory for events which occurred before the procedure (retrograde amnesia) and events which take place after it (anterograde amnesia). Delirium may also develop between treatments, particularly in patients who are taking concurrent psychotropic drugs, or those with pre-existing cognitive impairment or neurological conditions. If delirium occurs, changes to the drug regime and/or a change from bilateral to unilateral ECT may lessen the confusion.

There are no absolute contraindications to ECT,[26] but in individual patients it is important to balance the risks of ECT against the risks of not giving it. People with a wide range of physical illnesses have been successfully treated with ECT. If there is any doubt, this should be discussed with the anaesthetist and/or colleagues working in medicine for the elderly. Transcranial magnetic stimulation may eventually provide a better alternative to ECT, but its use in the UK is limited to research projects.

Prognosis

The recovery rate for an individual episode of depressive illness is good, and 75–80% of cases will improve over a 6-month period. The immediate prognosis for an episode of depressive illness in later life is therefore very good. In the longer term, only about 25% of cases will remain completely well. These patients seem to be a distinct subgroup, in that most of them will have responded rapidly to conventional treatments and are notable for their physical fitness. For approximately 60% of all patients, the prognosis in the longer term is 'quite good', in that they will either remain well or have relapses which can be successfully treated. However, a small proportion of patients with depression remain resistant to all conventional therapies. Even after recovery, relapses are common and tend to occur relatively early on. Two-thirds of such relapses occur within the first 18 months of follow-up, and careful follow-up plans are therefore an essential part of the management of older people with depression. Adverse prognostic factors include poor response to treatment, serious physical illness (either at initial contact or during follow-up), long duration of illness prior to presentation, and the presence of delusions. In addition, there are many physical causes of depression, and these have been described above. If such causes remain untreated, it is likely that the depression, despite adequate treatment, will be more resistant to therapy, and it is essential that physical causes of depression are vigorously treated. Physical disability and social isolation may also predispose to recurrence, and management plans should take this into account. Finally, even in patients who make a full recovery and are taking the full therapeutic dose of an antidepressant, the risk of relapse is much greater in those who had a psychotic depressive illness, and continuation of low doses of an appropriate antipsychotic may be justified.

MANIA

Manic illness is an important and serious illness in old age, but it is less common, less frequently recognised, and in general is given less attention than depression or dementia. Patients with mania often have a long history of psychiatric illness dating back to early adult life, and the presentation and course are highly variable. When mania presents for the first time in old age, the presentation can often be bizarre and it can frequently be mistaken for other conditions. In addition, physical illness (e.g. a frontal lobe tumour) is more often the underlying cause of manic illness presenting in late life.[29] As with depression, it is frequently misdiagnosed, but if the diagnosis can be accurately made, treatment is generally effective and can markedly improve the quality of life of patients with this condition. Although older people may have episodes of both depression and mania (bipolar disorder), recurrent depression is more common, and mania may occur separately either episodically or in a chronic unremitting form. For the sake of clarity, mania in old age will be considered separately in this chapter.

Epidemiology

One of the difficulties in trying to understand the epidemiology of mania in old age is that mania and depression are often assessed as if they were a single disease. In most cases, the first episode of an affective illness is depression, usually between the ages of 25 and 35 years. There is usually another peak in the fifth decade. Broadhead and Jacoby,[30] in a study of 35 elderly manic (manic-depressive) patients, found that on average the first episode of depression was at 44 years and the first manic attack was at 59 years of age. It is commonly observed that, with increasing age, the frequency of affective episodes increases, as does the duration, so that in very old age affective episodes may be extremely protracted and very difficult to treat. The prevalence and incidence of manic illness in older people have been less well studied than depression. When manic illness has been studied, it has usually been mixed with depression, making a precise estimate of prevalence more difficult than with depression. One of the first studies was that of Hopkinson,[27] who reported a prevalence of mania of 6.5% of patients with a first onset of affective disorder after the age of 50 years. Severe depression is about ten times more common than mania in elderly psychiatric patients.

Clinical features

The term 'hypomania' is used to describe milder forms of mania. In both mania and hypomania there is elevated mood with abnormalities of speech and cognition, as well as somatic, biological and behavioural symptoms. Moreover, in both the elevated mood is persistent and, especially in older people, irritability is a common feature. It is also not uncommon for a transient depression of mood to be intermingled with the symptoms. There is usually pressure of speech, increased tempo of thinking, and impaired concentration with 'flight of ideas'. Patients tend to be easily distracted, and may have an inflated self-image with grandiose and expansive ideas. They often report having increased drive and activity, particularly with regard to physical activity, social skills, work and libido. Increased activity may also be associated with risk-taking pursuits and social indiscretion. Insomnia may be a frequent and early sign of mania, but patients show no evidence of fatigue, and despite a very good appetite, weight loss may be evident. These are features typical of a younger person with mania, and all of them may to some extent be modified in older people. In particular, one is less likely to see flight of ideas, and there may be higher levels of depression and irritability. It has been suggested that older people tend to be more irritable, have a greater degree of cognitive impairment, have 'slow flight of ideas' and may be more garrulous. The clinical picture can also be complicated because in older people with mania there is a greater likelihood of an underlying organic aetiology, and other conditions such as delirium may be misdiagnosed as mania. The main types of manic illness are discussed below.

F30 Manic episode

F30.0 Hypomania

Hypomania is a milder form of mania, in which mood and behaviour are clinically abnormal but are not accompanied by hallucinations or delusions. The following are key features:
➤ persistent mild elevation of mood (for at least several consecutive days)
➤ increased energy and activity
➤ marked feelings of well-being
➤ a sense of physical and mental efficiency
➤ increased sociability, talkativeness, over-familiarity, increased sexual energy, and a decreased need for sleep are often present, but not to the extent that they lead to severe disruption of work or result in social rejection
➤ irritability, conceit and boorish behaviour may take the place of the more usual euphoric sociability
➤ concentration and attention may be impaired, thus reducing the ability to settle down to work or to relaxation and leisure pursuits, but this may not

prevent the appearance of interests in quite new ventures and activities, or mild over-spending.

Diagnostic guidelines. Several of the features mentioned above, consistent with elevated or changed mood and increased activity, should be present for at least several consecutive days, to a degree and with a persistence greater than that described for cyclothymia.

F30.1 Mania without psychotic symptoms

Mood is elevated out of keeping with the individual's circumstances, and may vary from carefree joviality to almost uncontrollable excitement. Elation is accompanied by increased energy, resulting in overactivity, pressure of speech, and a decreased need for sleep. Normal social inhibitions are lost, attention cannot be sustained, and there is often marked distractibility. Self-esteem is inflated, and grandiose or over-optimistic ideas are freely expressed.

Perceptual disorders may occur, such as the appreciation of colours as especially vivid (and usually beautiful), a preoccupation with the fine details of surfaces or textures, and subjective hyperacusis. The individual may embark on extravagant and impractical schemes, spend money recklessly, or become aggressive, amorous or facetious in inappropriate circumstances. In some manic episodes the mood is irritable and suspicious rather than elated. The episode should last for at least one week and should be severe enough to disrupt ordinary work and social activities more or less completely.

F30.2 Mania with psychotic symptoms

The clinical picture is that of a more severe form of mania as described above. Inflated self-esteem and grandiose ideas may develop into delusions, and irritability and suspiciousness may develop into delusions of persecution. In severe cases, grandiose or religious delusions of identity or role may be prominent, and flight of ideas and pressure of speech may result in the individual becoming incomprehensible. Severe and sustained physical activity and excitement may result in aggression or violence, and neglect of eating, drinking and personal hygiene may result in dangerous states of dehydration and self-neglect. If required, delusions or hallucinations can be specified as being congruent or incongruent with the mood. 'Incongruent' should be taken to include mood-neutral delusions and hallucinations (e.g. delusions of reference with no guilty or accusatory content, or voices speaking to the individual about events that have no special emotional significance).

F31 Bipolar affective disorder

This disorder is characterised by repeated (i.e. at least two) episodes in which the patient's mood and activity levels are significantly disturbed. This disturbance consists on some occasions of an elevation of mood and increased energy and activity (mania or hypomania), and on others of a lowering of mood and decreased energy and activity (depression). A number of different types are included here for completeness (*see* Box 5.2).

Box 5.2   Classification of bipolar affective disorders (ICD-10)

F31.0 Bipolar affective disorder, current episode hypomanic
F31.1 Bipolar affective disorder, current episode manic without psychotic symptoms
F31.2 Bipolar affective disorder, current episode manic with psychotic symptoms
F31.3 Bipolar affective disorder, current episode mild or moderate depression
F31.4 Bipolar affective disorder, current episode severe depression without psychotic symptoms
F31.5 Bipolar affective disorder, current episode severe depression with psychotic symptoms
F31.6 Bipolar affective disorder, current episode mixed
F31.7 Bipolar affective disorder, currently in remission

Aetiology

To a large extent, the aetiology of manic illness in old age is similar to that of depression (described earlier). However, two specific aspects of aetiology are worthy of further description, namely genetic and organic factors. As with depression, genetic loading is less important as an aetiological factor in later life. However, organic factors are significantly more important in later life. This is sometimes referred to as 'secondary mania', and it is defined as mania that arises in patients with no previous history of affective disorder, in close temporal relationship to a physical illness or during treatment. Examples include cerebral tumour, infections and treatment with steroids (*see* Case History 5.6).

There is still some debate as to whether or not the mania which results from this situation is directly caused by the physical illness, or whether it is the result of an interaction between the physical illness and a 'vulnerable or susceptible' individual. There is now considerable evidence for an association between the onset of mania and a history of cerebral organic disease, including dementia of the Alzheimer's type and stroke disease.[31] It is therefore extremely important that patients with onset of mania in old age receive a detailed and thorough assessment, including a detailed physical examination and a range of investigations to exclude underlying physical illness.

Case History 5.6

Mr P was an 83-year-old man admitted to a geriatric ward with severe chronic obstructive airways disease. He was treated with high-dose prednisolone (a steroid), and within 3 days he had made a very good recovery and was discharged with the plan to follow him up in the outpatient clinic. Shortly after discharge he became extremely irritable, verbally threatening and over-talkative. He became threatening towards his wife and neighbours, and the police were called after an altercation in his street. He was taken to the local police station, and was eventually sectioned under the Mental Health Act to the local psychiatric unit. After consultation with the geriatricians he was gradually withdrawn from his prednisolone and at the same time was treated with trifluoperazine. After 5 days he made a full recovery.

Management

As with the depressed patient, the manic patient will need a detailed medical, psychological and social assessment to identify clearly the precise aetiology and the most effective way in which the patient can be helped. Consideration will need to be given to medical, psychological and social aspects of treatment, as well as to management in both the immediate short term and the long term. An important aspect of treatment will be to identify any underlying physical cause of the mania, and this should be rigorously treated. Mood stabilisers were originally drugs that were used to treat mania and prevent its recurrence, although the definition has now become much broader. In the acute phase lithium remains an important treatment with proven efficacy, although its use has declined in recent years, partly because of risks associated with lithium and partly because of new safer and more effective drugs. Anticonvulsants also remain important treatments, including semisodium valproate, carbamazepine and, increasingly, lamotrigine. Gabapentin and pregabalin seem to have little benefit as mood stabilisers, although they are excellent treatments for various painful conditions and anxiety disorders. Antipsychotics are also widely and effectively used as mood stabilisers, including risperidone, olanzapine, quetiapine and aripiprazole. Benzodiazepines such as lorazepam can be useful for short-term use so that other drugs such as antipsychotics have a chance to 'get established'. Bipolar disorders can in part be associated with glutamate hyperactivity. Memantine is a weak NMOA glutamate-receptor antagonist, and as such is being investigated as an additional treatment. For an excellent summary of the consensus guidelines published by the British Association of Psychopharmacology (2009), see www.bap.org.uk (accessed 15 May 2012).

Lithium is now well established as an effective treatment both for acute manic illness and also as prophylaxis. A thorough assessment is necessary prior to commencing lithium. In particular, renal function should be reasonable. Lithium levels, renal function and thyroid function should be monitored on a regular basis (see above). Any developing renal or thyroid impairment must be recognised early on and managed appropriately. Serial charting of lithium levels may show trends to toxic levels. Toxicity is particularly likely to occur if patients become dehydrated for any of various reasons (e.g. lack of fluids, taking thiazide diuretics, or during the summer months). Lithium levels should be lower than in younger patients, and the typical therapeutic range is 0.4–0.6 mmol/L, although some patients may do better at slightly higher levels. Patients need clear information, and the use of written information is good practice. In severely disturbed patients, ECT may be effective in bringing the manic symptoms under control, although in practice this is only occasionally necessary. If lithium levels rise above the therapeutic range, then lithium should be stopped immediately and re-introduced when the levels have settled, probably at a reduced dose. Lithium levels of 1.5 mmol/L and above require urgent specialist assessment, as hospital treatment may be indicated.

Elderly patients who have recovered from an acute manic episode usually require long-term follow-up, either in the outpatient clinic or through the community mental health team. This will depend to some extent on aetiological factors. For example, the patient who develops a manic episode following the use of steroids to treat a chest problem may require a relatively short follow-up period once they have made a full recovery. Unfortunately, there is very little research evidence to indicate how long into the recovery phase the patient should take antipsychotic medication, and ultimately this has to be a clinical decision. In clinical practice, many clinicians will prescribe antipsychotics for 3 to 6 months after the manic episode has resolved, and medication should then be very cautiously withdrawn, and recommenced if symptoms appear to be recurring. Lithium is now widely used for the prophylaxis of mania and bipolar affective disorders in older people, but again research evidence is lacking. There is considerable variation in individual clinicians' willingness to use lithium after the first episode of mania. However, the seriousness of the underlying illness and an urgent sense that this should be treated has to be balanced against the potentially toxic effects of lithium in older people. Mania in older people is a serious illness. If the condition is accurately diagnosed and treated, most patients respond and some of the serious consequences can be averted. The Mental Health Act may have to be used, as patients are often unwilling to be treated voluntarily.

Older people with mania may be extremely vulnerable in terms of both their personal safety and their vulnerability to exploitation. It is therefore crucially important that older patients with manic illness are managed in an integrated way through the multidisciplinary team, and particularly with the help of social services.

Bipolar affective disorder and prophylaxis

Lithium is an effective prophylactic agent in bipolar affective disorder. For patients who cannot tolerate lithium, an increasing range of options is now available. Carbamazepine and sodium valproate are both used as alternative mood stabilisers, and lamotrigine may be particularly useful where most episodes are depressive. NICE guidance is now available on the management of bipolar disorders.[32] Olanzapine, risperidone, aripiprazole and quetiapine may also be useful as mood stabilisers. Lithium, valproate, olanzapine, quetiapine and aripiprazole are useful first-line drugs to consider if mania predominates, with carbamazepine being a second line. Quetiapine and lamotrigine should be considered as first-line treatments if depression predominates, with lithium as a second line. If these fail, combination therapy might need to be considered. Doses in older people should be 'substantially lower' for all classes of drugs and for all phases of the illness. There is no consensus about how long maintenance treatment should be continued. It should probably be continued for at least 3–12 months, and longer if clinically indicated, but patients should be reviewed on a regular basis (see the BAP website for a detailed review).

Prognosis

Systematic evidence for the prognosis of isolated mania in elderly patients is poor because studies have usually focused on the prognosis of patients with bipolar affective disorder. Moreover, the majority of episodes of mania in old age are themselves relapses of an affective disorder – that is, bipolar affective disorder – which has often stretched back many years into younger adult life. With increasing age, patients with affective disorders tend to have increasingly frequent and prolonged episodes of depression/mania. Because of a range of other factors, including poor physical health and a large number of losses, affective disorders may be more difficult to treat in older people. Elderly patients may also be significantly more likely to develop a separate depressive illness after recovery from mania, which suggests that their remission was more fragile than that in younger patients. The general consensus is that adherence to lithium treatment at adequate doses is probably the most effective means of minimising the risk of relapse.

CONCLUSION

Depression in older people is common. Staged approaches to treatment mean that less severe and more transient symptoms are dealt with in primary care. In more severe or prolonged disorder, the aetiology is complex and this necessitates a thorough assessment. Detailed physical, psychological and social assessment is often needed, as is multidisciplinary (and multi-agency) work. Risk assessment and risk management, particularly suicide risk assessment, are essential and should be updated as clinical circumstances change. Depression in older people responds to treatment. For less severe depression, psychological treatment is indicated, primarily using CBT. For more severe or prolonged disorder, antidepressants are indicated, often in combination with more intensive CBT. Sometimes ECT is needed, and it can be life-saving. If a pharmacological approach is used, the patient should be given an adequate dose for an adequate period, and a response to treatment may take as long as 12 weeks. No single pharmacological treatment is suitable for all patients on all occasions. It is therefore important to choose the most appropriate treatment that meets the needs of individual patients. If the decision is made to treat with an antidepressant, the newer drugs are safer and better tolerated than TCAs and should be considered first. Many older people are living alone, often in unacceptable social circumstances. If patients are to make a full recovery, it is important that their social situation is fully assessed and every effort made to improve it.

Mania in later life is less common than depression, but it is a serious illness and can have profound consequences for patients, especially in relation to their personal safety, health and vulnerability. It is most commonly associated with a long-standing affective disorder, but mania presenting for the first time in late life is frequently associated with an underlying physical illness. A range of physical treatments are available for the treatment of mania in later life, including antipsychotics, ECT and lithium. Antipsychotics should be chosen with great care, and in particular it is preferable to use a drug with a low incidence of anticholinergic side-effects, such as risperidone, olanzapine or quetiapine. If adequately treated, patients usually make a good recovery, but there is very little evidence to indicate how long patients should be treated after making a recovery. Although lithium is a very effective treatment for mania and bipolar affective disorder in old age, it should be used with caution and, when it is used, will require frequent and careful monitoring of kidney and thyroid function, as well as lithium levels. Other drugs, such as the antipsychotics olanzapine, quetiapine and aripiprazole, and the anti-epileptics semisodium valproate, carbamazepine and lamotrigine, have an increasing role in the long-term management of bipolar disorder.

REFERENCES

1 Baldwin RC (1995) Affective disorders. In: R Jacoby and C Oppenheimer (eds) *Psychiatry in the Elderly.* Oxford University Press, Oxford.
2 Kay DW, Beamish P and Roth M (1964) Old age mental disorders in Newcastle-upon-Tyne. Part I. A study of prevalence. *Br J Psychiatry.* **110**: 146–58.

3   Copeland JRM, Dewey ME, Wood N, Searle R, Davidson IA and McWilliam C (1987) Range of mental illness among the elderly in the community: prevalence in Liverpool using the SMG-AGECAT package. *Br J Psychiatry.* **150**: 815–23.

4   Morgan K, Dallosso HM, Arie T, Byrne EJ, Jones R and Waite J (1987) Mental health and psychological well-being among the old and very old at home. *Br J Psychiatry.* **150**: 801–7.

5   Burn WK, Davies KN, McKenzie FR, Brothwell JA and Wattis JP (1993) The prevalence of acute psychiatric illness in acute geriatric admissions. *Int J Geriatr Psychiatry.* **8**: 171–4.

6   World Health Organization (1992) *The ICD-10 Classification of Mental and Behavioural Disorders.* World Health Organization, Geneva.

7   Allen A and Busse EW (1994) Hypochondriacal disorder. In: JRM Copeland, MT Abou-Saleh and DG Blazer (eds) *Principles and Practice of Geriatric Psychiatry.* John Wiley & Sons, Chichester.

8   Winokur G, Morrison J, Clancy J and Crowe R (1973) The Iowa 500: familial and clinical findings favour two kinds of depression illness. *Compr Psychiatry.* **14**: 99–107.

9   Georgotas A (1983) Affective disorders in the elderly: diagnostic and research consideration. *Age Ageing.* **12**: 1–10.

10   Silverstone PH (1992) Is anhedonia a good measure of depression? *Acta Psychiatr Scand.* **83**: 248–50.

11   Alexopoulos GS (1992) Geriatric depression reaches maturity. *Int J Geriatr Psychiatry.* **7**: 305–6.

12   Yesavage JA, Brink TL, Rose TL *et al* (1983) Development and validation of the Geriatric Depression Screening Scale: a preliminary report. *J Psychiatric Res.* **17**: 37–49.

13   Jackson R and Baldwin B (1993) Detecting depression in elderly medically ill inpatients: the use of the Geriatric Depression Scale compared with nursing observations. *Age Ageing.* **22**: 349–53.

14   Shiekh J and Yesavage J (1986) Geriatric depression scale: recent findings and development of a short version. In: T Brink (ed.) *Clinical Gerontology: A Guide to Assessment and Intervention.* Howarth Press, New York.

15   Zigmond AS and Snaith RP (1983) The Hospital Anxiety and Depression Scale *Acta Psychiatr Scand.* **67**: 361–70.

16   Davies KN, Burn WK, McKenzie FR, Brothwell JA and Wattis JP (1993) Evaluation of the Hospital Anxiety and Depression Scale as a screening instrument in geriatric medical inpatients. *Int J Geriatr Psychiatry.* **8**: 165–9.

17   Wattis JP, Butler A, Martin C and Summer T (1994) Outcome of admission to an acute psychiatric facility for older people: a pluralistic evaluation. *Int J Geriatr Psychiatry.* **9**: 835–40.

18   Evans M and Mottram P (2000) Diagnosis of depression in elderly patients. *Adv Psychiatr Treat.* **6**: 49–56.

19   Patten SB and Barbui CC (2004) Drug-induced depression: a systematic review to inform clinical practice. *Psychotherapy and Psychosomatics.* **73**: 207–15.

20   Lovestone S and Howard R (1997) *Depression in the Elderly.* Martin Dunitz, London.

21   Murphy E (1983) The prognosis of depression in old age. *Br J Psychiatry.* **142**: 111–19.

22   Wilson KCM, Copeland JRM, Taylor S, Donoghue J and McCracken CFM (1999) Natural history of pharmacotherapy of older depressed community residents. *Br J Psychiatry.* **175**: 439–43.

23 Curran S and Wattis JP (2008) *Practical Management of Affective Disorders in Older People*. Radcliffe, London.

24 Waern M, Beskow J, Runeson B and Skoog I (1996) High rate of antidepressant treatment in elderly people who commit suicide. *BMJ*. **313**: 1118.

25 Anderson IM, Ferries IN, Baldwin RC *et al* (2008) Evidence-based guidelines for treating depressive disorders with antidepressants: a revision of the 2000 British Association for Psychopharmacology guidelines. *J Psychopharmacol*. **22**: 343–96.

26 Benbow SM (2008) Electricity, magnetism and mood. In: S Curran and J Wattis (eds) *Practical Management of Affective Disorders in Older People*. Radcliffe Publishing, London.

27 Hopkinson G (1964) A genetic study of affective illness in patients over 50. *Br J Psychiatry*. **110**: 244–54.

28 Shelly R (2004) Affective disorders: lithium and anticonvulsants. In: DJ King (ed.) *Seminars in Clinical Psychopharmacology*. Radcliffe Publishing, London. pp. 244–77.

29 Shulman K and Post F (1980) Bipolar affective disorders in old age. *Br J Psychiatry*. **136**: 26–32.

30 Broadhead J and Jacoby RJ (1990) Mania in old age: a first prospective study. *Int J Geriatr Psychiatry*. **5**: 215–22.

31 Stone K (1989) Mania in the elderly. *Br J Psychiatry*. **155**: 220–4.

32 National Institute for Health and Clinical Excellence (2006) *The Management of Bipolar Disorder in Adults, Children and Adolescents in Primary and Secondary Care* (CG38). Available at www.nice.org.uk/CG38.

FURTHER READING

➤ Curran S and Wattis JP (eds) (2008) *Practical Management of Affective Disorders in Older People*. Radcliffe Publishing, London.

6

Late-life psychotic disorders

INTRODUCTION

There is some confusion about how non-affective, non-dementing psychotic disorders in the elderly should be classified. Fortunately, diagnosis and treatment are more straightforward. Although there are some similarities between schizophrenia in younger people and paranoid states in older people, there has been reluctance, especially in Europe, to use the term 'schizophrenia' for disorders with onset in old age. The term 'paraphrenia' was introduced into the psychiatric literature by Kraepelin in 1909. Patients with paraphrenia had delusions and hallucinations, with relatively well-preserved personality, and the symptoms appeared later than in those with schizophrenia. However, controversy over the concept of paraphrenia began to develop soon after that concept became more widely known. The term 'paraphrenia' became less popular and was replaced by a broader concept of schizophrenia in the 1940s. In 1955, Sir Martin Roth reintroduced the term 'paraphrenia' and added the adjective 'late' to describe hallucinations and delusions, with well-preserved personality, with the first onset at or after the age of 60 years.[1] Since that time, the term 'late paraphrenia' has been most widely used in the UK, but it has not found its way into the *International Classification of Diseases, Tenth Edition (ICD-10)*.[2] A consensus group in 1998 suggested that the terms late onset (or middle-aged, 40–60 years) and very late onset (over 60 years) described syndromes that were sufficiently different from young-onset schizophrenia to deserve separate subcategories within the overall category of schizophrenia. It remains to be seen whether this sensible suggestion will be adopted in *ICD-11* or *DSM-V*. The distinguishing characteristics of very-late-onset schizophrenia are a very high female:male ratio (8:1), sensory deficits, structural brain abnormalities, response to relatively low doses of antipsychotic and higher risk of developing tardive dyskinesia (see below). These patients also have less abnormal premorbid personalities, less family history of schizophrenia, less thought disorder and less negative symptoms.[3] The term 'paranoia' has also gone through similar changes. It was originally used by Kraepelin to describe patients with delusions in the absence of hallucinations. To some extent it is still used in this sense today, but it has not been a popular diagnostic label, the term 'delusional disorder' generally being preferred. Patients with late-onset delusional disorders may have a preoccupation with (often non-bizarre) delusions with preserved affective personality and cognitive functions.[3]

EPIDEMIOLOGY

There is much variation in the prevalence and incidence of these disorders in old age. This depends partly on the definition used and partly on the diagnostic criteria. The rates change when patients with organic disorders are included. The population studied also has an impact on the prevalence figures (e.g. community studies vs. hospital inpatients).

There have been relatively few studies of these disorders in old age compared with studies of other disorders such as dementia. The research that has been conducted is often difficult to interpret because of the wide variation in diagnostic criteria and terminology. About 10% of first psychotic admissions over the age of 60 years are non-affective psychotic disorders. Because it is assumed that schizophrenia is a serious disorder, likely to lead to hospital admission, first-admission rates are sometimes used as a rough surrogate for incidence (the number of new cases in a given population over a standard period, usually a year). The Department of Health reported that the annual age-specific first-admission rate for schizophrenia was 8.7 per 100000 in the 65–74 years age group, and increased to 14.5 per 100000 in the ≥ 75 years age group.[4] Age- and gender-specific first-admission rates suggest a peak incidence for males in young adulthood, with a secondary peak in old age. For women there is a relatively small peak in mid-life with another larger peak in late life. Holden[5] estimated the annual incidence of late paraphrenia to be 17–26 per 100000, depending on whether or not cases thought to have an organic aetiology were included.

The incidence figures for schizophrenia in patients aged 65 years or older, usually based on the diagnostic interviews schedule, were approximately 0.1% for males, but were as high as 0.9% for females.[6] In a further study involving the total population of Denmark,[7] over a 6-month period, for individuals aged 65 years or over, the rate for female patients was 0.4–0.6%. For community samples in the elderly, prevalence rates of schizophrenia and paranoid psychosis of 1–2.5% have been reported.[8] These higher rates include patients with long-term schizophrenia who have grown old, as well as those with late-onset (or very-late-onset) 'schizophrenia'.

CLINICAL DESCRIPTION

Delusions and hallucinations are the hallmarks of these disorders. *Delusions* are fixed false beliefs that are held in the face of evidence to the contrary, and that are not consistent with the patient's social, cultural and educational background. In addition, they are held unshakeably, they are not modified by reason or experience, and their content is often bizarre. *Hallucinations* are perceptions that arise in the absence of any external stimulus. These phenomena are not distortions of real perceptions (illusions). They are perceived as being located in the external world and as having the same qualities as normal perceptions (i.e. patients perceive them as real). In addition, hallucinations are not subject to conscious manipulation. Box 6.1 summarises the classification of schizophrenia and related disorders according to the *International Classification of Diseases, ICD-10*.[2]

Two excellent clinical reviews of schizophrenia in older people were published in 2000.[9,10] A useful flow chart that can be used for the diagnosis of hallucinations is summarised in Figure 6.1.

Box 6.1   Classification of schizophrenia, schizotypal and delusional disorders *(ICD-10)*

F20	Schizophrenia
F20.0	Paranoid schizophrenia
F20.1	Hebephrenic schizophrenia
F20.2	Catatonic schizophrenia
F20.3	Undifferentiated schizophrenia
F20.5	Residual schizophrenia
F21	**Schizotypal disorder**
F22	**Persistent delusional disorders**
F22.0	Delusional disorder
F23	**Acute and transient psychotic disorders**
F25	**Schizoaffective disorders**

F20 Schizophrenia

According to *ICD-10*, the schizophrenia disorders are generally characterised by fundamental and characteristic distortions of thinking and perception, and by inappropriate or blunted affect. Clear consciousness and intellectual capacity are usually maintained, although certain cognitive deficits may evolve in the course of time. However, for 'late onset' and especially 'very late onset' (over 60 years) the reservations discussed earlier must be borne in mind.

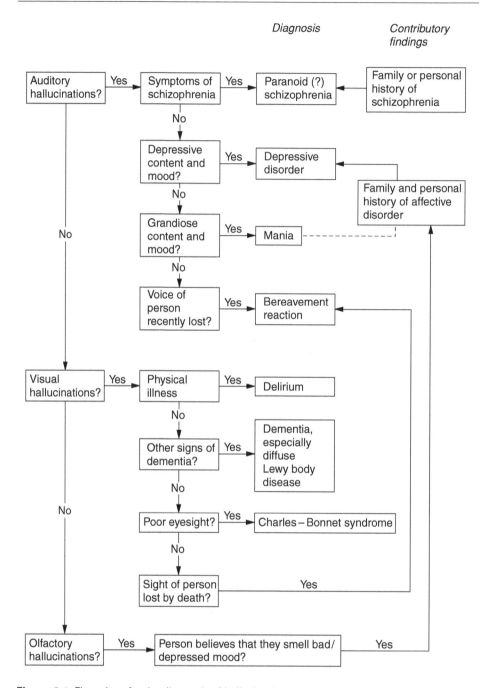

Figure 6.1 Flow chart for the diagnosis of hallucinations.

For practical purposes it is useful to divide these symptoms into groups that have special importance for the diagnosis and often occur together. These are as follows:

(a) thought echo, thought insertion or withdrawal, and thought broadcasting

(b) delusions of control, influence or passivity, clearly referred to body or limb movements or specific thoughts, actions or sensations; delusional perception

(c) hallucinatory voices giving a running commentary on the patient's behaviour, or discussing the patient among themselves

(d) persistent delusions that are culturally inappropriate and completely impossible

(e) persistent hallucinations in any modality

(f) breaks or interpolations in the train of thought, resulting in incoherence or irrelevant speech

(g) catatonic behaviour, such as excitement, posturing or waxy flexibility, negativism, mutism and stupor

(h) 'negative' symptoms such as marked apathy, paucity of speech, and blunting or incongruity of emotional responses

(i) a significant and consistent change in the overall quality of some aspects of personal behaviour.

Diagnostic guidelines

The normal requirement for a diagnosis of schizophrenia is that a minimum of one very clear symptom (and usually two or more if symptoms are less clear-cut) belonging to any one of the groups listed as (a) to (d) above, or symptoms from at least two of the groups listed as (e) to (h), should have been clearly present for most of the time *during a period of 1 month or more*. Figure 6.2 provides an algorithm for diagnosing persecutory states.

F20.0 Paranoid schizophrenia

This is the commonest type of schizophrenia in most parts of the world. The clinical picture is dominated by relatively stable, often persecutory delusions, usually accompanied by hallucinations, especially of the auditory variety. This is the type of schizophrenia that is most often seen in late onset or very late onset.

Delusions are central to the phenomenology of late-onset disorder. Sexual themes are common, as are delusions of self-reference and persecution. Delusions of influence and passivity phenomena are reported in approximately 40% of cases.[11] Other first-rank symptoms (including thought insertion, thought withdrawal and thought broadcasting) are relatively rare, and formal thought disorder is virtually non-existent in very-late-onset schizophrenia.

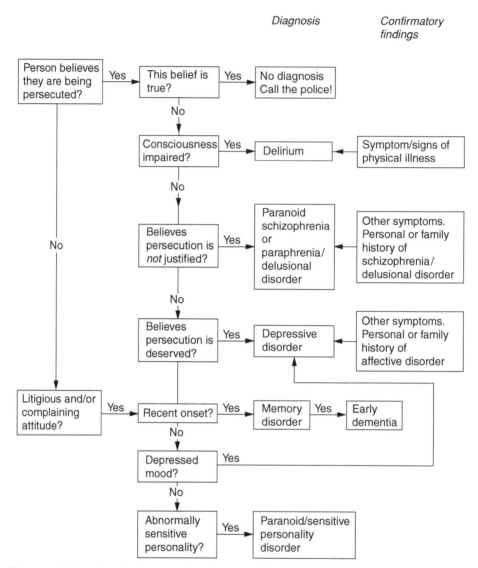

Diagnosis   *Confirmatory findings*

Figure 6.2 Flow chart for the diagnosis of persecutory states.

Hallucinations are found in the majority of patients. Auditory hallucinations are by far the commonest type, and these are mostly accusatory and/or insulting, and the voices concerned are usually in the second or third person. Running commentary is also occasionally encountered. Hallucinations of bodily sensation may also be present, and as many as 25% of cases may report tactile hallucinations.[1] Olfactory hallucinations are also encountered, and are typically described as 'an unpleasant smell', or may be described as 'a poisonous gas'.

Olfactory hallucinations of body odour or rotting flesh are perhaps more common in psychotic depression.

F20.1 Hebephrenic schizophrenia

This is a form of schizophrenia in which affective changes are prominent, delusions and hallucinations are fleeting and fragmentary, behaviour is irresponsible and unpredictable, and mannerisms are common.

F20.2 Catatonic schizophrenia

Prominent psychomotor disturbances are essential and dominant features, and may alternate between extremes such as hyperkinesis and stupor, or automatic obedience and negativism. Constrained attitudes and postures may be maintained for long periods. Episodes of violent excitement may be a striking feature of the condition.

F20.3 Undifferentiated schizophrenia

This term is used for conditions that meet the general diagnostic criteria for schizophrenia but do not conform to any of the above subtypes, although they may exhibit features of more than one of them without a clear predominance of a particular set of diagnostic characteristics.

Hebephrenic, catatonic and undifferentiated schizophrenia are more common in early-onset cases.

F20.5 Residual schizophrenia

This is a chronic stage in the development of a schizophrenic disorder in which there has been a clear progression from an early stage (consisting of one or more episodes with psychotic symptoms meeting the general criteria for schizophrenia described above) to a later stage characterised by long-term, although not necessarily irreversible, 'negative' symptoms. This form is also relatively common in old age in people who have grown old with the disease.

F21 Schizotypal disorder

This is a disorder characterised by eccentric behaviour and anomalies of thinking and affect which resemble those seen in schizophrenia, although no definite and characteristic schizophrenic anomalies are evident.

F22 Persistent delusional disorders

This group includes a variety of disorders in which long-standing delusions constitute the only or the most conspicuous clinical characteristic, and which cannot be classified as organic, schizophrenic or affective. They are probably heterogeneous, and have uncertain relationships to schizophrenia.

F22.0 Delusional disorder

This group of disorders is characterised by the development of either a single delusion or a set of related delusions which are usually persistent and sometimes lifelong. The delusions are highly variable in content. Often they are persecutory, hypochondriacal or grandiose, but they may be concerned with litigation or jealousy, or express a conviction (e.g. that the individual's body is misshapen, or that others think that he or she smells or is homosexual). Clear and persistent auditory hallucinations (voices), schizophrenic symptoms such as delusions of control and marked blunting of affect, and definite evidence of brain disease are all incompatible with this diagnosis.

Delusions constitute the most conspicuous or the only clinical characteristic. They must be present for at least 3 months and be clearly personal rather than subcultural.

F23 Acute and transient psychotic disorders

To avoid diagnostic confusion, a diagnostic sequence should be constructed that reflects the order of priority given to selected key features of the disorder. The order of priority used here is as follows:
(a) an acute onset (within 2 weeks) as the defining feature of the whole group
(b) the presence of typical syndromes
(c) the presence of associated acute stress.

Acute onset is defined as a change from a state without psychotic features to a clearly abnormal psychotic state within a period of 2 weeks or less. There is some evidence that acute onset is associated with a good outcome, and it may be that the more abrupt the onset, the better the outcome. It is therefore recommended that, whenever it is appropriate, *abrupt onset* (within 48 hours or less) is specified.

F25 Schizoaffective disorders

These are episodic disorders in which both affective and schizophrenic symptoms are prominent within the same episode of illness, preferably simultaneously, but at least within a few days of each other. Patients who suffer from recurrent schizoaffective episodes, particularly those whose symptoms are of the manic type rather than the depressive type, usually make a full recovery and only rarely develop a defect state. Late-onset schizoaffective disorders have not been extensively studied.

DIFFERENTIAL DIAGNOSIS

A differential diagnosis of very-late-onset schizophrenia includes depression, dementia, schizoaffective disorders, acute paranoid reactions, paranoid personality disorder and other organic paranoid psychoses, including temporal lobe epilepsy, psychotic reactions following head injury, and a number of toxic and metabolic states, including hyperthyroidism. These can usually be differentiated from very-late-onset schizophrenia by a careful medical and psychiatric history, physical examination, appropriate laboratory investigations and special investigations such as CT scan, where these are indicated. A fuller description and discussion of the differential diagnosis of paraphrenia can be found in a review by Anderson.[12]

AETIOLOGY

The precise aetiology of very-late-onset schizophrenia remains largely unknown. Aetiological research is complicated by the different diagnostic terms used over the years, and especially by the use of 'late onset' to refer to onset over 40 years in some cases. The following factors may be important:

➤ a paranoid and/or schizoid premorbid personality (especially in late onset: 40–60 years)
➤ genetic factors (more important in late onset than very late onset: ≥60 years)
➤ cerebral disease (more important in very late onset)
➤ social isolation
➤ female gender (F:M 2:1 in late onset, 8:1 in very late onset)
➤ sensory impairment, particularly deafness.

A premorbid paranoid and/or schizoid personality is frequently found in patients with late or very late onset. Paranoid personalities are characterised by morbid suspicion, extreme sensitivity to disappointments, preoccupation with what other people think about them, and a tendency to be distrustful and hostile, and to have feelings of inadequacy. There have been a number of studies in which a premorbid paranoid personality has subsequently developed into a 'late paraphrenic' illness.[13]

Social isolation is also an important factor, but sometimes it can be difficult to disentangle cause and effect. Many patients have always tended to be somewhat socially isolated, have never married, and have few family or personal attachments. As the disease progresses, this social isolation may intensify.[1] There has also been a considerable amount of research confirming that patients with very-late-onset schizophrenia have an increased incidence of deafness. This tended to be conductive deafness contracted early in life and of a degree that impeded social interaction (social deafness).[14] Organic factors may also be an important contributory factor. However, when organic factors are clearly responsible for the illness, it may be more appropriate to classify the latter as secondary to the organic factors, rather than as 'pure' late paraphrenia.

Neuropathological and neuroimaging studies are beginning to contribute to our understanding of the relationship between late-onset schizophrenia, very-late-onset schizophrenia, other types of schizophrenia and various forms of dementia. One study[15] showed neurofibrillary tangles (tau pathology Braak stages III and IV) to be present in 11% of controls, 37% of people with schizophrenia with onset before the age of 40 years, and 59% of people with onset over 40 years. Amyloid deposits were relatively rare. The investigators concluded that restricted limbic tauopathy affected the majority of patients with 'late'-onset schizophrenia but also affected a third of elderly schizophrenics with 'early' (before 40 years) onset. They suggest that their neuropathological findings define a subtype of a schizophrenia-like condition where the flow of information through the hippocampus is disrupted. Gross measurement of white matter hyperintensity and volume in late- and early-onset schizophrenia compared with controls showed no significant differences on neuroimaging.[16] However, more localised imaging of medial temporal lobe atrophy[17] did enable reasonable distinctions to be made between Alzheimer's disease on the one hand and very-late-onset schizophrenia and vascular dementia on the other. A neuropsychopharmacological review[18] suggests that affect-laden paraphrenia may be a distinct treatment-related subpopulation in the biologically heterogeneous group of conditions labelled schizophrenia.

MANAGEMENT

The general principles of management are similar to those for other psychiatric disorders in old age. It is important that patients have a thorough psychiatric history, physical examination and appropriate investigations to rule out organic causes of the illness. Social issues will often need to be addressed. Formal psychological therapy (e.g. CBT) for this group is in its infancy.

Patients often come to the attention of the GP as a result of complaints by neighbours, the police or other public bodies, who have often been bombarded by sometimes convincing accusations, often over long periods of time. Initial assessment is usually in the patient's home, as they invariably refuse to come to hospital, claiming that there is nothing wrong with them. Gaining access to the patient's home is usually no easy task. It may be necessary to be extremely persistent, and interviews may have to be conducted through the letterbox in the first instance. With perseverance, patients will often agree to let you enter their home, and this is often the first stage in the important process of developing a trusting working relationship with the patient. A brief assessment of the patient's home will often give a very good indication of the degree of illness. For example, the windows may be barricaded and there may be considerable disorder in the home and lack of food and other resources, because of the degree of social isolation. Hearing impairment can interfere with the assessment. The mainstay of treatment in the early stages is pharmacological. The patient may accept oral medication, but not infrequently treatment has to be administered under the Mental Health Act (1983). The general principles of antipsychotic use in older people have been described in Chapter 3. Two cases are described in Case Histories 6.1 and 6.2 to illustrate the management of two patients with very-late-onset schizophrenia.

Case History 6.1

Mrs A was an 88-year-old woman living with her son. She was physically well but had had impaired hearing and vision for several years. She was able to do most things for herself with assistance from her son, and there was no past history of psychiatric illness. Over the past 12 months she had become suspicious that her son was bringing 'prostitutes' into her home and hiding them in various rooms for 'weeks at a time'. She had heard various women talking and saying 'unkind things' about her, but despite searching her home she had been unable to find anyone. She believed that women were being brought into her home to have sex with her son, and this was causing her considerable distress. She had tried to involve a number of other people to help her, including her neighbours, her general practitioner, a community psychiatric nurse, social services and the police. The police had been called to her house several times, and on one occasion they were led to believe that Mrs A was being held 'hostage', and several police cars attended the scene along with eight officers in full 'riot gear'. In addition, in recent months her relationship with her son had deteriorated and she believed that he wanted to 'poison' her. The psychiatric team made an assessment at home. Mrs A was found to be physically well, with no evidence of depression or cognitive impairment, but she had clear evidence of delusional beliefs and auditory hallucinations at interview. She was initially very reluctant to take any medication, saying that her son wanted to poison her. However, after 3 or 4 weeks of input and persuasion by the community psychiatric nurse, she eventually agreed to take risperidone (gradually increased to 2 mg at night), and after 3 weeks there was a significant improvement in her symptoms. She then agreed to attend the local day hospital.

The selection of the antipsychotic should be individualised, since there is no clear systematic evidence base for antipsychotic treatment of late-onset schizophrenia.[19] When selecting an antipsychotic, the prescriber should take into account the patient's physical health, concomitant medications and the expected side-effects. Most of the currently available antipsychotics are equivalent with regard to their clinical efficacy, but they vary greatly in terms of their side-effects, some of which are particularly troublesome in older people. The daily dose may be slowly titrated upwards until a therapeutic effect is observed or intolerance of side-effects occurs. After the desired response has been achieved, the dose should be gradually reduced to maintain the elderly patient on the minimum effective dose. However, although general guidelines on the use of antipsychotics in the elderly do exist, studies on the pathophysiology and treatment of psychotic disorders in late life are still urgently needed.[20]

Case History 6.2

Mrs D was a 71-year-old woman with a 2-year history of gradual decline. Her neighbours had become concerned about her. She had closed all her curtains, she seldom left the house and would let no one into her home, including her daughter. She was doing less and less for herself, she was extremely unkempt and her house was very untidy and dirty. Frequent calls by her GP and community psychiatric nurse had been unsuccessful, and neither was able to gain entry. Mrs D said that she was 'perfectly well' and didn't want 'any help'. The local old age psychiatrist was asked to see her, and initially the examination was conducted through Mrs D's sitting-room window. Mrs D was noted to be very agitated, pacing up and down her sitting-room and shouting at the psychiatrist. She also appeared to be having a conversation with herself. She adamantly denied that she had any problems, and refused to let anyone into her home. A second visit with the approved social worker, psychiatrist, GP and her daughter resulted in successful entry into her home. She denied that she was ill, but she did say that the neighbours were listening to her telephone conversations, plotting to gas her and were 'spying' on her and commenting on her day-to-day activities. On examination she had evidence of clear delusional beliefs and auditory hallucinations, but with no evidence of depression or cognitive impairment. She was invited to come into hospital as a voluntary patient but she refused, and she was then detained under Section 2 of the Mental Health Act (1983) and brought to an acute ward. Once in hospital she enjoyed a good diet, she had a good rest and her personal hygiene needs were attended to. There was some improvement in her mental state over a 3-day period, despite the fact that she refused to take any medication, but she then agreed to take an oral antipsychotic drug with good effect. She responded very well to treatment and was discharged with community follow-up after approximately 3 months.

Although there have been a large number of randomised controlled trials examining the clinical efficacy of antipsychotic medication in younger patients with schizophrenia and related disorders, there have been no randomised controlled trials of treatment of very-late-onset schizophrenia, even though there have been numerous case studies and open trials. In addition, antipsychotic drugs are used for a wide variety of purposes in older people, not just for those with psychotic symptoms. Some of these uses include the following:

➤ treatment of acute schizophrenia, paranoid illnesses
➤ maintenance treatment in patients with persistent schizophrenia
➤ treatment of negative symptoms in schizophrenia
➤ treatment of psychotic symptoms in depression
➤ treatment of mania.

Where possible, these drugs should be avoided, but if they are used it is helpful to prescribe them taking into account the following principles.

➤ Use one antipsychotic drug (usually risperidone, aripiprazole, olanzapine or quetiapine).
➤ Adjust the dose according to the individual patient's response.
➤ Avoid older antipsychotic drugs.
➤ Use the drug for the minimum period necessary (in schizophrenia often for life).
➤ Discontinue the drug gradually.
➤ Appropriate follow-up is needed after stopping the drug.[21]

PSYCHOPHARMACOLOGY OF ANTIPSYCHOTIC DRUGS

A basic understanding of antipsychotic drugs is essential if these drugs are to be used in a rational manner. Antipsychotic drugs have a number of important actions, including non-specific sedation (immediate), an antipsychotic effect (within days or weeks) and the production of extrapyramidal symptoms/signs (EPSE). A number of different terms have been used to describe these drugs, including 'neuroleptics', 'major tranquillisers' and 'antipsychotics', the last being the preferred term. The common antipsychotic drugs are listed in Table 6.1 on the basis of their chemical structures.

Conventional antipsychotics share the primary pharmacological property of D2 antagonism, which is responsible for their antipsychotic efficacy as well as many of their side-effects, such as extrapyramidal symptoms (EPS) and tardive dyskinesia. Atypical antipsychotics are more difficult to define. Clinically they have a low propensity to cause EPS and they are effective for 'negative symptoms'. Pharmacologically they have several mechanisms, including the following:

➤ serotonin–dopamine antagonists (e.g. clozapine, risperidone, paliperidone, olanzapine, quetiapine)

➤ D2 antagonists with rapid dissociation (e.g. clozapine, quetiapine)

➤ D2 partial agonists (e.g. amisulpride, aripiprazole)

➤ serotonin partial agonists (e.g. quetiapine, clozapine, aripiprazole).

Table 6.1 Conventional and atypical antipsychotics[22-25]

Conventional	Atypical
Chlorpromazine	Amisulpride
Flupenthixol	Aripiprazole
Fluphenazine	Clozapine
Haloperidol	Olanzapine
Pimozide	Risperidone
Sulpiride	Quetiapine
Trifluoperazine	Ziprasidone
Zuclopenthixol	

MODE OF ACTION

There are three principal dopamine-containing tracts in the brain. These are the *nigrostriatal tract* (substantial nigra to caudate nucleus and putamen), the *mesolimbic tract* (ventral tegmental area to the amygdala, pyriform cortex, lateral septal nuclei, nucleus accumbens, frontal cortex and septohippocampal regions) and the *tuberoinfundibular tract* (arcuate nucleus of the hypothalamus to the median eminence). The essential point is that antagonism (blocking) of dopamine activity (at receptors) in these sites is associated with EPS and antipsychotic effects.

THE DOPAMINE HYPOTHESIS OF SCHIZOPHRENIA

The exact biological basis of schizophrenia and related disorders remains unknown. However, the monoamine neurotransmitter dopamine still remains central in the hypothesis of schizophrenia,[26] and dopamine antagonism is the principal mechanism of the conventional antipsychotics. We now know that dopamine is only one of the neurotransmitters affected in schizophrenia, and the wide range of pharmacological mechanisms associated with atypical antipsychotics (*see* table 6.1) underlines this complexity.

CLASSIC ANTIPSYCHOTIC DRUGS

Classic antipsychotics (e.g. chlorpromazine, haloperidol, trifluoperazine, thioridazine) have had a profound impact on the treatment of schizophrenia and related disorders, and until relatively recently they were the mainstay of treatment. These drugs are very effective for the treatment of psychotic symptoms, but they are associated with significant side-effects, including sedation, acute movement disorders, parkinsonism, weight gain and seizures. They are also more likely to cause tardive dyskinesia, and they are dangerous in overdose due to cardiotoxicity. Side-effects are usually dose related, but with careful monitoring they can be easily detected.

ATYPICAL ANTIPSYCHOTIC DRUGS

Atypical antipsychotics are usually defined as drugs with antipsychotic properties but 'devoid' of extrapyramidal side-effects. They are at least as effective as classic antipsychotics, but are associated with significantly fewer extrapyramidal side-effects.[27] However, although atypical antipsychotics have fewer side-effects than classic antipsychotics, they are certainly not free of side-effects (e.g. clozapine, a drug used for treatment-resistant schizophrenia, may cause neutropenia).

In the absence of robust studies of sufficient power to give clear answers about which atypical antipsychotics to use, the consensus of experts suggests that risperidone, aripiprazole, olanzapine and quetiapine are all appropriate.[20] Clozapine may also be indicated in resistant schizophrenia, with the usual precautions.

For more information on prescribing antipsychotics, the reader is referred to *The Maudsley Prescribing Guidelines in Psychiatry*.[21]

SIDE-EFFECTS OF ANTIPSYCHOTICS

Atypical antipsychotics cause fewer and less serious side-effects than classic antipsychotics, but weight gain is common, especially with clozapine and olanzapine.[28] Concerns have also been expressed about cardiac arrhythmias and cerebrovascular accidents, the latter particularly in the context of behavioural and psychological symptoms in dementia.

The main effects of classical antipsychotics include the following:

➤ sedation
➤ anticholinergic side-effects (e.g. dry mouth, blurred vision, memory impairment)
➤ extrapyramidal side-effects
➤ cardiac arrhythmias.

Extrapyramidal side-effects

Even though classic antipsychotics are rarely used in older people, their side-effects are briefly described below.

Parkinsonism

This consists of symptoms mimicking Parkinson's disease, with akinesia, rigidity and tremor. Parkinsonism is more common in older people and women. Anticholinergic drugs should only be used when indicated, and may cause an acute confusional state or increase the risk of tardive dyskinesia. They can be fatal in overdose and are abused. Patients with Lewy body disease are particularly sensitive to antipsychotic-induced EPS. Anticholinergics should be introduced cautiously. Tolerance to EPS may develop, and after 6 months only 10% of cases should need an anticholinergic drug.

Acute dystonias

These are abnormal drug-induced movement disorders involving specific muscle groups (e.g. those of the face, tongue, eye or neck). The onset can be acute and alarming for the patient, and it should be treated as a medical emergency, often requiring emergency treatment with anticholinergic drugs. Acute dystonias are more commonly seen in younger people.

Akathisia

This is the most common reaction, and it occurs in approximately 50% of patients. It is characterised by motor restlessness and subjective agitation, dysphoria or intolerance of inactivity. Shifting of the legs, tapping, rocking or shifting of the weight are common. Internal anxiety can be intense. The underlying mechanism is unclear, and the response to anticholinergic treatment is highly variable.

Tardive dyskinesia

This condition is very difficult to treat, so prevention is important. The average prevalence in people treated with long-term antipsychotics is 15%.[22] Tardive dyskinesia was first described over 30 years ago, and is characterised by orofacial and buccal–lingual involuntary movements, especially in the elderly. Choreoathetoid movements of the upper and lower limbs can also occur. It has a higher incidence, greater severity and poorer prognosis with increasing age, female gender and the presence of brain damage. The link with the amount of antipsychotic is not established, and it appears to have a multifactorial origin. It may be worsened by anticholinergic drugs, and is more likely to occur with rapid antipsychotic drug withdrawal. The mechanism is dopamine-receptor hypersensitivity, and an increase in the dose of antipsychotic is usually associated with a reduction in symptoms. A wide range of treatments have been tried, with limited success. Recovery is more likely in younger people. The antipsychotic drug should be very gradually withdrawn. Anticholinergic drugs should be avoided, and benzodiazepines may occasionally be helpful.

Because of these side-effects the older antipsychotics are rarely used in older people. A special case arises in those who grow old with an established diagnosis of schizophrenia on these drugs. Many old age psychiatrists will seek to transfer these patients on to newer drugs or even to wean them off antipsychotic medication altogether. This must be done with great caution. The aim must always be to ensure that the patient is left with the best possible control of symptoms and the fewest possible side-effects.

Metabolic dysregulation

Atypical antipsychotics differ markedly in their potential to cause metabolic disturbances, including dyslipidaemia, obesity and diabetes[27]. Clozapine and olanzapine carry the greatest risks, whereas risperidone and quetiapine have the lowest risks. Aripiprazole, a relatively new antipsychotic, is associated with minimal metabolic risk, but further research and guidance are needed in this area.[28]

NEUROLEPTIC MALIGNANT SYNDROME (NMS)

Neuroleptic malignant syndrome (NMS) is a serious side-effect of antipsychotics and is potentially lethal. Symptoms and signs include muscle rigidity, elevated temperature, autonomic instability, fluctuating levels of consciousness (sometimes mistaken for delirium), elevated CPK and white blood cell count. NMS can be seen with all antipsychotics but is more commonly associated with conventional/typical drugs, especially haloperidol. The aetiology is unknown. It is an idiosyncratic reaction rather than an allergic one, and is unrelated to dose/ length of treatment. Re-exposure to antipsychotics is uneventful in two-thirds of cases, but this is NOT recommended. Treatment involves the immediate discontinuation of treatment, and administration of dantrolene or a dopamine agonist (e.g. bromocriptine) may be considered. Supportive measures may be necessary. Psychotic symptoms may be treated with benzodiazepines, lithium or ECT. Drugs with minimal potential for EPSE might be tried with caution.

PROGNOSIS OF VERY-LATE-ONSET SCHIZOPHRENIA

Very little has been written about the prognosis of very-late-onset schizophrenia or other paranoid disorders in old age. Improvement is frequently achieved, but a long-term follow-up study[29] has shown that continuing mild impairment is not uncommon. Although patients with late paraphrenia may be extremely difficult to engage in the early stages of treatment, they often show a good response to treatment, and the management of these patients can be very rewarding. However, not many detailed follow-up studies of their prognosis have been undertaken, and this would be a useful area for further investigation.

CONCLUSION

Delusions and hallucinations in older people are common and distressing. They can occur in a variety of disorders, including schizophrenia and related disorders, affective disorders (*see* Chapter 5) and dementia and delirium (*see* Chapter 4). This chapter has concentrated on schizophrenic disorders in later life. These disorders are not common but, with careful assessment and appropriate treatment, patients usually have a reasonable prognosis. There is now a wide variety of antipsychotic drugs available, but care must be taken when choosing antipsychotic drugs to ensure that their side-effects do not exacerbate coexisting medical conditions or interact with other drugs. In general, the newer antipsychotic drugs (e.g. risperidone, aripiprazole, olanzapine, quetiapine) have the same clinical efficacy as the older antipsychotic drugs, but fewer serious side-effects. The National Institute for Health and Clinical Excellence has produced national guidelines on the use of atypical antipsychotics in schizophrenia, and recommends that these drugs are used as first-line treatment.[30] Finally, patients are frequently reluctant to accept treatment, and they often have little or no insight into their mental illness. Sometimes distrust can be overcome by a doctor or nurse working hard to get to know the patient. Often the Mental Health Act (1983) has to be invoked, making close cooperation with primary care and social services (and other healthcare professionals) of vital importance.

REFERENCES

1   Naguib M and Levy R (1995) Paranoid states in the elderly and late paraphrenia. In: R Jacoby and C Oppenheimer (eds) *Psychiatry in the Elderly.* Oxford University Press, Oxford.

2   World Health Organization (1992) *The ICD-10 Classification of Mental and Behavioural Disorders.* World Health Organization, Geneva.

3   Lanoutte NM, Eyler LT and Jeste DV (2011) Late-life psychotic disorders: nosology and classification. In: MT Abou-Saley, C Katona and A Kumar (eds) *Principles and Practice of Geriatric Psychiatry* (3e). John Wiley & Sons, Chichester.

4   Department of Health and Social Security (1985) *Mental Health Statistics.* HMSO, London.

5   Holden N (1987) Late paraphrenia or the paraphrenias? *Br J Psychiatry.* 150: 635–9.

6   Myers JK, Weissman MM, Tischler GL *et al* (1984) Six-month prevalence of psychiatric disorders in three communities. *Arch Gen Psychiatry.* 41: 959–67.

7   Nielsen JA and Nielsen J (1989) Prevalence investigation of mental illness in the aged in 1961, 1972 and 1977 in a geographically delimited Danish population group. *Acta Psychiatr Scand.* 79: 95–104.

8   Blazer D (1980) The epidemiology of mental illness in late life. In: EW Busse and DG Blazer (eds) *Handbook of Geriatric Psychiatry.* Van Nostrand Reinhold, New York.

9   Cohen CI, Cohen GD, Blank K *et al* (2000) Schizophrenia and older adults. *Am J Geriatr Psychiatry.* 8: 19–28.

10 Howard R, Rabins PV, Seeman MV and Jeste DV (2000) Late-onset schizophrenia and very-late-onset schizophrenia-like psychosis: an international consensus. *Am J Psychiatry.* **157**: 172–8.

11 Levy R and Naguib M (1985) Late paraphrenia. *Br J Psychiatry.* **146**: 451.

12 Anderson D (2011) Clinical assessment and differential diagnosis. In: MT Abou-Saley, C Katona and A Kumar (eds) *Principles and Practice of Geriatric Psychiatry* (3e). John Wiley & Sons, Chichester.

13 Post F (1966) *Persistent Persecutory States of the Elderly.* Pergamon, Oxford.

14 Cooper AF, Kay DWD, Curry AR, Garside RF and Roth M (1974) Hearing loss in paranoid and affective psychoses of the elderly. *Lancet.* ii: 851–61.

15 Casanova MF, Stevens JR, Brown R *et al* (2002) Disentangling the pathology of schizophrenia and paraphrenia. *Acta Neuropathol.* **103**: 313–20.

16 Rivkin P, Kraut M, Barta P *et al* (2000) White matter hyperintensity volume in late-onset and early-onset schizophrenia. *Int J Geriatr Psychiatry.* **15**: 1085–9.

17 Denihan A, Wilson G, Cunningham C *et al* (2004) CT measurement of medial temporal lobe atrophy in Alzheimer's disease, vascular dementia, depression and paraphrenia. *Int J Geriatr Psychiatry.* **15**: 306–12.

18 Ban TA (2004) Neuropsychopharmacology and the genetics of schizophrenia: a history of the diagnosis of schizophrenia. *Prog Neuropsychopharmacol Biol Psychiatry.* **28**: 753–62.

19 Arunpongpaisal S, Ahmed I, Ageel N *et al* (2003) Antipsychotic drug for elderly people with late-onset schizophrenia. *Cochrane Database of Systemic Reviews.* 2: CD004162.

20 Connelly P and Prentice N (2011) Treatment of late-life psychosis. In: MT Abou-Saley, C Katona and A Kumar (eds) *Principles and Practice of Geriatric Psychiatry* (3e). John Wiley & Sons, Chichester. pp. 604–8.

21 Taylor D, Paton C and Kapur S (2012) *The Maudsley Prescribing Guidelines in Psychiatry* (11e). Wiley Blackwell, Chichester.

22 King DJ and Waddington JL (2004) Antipsychotic drugs and the treatment of schizophrenia. In: DJ King (ed.) *Seminars in Clinical Psychopharmacology* (2e). Gaskell, London. pp. 316–80.

23 Stahl S (2009) *Stahl's Essential Psychopharmacology* (3e). Cambridge University Press, Cambridge. pp. 327–451.

24 Buckley P and Naber D (2000) Quetiapine and sertindole: clinical use and experience. In: PF Buckley and JL Waddington (eds) *Schizophrenia and Mood Disorders.* Butterworth-Heinemann, Oxford.

25 Potkin S and Cooper S (2000) Ziprasidone and zotepine: clinical use and experience. In: PF Buckley and JL Waddington (eds) *Schizophrenia and Mood Disorders.* Butterworth-Heinemann, Oxford.

26 Lopez-Munoz F and Alamo C (2011) Neurobiological background for the development of new drugs in schizophrenia. *Clin Neuropharmacol.* **34**: 111–26.

27 Brown CS, Markowitz JS, Moore TR and Parker NG (1999) Atypical antipsychotics – Part II. Adverse effects, drug interactions and costs. *Ann Pharmacother.* **33**: 210–17.

28 Casey DE (2005) Metabolic issues and cardiovascular disease in patients with psychiatric disorders. *Am J Med.* **118 (Suppl 2)**: 15–22.

29 Hymas N, Naguib M and Levy R (1989) Late paraphrenia – a follow-up study. *Int J Geriatr Psychiatry.* **4**: 23–9.

30 National Institute for Health and Clinical Excellence (2002) *Schizophrenia: Core Interventions in the Treatment and Management of Schizophrenia in Adults in Primary and Secondary Care.* Nice Clinical Guidelines CG82. Available at www.nice.org.uk

7

Neurotic (anxiety) disorders

INTRODUCTION

The concept of 'neurotic disorders' is a difficult one with a tangled history.[1] A potential underlying factor is a tendency to experience (and sometimes defend against) anxiety at a higher than normal level. There is considerable overlap with depressive disorders (milder, prolonged depression, now called dysthymia, used to be called 'neurotic depression'). Although neuroses were originally thought to be psychogenic in nature, there is no mistaking the fact that they can be extremely disabling and may sometimes respond to pharmacological as well as psychological treatment. They are common in older people, and they are a frequent source of referral to specialist psychiatric teams. Helping patients with neurotic disorders can be frustrating because of the mixture of symptoms, the complexity of presentations, and the tendency for problems to persist. Patients who present with neurotic disorders need a careful medical, psychological and social assessment in order to identify diagnostic categories *and* problems as perceived by the patient. Although they can be very challenging, they often respond well to appropriate management. Because of the pressure from other disorders such as dementia, depression and delirium, and the limited resources available, neurotic disorders in older people have been a relatively low clinical priority. The amount of research relating to older people published in this area compared with that on the dementias is limited.

In the past, neurotic disorders were considered to be less severe than psychotic disorders, but it is now clear that neurotic disorders can be extremely severe and disabling. In addition, the term 'neurotic' has many negative associations and this, combined with ageist views, can lead to older people with neurotic disorders being severely disadvantaged. There is a wide range of neurotic disorders. For the purposes of continuity, this chapter will focus on neurotic disorders as described in *ICD-10*,[2] although this is by no means the only or necessarily the best classification of neurotic disorders.

Neurotic disorders are mental disorders that were historically considered to have no demonstrable organic basis. The patient usually has considerable insight into their illness, and there is no evidence of psychotic features. In general, neurotic disorders include a range of anxiety disorders, hysteria, phobic disorders, obsessive-compulsive disorder, neurasthenia and depersonalisation syndrome. These will be discussed in greater detail below. Neuroticism as a trait can be measured and is essentially stable in mid to late life.[3]

EPIDEMIOLOGY

The epidemiology of neurotic disorders is plagued by variations in definitions and diagnostic criteria, making it very difficult to establish the precise prevalence. Early studies suggested that neurotic disorders tend to decrease in prevalence with increasing age. However, Bergmann reported a prevalence of 11% in a community sample of 300 people over the age of 60 years.[4] These studies tended to group neurotic disorders together, and the variations are as much to do with variations in diagnostic criteria as with anything else. More recently, Copeland *et al* undertook a survey of 1070 elderly people aged 65 years or over and administered the Geriatric Mental State instrument.[5] The overall level of neurotic disorders in the elderly was found to be considerably lower, at 2.4%, than in the previous studies. Hypochondriasis and obsessive-compulsive disorder were found in approximately 0.5% and 0.2% of cases, respectively. The remaining 1.7% of cases were due to various forms of anxiety disorder, including phobic disorder. It was also found that women were more likely to be cases than were men, and this finding has been confirmed by a number of other studies.

CLASSIFICATION OF NEUROTIC DISORDERS

For consistency we have chosen to use *ICD-10*,[2] but the *DSM-IV* is an important alternative classification and differs in a number of minor but not crucial details. These disorders are classified in *ICD-10*[2] under F40–F48 beneath the general heading 'neurotic, stress-related and somatoform disorder'. Somatoform disorders and hypochondriasis are discussed in greater detail in Chapter 9. The main disorders under this heading include the following:
➤ **F40 Phobic anxiety disorders** (agoraphobia, social phobias, specific phobias).
➤ **F41 Other anxiety disorders** (panic disorder, generalised anxiety disorder).
➤ **F42 Obsessive-compulsive disorder** (with predominant obsessional thoughts or ruminations, with predominant compulsive acts, mixed obsessional thoughts and acts).

➤ F43 **Reaction to severe stress and adjustment disorders** (acute stress reaction, post-traumatic stress disorder, adjustment disorders).

➤ F44 **Dissociative disorders** (dissociative amnesia, dissociative fugue, dissociative stupor, trance and possession disorders, dissociative motor disorders, dissociative convulsions and dissociative anaesthesia/sensory loss).

➤ F45 **Somatoform disorders** (somatisation disorder, hypochondriacal disorder, persistent somatoform pain disorder).

➤ F45.8 **Other neurotic disorders** (neurasthenia, depersonalisation/ derealisation syndrome).

The grouping together of this seemingly heterogeneous group of disorders under one classificatory heading is an attempt to solve a nosological conundrum dating back to the last century. Initially, neurasthenia, anxiety neuroses and hypochondriacal disorder were classified as 'neuroses'. In contrast, hysteria, obsessive neurosis and psychoses were classified as 'psychoneuroses'. It was thought that both forms of neurosis were related to sexual disturbance, but that 'neuroses' were the direct physical consequences of misdirected sexual energy. The 'psychoneuroses', in contrast, were said to be caused by unconscious conflict between instinctual and counterinstinctual forces. Eventually, the psychoses were classified independently, and in 1952 the American Psychiatric Association grouped a range of disorders, including anxiety, dissociative, conversion, phobic, obsessive-compulsive and certain depressive reactions, under the general heading psychoneurotic disorders. In *ICD-10*,[2] neurotic and related disorders are grouped under the same heading, whereas in *DSM-IV* different categories are classified with the appropriate major disorder (e.g. with affective disorders where this is appropriate). For a more detailed discussion of the nosology and classification of neurotic disorders, the reader is referred to Bienenfeld.[1]

CLINICAL FEATURES

In *ICD-10*,[2] the neurotic, stress-related and somatoform disorders have been brought together in one group primarily because of this historical association with the concept of 'neurosis', and because of the general belief that these disorders have a psychological causation. Although disorders are described individually below (e.g. obsessive-compulsive disorder), patients commonly have a mixture of symptoms, and it may sometimes be very difficult to diagnose 'pure' neurotic disorders (*see* Case History 7.1).

Case History 7.1

Miss AT was a 69-year-old woman with a wide range of neurotic symptoms, including depression, agoraphobia, panic attacks and generalised anxiety. These symptoms had been present for many years and had not changed significantly despite numerous pharmacological interventions. Her life was affected in many ways. She had little confidence and her social life was very poor. She also found it very difficult to do her shopping and collect her pension, and she believed that she was disliked by 'everyone'. Detailed questioning revealed that she had been sexually abused as a child and her self-esteem was extremely low. She had found this very difficult to talk about. Following a period of assessment she was referred to psychodynamic psychotherapy and she made slow but very good progress. She is now functioning very much better. Her self-esteem has improved, she is socialising more and she takes an active interest in her life.

The main neurotic disorders are described below. This is not an exhaustive summary of all the possible neurotic disorders described in *ICD-10*.[2] If the reader requires more detailed information, it is recommended that they consult *ICD-10*.[2]

F40 Phobic anxiety disorders

In this group of disorders, anxiety is evoked only or predominantly by specific well-defined objects or situations which to most individuals would not be perceived as dangerous. Consequently, these objects or situations are invariably avoided. The anxiety resulting from these situations is physiologically, subjectively and behaviourally indistinguishable from anxiety occurring in a frightening situation (e.g. meeting a lion in the local post office). The three important forms of phobic anxiety include agoraphobia, social phobia and specific phobias.

F40.0 Agoraphobia

Although traditionally agoraphobia has been taken to mean 'a fear of open spaces', it also relates to fear in the presence of crowds or in any situation where there might be difficulty in escaping to a safe place (usually the patient's home). It therefore relates to a group of phobias including fear about leaving home, entering shops, crowds and public places, or travelling on a variety of different forms of transport. The diagnostic criteria include the following:

➤ The anxiety is not secondary to other disorders.

➤ The anxiety must be restricted to at least two of the following situations: crowds, public places, travelling away from home and travelling alone.

➤ Avoidance of the phobic situation must be a predominant feature (*see* Case History 7.2).

Case History 7.2

Mrs BR was a 77-year-old woman living alone in a block of flats near to a busy city centre. Her husband had died several years previously and she had one daughter who lived approximately 5 miles away. Every week she walked to her local post office to pick up her pension and do her weekly shopping. On one occasion she returned to the block of flats but was attacked as she entered the lift. She had her purse and all of her shopping stolen. She was not physically injured and she was able to return to her flat. After this she became low in mood and anxious about leaving her flat, and this situation became gradually worse over 3 to 4 months, despite support and encouragement from her daughter. She had symptoms of depression but no significant symptoms of post-traumatic stress disorder. However, she was very anxious about leaving the flat, and eventually she was unable to go out. After an initial psychiatric assessment she was referred to the community mental health team and she commenced a behaviour therapy programme with supervision from the community psychiatric nurse. After 2 months she was able to return to her 'normal life' and continue to collect her own pension, do her own shopping and use the lift.

F40.1 Social phobias

These essentially centre on a fear of scrutiny by other people, usually in comparatively small groups, and this leads to avoidance of social situations. Unlike most other phobias, social phobias are equally common in women and men. These phobias may be either generalised (e.g. involving almost all social situations outside the family) or discrete (e.g. fear of eating or signing cheques in public).

The diagnostic criteria are very similar to those for agoraphobia. The anxiety must not be secondary to other symptoms, and it must be restricted to particular social situations. In addition, there is avoidance of a specific social situation and this must be a prominent feature.

F40.2 Specific phobias

These are phobias that are restricted to very specific situations. Phobias that are common in children may be prominent (e.g. fear of certain animals, heights, thunder or darkness). However, virtually any object can be the stimulus for a phobic reaction, and a bizarre example encountered by one of the authors was a fear of black coat-hangers. Specific phobias usually commence in early childhood and may persist for many years if they are not appropriately managed. The diagnostic criteria include anxiety that is not secondary to other disorders, anxiety restricted to the specific phobic's object or situation, and the patient invariably avoiding the phobic object or situation. Specific phobias are relatively uncommon in old age.

F41 Panic disorder

This is also sometimes referred to as 'episodic paroxysmal anxiety'. The principal features include recurrent attacks of severe anxiety which tend not to be restricted to any particular situation or set of circumstances, and for this reason the anxiety attack is unpredictable. This invariably leads the patient to become extremely anxious as they have 'no control' over the development of their attacks. Patients develop a variety of symptoms which vary from one individual to another. The range of symptoms include palpitations, chest pain, choking sensations, dizziness, depersonalisation and derealisation, fear of dying and fear of losing control; sometimes patients may worry that they are 'going mad' (*see* Table 7.1). Individual attacks usually last for several minutes, but it is not uncommon for them to last for approximately 20 minutes. Both the frequency and the cause of the disorder are highly variable. It is common for individual patients to focus on specific symptoms (e.g. palpitations), and they may be convinced that 'they are going to die'.

The diagnosis depends upon the presence of several severe attacks of anxiety with autonomic features (e.g. sweating) over the course of a 1-month period.

Table 7.1 Multidimensional symptoms of anxiety (adapted from Sheikh *et al*)[6]

Cognitive symptoms	Behavioural symptoms	Physiological symptoms
Nervousness	Hyperkinesis	Muscle tension
Apprehension	Repetitive motor acts	Chest tightness
Worry	Phobias	Palpitations
Fearfulness	Pressured speech	Hyperventilation
Irritability	Startled response	Paraesthesiae
Distractibility		Light-headedness
		Sweating
		Urinary frequency

These should develop in situations where there is no objective danger, and there should be no underlying cause of the anxiety. In addition, patients are usually in good health between attacks, although they can become agoraphobic because of fears of developing attacks if they leave the house.

Panic attacks can also emerge as part of a depressive illness. Detailed questioning will usually reveal a range of depressive symptoms (*see* Chapter 5), as well as symptoms of panic disorder (described earlier). However, the panic symptoms may be so severe that depressive symptoms are obscured, with a consequent failure to diagnose and treat the condition (*see* Case History 7.3).

Case History 7.3

Mr CS was a 79-year-old man referred by his GP and seen at home. He had a full range of panic symptoms, including sweating, facial flushing, hyperventilation, numbness and tingling in his fingers, diarrhoea, dizziness and a feeling that he was 'going to die'. The symptoms had first started during a bus journey when he thought he was having a heart attack and he was unable to get off the bus. He had a desperate urge to get home. Following this he had a number of further 'attacks', each lasting approximately 15 minutes, in various places outside his home, and he was becoming increasingly frightened about leaving the house and was low in mood. He had previously been tried on an antidepressant (fluoxetine), but this had to be stopped because of nausea. We commenced him on citalopram drops, 5 mg/day for 1 week increased to 10 mg/day for 1 week and then 20 mg/day. He was able to tolerate this with no side-effects, and within 3 weeks there were noticeable improvements. By 3 months he was fully recovered and 'back to his normal self'.

F4l.l Generalised anxiety disorder

The principal feature of generalised anxiety disorder is anxiety that is generalised and persistent but not restricted to any particular environmental situation or object. It is sometimes described as 'free-floating'. The predominant symptoms in individual patients are variable, but include a continuous feeling of nervousness, trembling, muscular tension, sweating, light-headedness, palpitations, dizziness and dyspepsia. The disorder is more common in women, but individual patients may, as in panic disorder, concentrate on individual symptoms (e.g. muscular tension). To fulfil the criteria for a diagnosis of generalised anxiety disorder, the symptoms of anxiety as described above must be present on most days for at least several weeks, and usually for several months. In addition, there should be evidence of apprehension, motor tension and autonomic overactivity (e.g. light-headedness, tachycardia, sweating, increased respiratory rate, dyspepsia, dry mouth and dizziness). There is considerable comorbidity with major depressive disorder and dysthymia.

F42 Obsessive-compulsive disorder

The main feature of this disorder is recurrent obsessional thoughts and/ or compulsive acts. Obsessional thoughts are ideas, images or impulses that intrude into the individual's mind over and over again. They are invariably distressing to the patient (e.g. because they are violent or obscene), and they are usually perceived by them as 'silly'. The patient usually tries unsuccessfully to resist thinking about them, but this resistance leads to anxiety. Compulsive acts are similar to obsessions in that they are stereotyped behaviours that are repeated over and over again. They are not enjoyed by the patient, who feels compelled to undertake the task, and again usually regards it as 'silly'. As with obsessions, resistance leads to severe anxiety, and the only way in which the patient is able to relieve the anxiety is by undertaking the compulsive act (e.g. handwashing). In very long-standing cases, resistance to both obsessions and compulsions may be absolutely minimal. There is also a very close relationship between obsessional symptoms and compulsions and depression, and the prevalence of the disorder is the same in men and women.

For a diagnosis of obsessive-compulsive disorder, obsessional symptoms and/or compulsive acts must be present on most days for at least 2 weeks and be a source of distress to the patient (and usually their family). The patient must recognise that these thoughts are their own, and they must derive no pleasure from their obsessional thoughts or compulsions. In both types, resistance must be associated with anxiety (*see* Case History 7.4).

F43.0 Acute stress reaction

This is a transient disorder of significant severity. It can develop in an individual without any previous history of mental disorder, and it occurs in response to physical and/or mental stress of an 'exceptional' nature. For example, the stressor may be an overwhelming traumatic experience involving serious 'threat' to the security or physical integrity of the individual or of a 'loved person'. The risk of this disorder developing is increased in physical exhaustion and/or if organic factors are also present, and this is particularly pertinent to older people.

For a diagnosis there must be an immediate and clear temporal association between the stressor and the onset of symptoms, and this usually occurs within a few minutes if not immediately. The symptoms may change over a relatively short period of time, and include an initial state of 'daze', depression, anxiety,

---

Case History 7.4

Mrs EF was a 67-year-old woman who had recently retired from work. She was finding it increasingly difficult to adjust to her new life and roles, and she became low in mood. She had always been rather 'houseproud', and noticed that since she had retired she had been doing 'less around the house'. She decided that she would do 'an hour or so' cleaning every day, and over several months this gradually increased. After approximately 4 months she was cleaning for 8–10 hours each day, and often she would clean the same thing several times. She then had her carpets removed and linoleum put in every room so that she could wash the floors regularly. She recognised that the compulsion to do these tasks came from within herself and that the tasks were 'senseless'. She admitted that she had tried to stop doing the tasks, but this 'only made me more anxious'. These activities were now affecting all aspects of her life. She felt exhausted and low in mood, she was unable to go out because of her rituals, and she was reluctant to let people into her home in case they made her house 'dirty'. She was not eating properly, and it was taking her an hour to use the lavatory. She sought help, and this was provided in the form of a behavioural programme of exposure to normal 'household dirt' and response prevention. After 10 weekly sessions in her home with the community psychiatric nurse she made a full recovery without the need for pharmacological treatments.

---

anger, despair, overactivity and withdrawal. The symptoms usually resolve very rapidly, and they seldom persist for more than 3 days.

F43.I Post-traumatic stress disorder (PTSD)

This is similar to an acute stress reaction, but it usually develops as a delayed and/ or protracted response to a stressful event or situation, again of an exceptionally catastrophic or threatening nature. It is likely that such stressors would cause significant distress in almost any individual. The diagnostic guidelines can be summarised as follows.

The disorder should not usually be diagnosed unless there is evidence that it developed within approximately 6 months of the traumatic event as described here. In addition to the traumatic event, there must be evidence of repetitive and intrusive recollections of the traumatic event with distressing imagery and/ or dreams. There is usually a sense of emotional detachment and numbing, as well as avoidance of stimuli that might be associated with the traumatic event. There is also usually autonomic disturbance with hypervigilance, mood disorder and behavioural abnormalities. In older people, these symptoms can develop in response to circumstances that younger adults would not perceive as threatening, but which in older individuals with cognitive impairment, physical illness and frailty, as well as sensory impairment, may induce severe stress reactions (e.g. being burgled). In addition, older people who experienced psychological trauma during World War Two, especially concentration camp survivors, may experience 'postponed' PTSD in later life. Although part of the treatment for PTSD involves talking about the experience, older people are often very reluctant to discuss such experiences, and this can significantly worsen the prognosis. It is important to deal with such issues very sensitively and at a pace that the older person can manage.

F43.2 Adjustment disorders

These are states of subjective distress and emotional disturbance that interfere with social functioning and performance. They develop in response to a significant life change (e.g. a move into a nursing home) or a stressful life event (e.g. the development of a serious physical illness or the loss of a partner). The onset of symptoms is usually within approximately 1 month of the occurrence of the stressful event or life change, and the duration of symptoms does not usually exceed 6 months.

F44 Dissociative (conversion) disorders

There are a number of different forms of dissociative disorder, but a common theme runs through them all. In essence, there is a partial or complete loss of the normal integration between memories of the past, awareness of identity and immediate sensations and the control of bodily movements. In dissociative disorders, there is a reduced ability to exercise a conscious and selective control over one's memory, sensations or bodily movement, but the impairment may vary in intensity from day to day or even from hour to hour. It is frequently associated with severe stress or conflict, but this may be difficult to identify in the early stages. These disorders were previously classified as 'hysteria', but because this term is now used in a variety of different ways, some of which have negative associations, it is generally avoided. In addition, patients with dissociative disorders often show a marked denial of problems or difficulties, and they may not be particularly anxious about their symptoms (e.g. a paralysed leg). The diagnostic criteria include those for individual disorders (e.g. dissociative amnesia), no evidence of a physical disorder that might explain the symptoms, and evidence for a psychological causation.

The main forms of dissociative disorders include dissociative amnesia, dissociative fugue, dissociative stupor, dissociative motor disorders, dissociative convulsions and dissociative sensory loss. If these conditions arise for the first time in late life, an underlying neurological disorder must always be rigorously excluded.

F44.0 Dissociative amnesia

For a diagnosis of dissociative amnesia, the amnesia can be either partial or complete, and it is usually for recent events that are of a traumatic or stressful nature. There should be no evidence of organic brain disorders, intoxication or excessive fatigue.

F44.1 Dissociative fugue

Dissociative fugue has all the clinical features of dissociative amnesia. In addition there is usually an apparently purposeful journey away from home or the place of work during which the patient is able to maintain their self-care. In a few patients, a new identity may be assumed. This usually only lasts for a few days, but occasionally may last for longer periods. During these purposeful journeys the patient is able to undertake simple social interactions with strangers (e.g. buying petrol).

F44.2 Dissociative stupor

In this condition there is a marked diminution or absence of voluntary movement and normal responsiveness to external stimuli (e.g. touch or noise). The individual lies or sits largely motionless for long periods of time. Speech and spontaneous (purposeful) movement are almost completely absent. Although there may be a degree of disturbance of consciousness, it is clear from the clinical observation that the patient is neither asleep nor unconscious. For a diagnosis of dissociative stupor, there should be evidence of stupor as described above, but with no evidence of physical and/or psychiatric disorder, and there should be evidence of a recent stressful event.

F44.4 Dissociative motor disorders

The commonest presentation involves a loss of ability to move the whole or a part of a limb or limbs. Paralysis may be partial or complete. There may be various degrees of incoordination, bizarre gait and exaggerated trembling or shaking. For a diagnosis there should be no organic aetiology, no other psychiatric disorder, and evidence of a recent stressful life event or conflict.

F44.5 Dissociative convulsions

Dissociative convulsions are sometimes referred to as pseudoseizures, and they may closely mimic epileptic seizures. However, it is very rare for patients with dissociative convulsions to bite their tongue, they rarely seriously injure themselves, and there is usually no evidence of incontinence. It is also unusual for patients with dissociative convulsions to lose consciousness. The diagnosis is based on the above clinical symptoms. There should be no physical and/or other psychiatric disorder that could be responsible for these 'seizures', and there should be evidence of a recent stressful life event or conflict.

F44.6 Dissociative anaesthesia and sensory loss

In this condition, areas of the skin are described as being without sensation, but usually these areas of loss of sensation do not conform to known dermatomes (i.e. areas of skin innervated by specific sensory nerves). It is not usually possible to explain the sensory loss in neurological terms and, as with other dissociative disorders, one has to exclude physical causes and other psychiatric illnesses, and there should be a clear association with a stressful life event or conflict.

AETIOLOGY

The aetiology of neurotic disorders is poorly understood. There are many possible factors, and early lifetime experiences are particularly important. These include prolonged maternal separation, undue emphasis on achievement, and parental demands for excessive conformity, as well as traumatic experiences such as sexual abuse and exposure to other frightening situations and experiences. Genetic factors may also be important, but again these are not well understood. In particular, if one monozygotic (identical) twin has a neurotic disorder, the other twin has a four times higher risk of neurotic disorders compared with dizygotic (non-identical) twins. A number of biological factors may predispose to neurotic disorders, and the best-described association is between panic disorder and mitral valve prolapse. In most patients the aetiological factors are complex, and may have occurred in childhood and be either 'distant memories' or repressed and thus not available to consciousness. The underlying mechanism for many neurotic disorders appears to be excessive anxiety, and often this responds to treatments that also work for depression.[7]

MANAGEMENT OF ANXIETY AND PHOBIC DISORDERS

A staged approach to the management of anxiety disorders

The National Institute for Health and Clinical Excellence (NICE) recommends a stepped approach to the management of generalised anxiety disorder[8] and panic disorder.[9] The advice for generalised anxiety disorder is summarised here, but in essence the steps are similar for other conditions. Once the condition is diagnosed it is important to identify and treat any comorbid depressive disorder or medical illness. Where the comorbid disorder is depressive (or another anxiety disorder), priority should be given to the one that is judged to be 'primary'. The first step in treatment (generally in primary care) is education, including self-help material and monitoring. Failure to respond leads to low-intensity psychological intervention (Step 2). This includes self-help, guided self-help and psychoeducational groups. Step 3 is for those who have marked functional impairment or fail to improve with Step 2. This includes high-intensity psychological interventions and drug treatment. Williams' 5-area approach is a useful guide to CBT in these conditions.[9] If, at any stage, there is a risk of self-harm or suicide, or where there is significant physical or psychiatric comorbidity, where there is self-neglect or where there is an inadequate response to Step 3, specialist mental health services (usually the community mental health team) should be called in (Step 4). Anxiety disorders are among the commonest psychiatric disorders occurring in older people. Most tend to be rather chronic in nature, but acute exacerbations are also extremely common. The goal of management is the relief of marked distress, and this can be broadly divided into pharmacological and psychological approaches. However, there are some general principles that are appropriate to the management of all 'neurotic' disorders. During states of severe anxiety, patients may have impaired judgement and may appear to be suffering from a psychotic condition. In addition, they may be unable to take in any advice that is given to them. Where possible it is helpful to give patients something in writing (e.g. an information leaflet). It is important to foster a supportive interaction with the patient and adopt a calm and reassuring manner. It is also important to have a good understanding of the unique medical, psychological and social issues that affect older people.

Psychological approaches

Anxiety can be understood to have three core components, namely psychological (e.g. cognition), physiological (e.g. palpitations) and behavioural (e.g. avoidance behaviours) aspects. Patients with severe anxiety tend to show maladaptive functioning and psychological disturbance. The way in which the patient perceives and understands the anxiety can be shaped by a number of factors, including coping mechanisms, personality, social/environmental factors and past trauma. Cognitive behavioural principles are very effective for a variety of anxiety-related symptoms.[9] There is also an important role for education, relaxation and general support.

Psychopharmacological treatment of anxiety disorders

Prior to commencing any pharmacological treatment, the patient should have a full medical assessment to rule out any medical conditions that might complicate treatment with psychoactive drugs. In addition, it is important to prescribe drugs only where the indications have been clearly met. There are a number of possible pharmacological interventions, which will be briefly discussed below.

SSRI antidepressants are now the first-line pharmacological treatment for many anxiety disorders. Sertraline, for example, is listed in the *BNF* as a treatment for obsessive-compulsive disorder, panic disorder, post-traumatic stress disorder and social anxiety, as well as for its primary indication as an antidepressant. NICE guidance[8] also suggests that it is an appropriate treatment for generalised anxiety disorder (GAD), although it is not presently licensed for that indication. Failure to respond to an adequate trial of sertraline (in combination with appropriate psychological measures) should lead to a trial of another SSRI or an SNRI. Pregabalin, an anti-epileptic, is an alternative for those with GAD who fail to respond to SSRI or SNRI treatment, but it should be used with caution, and renal function should be assessed before treatment. Older tricyclics such as imipramine and clomipramine which were once the mainstay of treatment are rarely used these days. Buspirone is effective in GAD, but is only recommended short term. Benzodiazepines and propranolol are not generally recommended, although they may still have a place in specialist practice. Antipsychotics should usually be avoided.

A number of drugs are currently licensed for the treatment of anxiety disorders, and these are summarised in Table 7.2. Further details are available at www.bnf.org.

Table 7.2 Licensed drugs for specific anxiety disorders

Drug	PAD	OCD	SAD	PD	GAD
Clomipramine	*	*			
Moclobemide			*		
Citalopram				*	
Escitalopram		*	*	*	*
Fluoxetine		*			
Fluvoxamine		*			
Paroxetine		*	*	*	*
Sertraline		*		*	
Duloxetine					*
Venlafaxine					*
Pregabalin					*

PAD, phobic anxiety disorder; OCD, obsessive-compulsive disorder; SAD, social anxiety disorder; PD, panic disorder; GAD, generalised anxiety disorder.

MANAGEMENT OF SPECIFIC DISORDERS

Panic disorder

Self-help and cognitive and behavioural therapies[9,10] can also be extremely effective in the treatment of panic disorder. Patient information is essential, and breathing/muscle relaxation techniques have an important place in the management of this disorder.

Antidepressants are effective in patients with panic disorder. The SSRIs are the first line pharmacologically. Benzodiazepines are no longer recommended even for short-term treatment.

Social phobia, simple phobia and agoraphobia

CBT, often with the added refinement of relaxation with graded exposure, is the mainstay of psychological approaches. SSRIs are the first-line pharmacological approach for these disorders, especially social phobia. Again, self-help guides are available for social anxiety,[11] simple phobia[12] and agoraphobia.[13]

Obsessional disorders

Although obsessive-compulsive disorder (OCD) clearly occurs in older people, it is largely ignored in the literature. However, it is fairly unusual for OCD to occur for the first time after the age of 50 years, and as few as 5% of cases have their first episode after the age of 40 years.[14] The clinical symptoms of OCD have been discussed above. However, it is important to note that the disorder rarely disappears without specific treatment, and it is therefore important that patients with suspected OCD are carefully assessed to establish the diagnosis and provide a sound basis for initiating treatment.

As with other neurotic disorders there are two broad strands to treatment, namely pharmacological and psychological approaches. Cognitive and behavioural therapies are the main psychological approaches and, although education and support for patients have an important role, the core element of treatment includes exposure to the feared situation or object (e.g. a dirty floor) and response prevention (e.g. the patient being prevented from washing the floor). Although this approach is associated with intense anxiety, if the patient is prevented from engaging in a compulsive act or obsessive thought, there will eventually be a gradual diminution of anxiety.[15] Traditional psychodynamic psychotherapy is not an effective treatment for obsessions and/or rituals.

Pharmacological treatment is principally with antidepressants, but these may have a dual action. OCD is commonly associated with depression, and the successful treatment of the underlying depression may result in complete resolution of the OCD. However, antidepressants such as the SSRIs are also effective specifically for the treatment of OCD in the absence of depression. If the obsessional symptoms are secondary to depression, the response to treatment is usually quicker and the prognosis is better. There is no clinical evidence that lithium carbonate or ECT is effective in the treatment of OCD (in the absence of depression). Buspirone can also be helpful in OCD.

Dissociative disorders

The clinical features of dissociative disorders were described earlier. They are not commonly reported in the elderly, although they do occasionally occur, and psychogenic amnesia in particular must be distinguished from post-concussional syndromes, cognitive impairment due to dementia and depressive pseudodementia. For this reason it is important that patients have a thorough medical assessment to rule out any underlying organic aetiology. It is also important to undertake a detailed psychosocial history, and this may reveal the source of the underlying stress that caused the dissociative disorder in the first place. Patients are often surprisingly calm about their predicament, and frequently do not present with any symptoms of depression. However, if the patient is motivated and is able to discuss in detail the stresses and conflicts that led to the dissociative disorder and, through supportive work, can find a solution to this, there is a good prospect that they will recover. The prognosis is less good if the disorder has been present for an extended period of time.

PROGNOSIS OF NEUROTIC DISORDERS

In general, neurotic disorders tend to begin in early adulthood, although later onset is not rare. In general, these disorders seem to have a relatively protracted course, although fluctuations in symptomatology and intensity are very common. Unfortunately, there has been relatively little research in this area in younger patients, let alone in older people with neurotic disorders.

Generalised anxiety disorder

Treatment interventions are reasonably effective in the short term (as described earlier), but the prognosis of generalised anxiety disorder (GAD) in older people in the longer term has been poorly studied. However, one study reported a remission rate of only 18% over 5 years in older patients with GAD who had previously received drug treatment,[16] a significantly lower remission rate than for panic disorder in older people (*see* p. 187).

Social phobia

Younger patients with social phobia tend to have lifelong problems and these tend to persist into old age.[17] Social phobia does tend to respond to cognitive behaviour therapy and pharmacological treatments in the short term (as discussed earlier), but information about the long-term prognosis using these treatment strategies is unavailable. Systematic studies of this disorder in older people have not been undertaken.

Simple phobia

This disorder also tends to have a fairly chronic course in younger patients,[18] but no studies have been conducted in older people with simple phobia.

Panic disorder

Again this disorder usually has a chronic course with fluctuating symptomatology and periods of partial or complete remission.[19] Although pharmacological and cognitive behavioural interventions appear to be effective (as discussed earlier) in the short term, the long-term effect of these treatments on the natural history of the disorder has not been extensively researched. In patients treated with pharmacological interventions in a clinical trial context, the remission rate over a 5-year period has been reported to be 45%. This is significantly better than for GAD. In addition, patients with panic disorder had a later onset and shorter duration of illness compared with GAD patients.[16] Depression is frequently associated with panic disorder, and this can significantly complicate the illness if it is left untreated. In addition, untreated panic disorder may lead to alcohol abuse, increased risk of suicide and increased cardiovascular mortality.[20]

Obsessive-compulsive disorder

The prognosis of this disorder can be significantly improved if any underlying depressive disorder is adequately treated. OCD generally responds to treatment, and with appropriate treatment there is a good prospect of remission in the short term. However, as with the other neurotic disorders described in this chapter, there is very little information available on the long-term prognosis of OCD in younger patients, and especially in older people with the condition. Because SSRIs are well tolerated in older people, this may be a useful starting point, usually in smaller doses than those recommended for depression in the early stages, but the dose can then be gradually increased.

CONCLUSION

Neurotic disorders in older people can present in many complex ways and can be either mild or severely disabling. They are frequently amenable to treatment, but this requires a thorough medical, psychological and social assessment to identify clearly the main problems, understand possible aetiological factors and engage the patient in the most appropriate treatment. A multiprofessional approach is particularly important, gaining the patient's trust is vital, and expectations should be realistic. Moreover, the patient's problems should be taken seriously and not 'dismissed'. Successful treatment may take time. It is important not to become disillusioned if treatment does not seem to be working after 'a few weeks'. Not 'abandoning' the patient can have a significant positive effect. It is also important for the patient to recognise that their condition is primarily psychological in nature. This, combined with education and a range of psychological approaches, can significantly improve the quality of life of patients with neurotic disorders.

REFERENCES

1 Bienenfeld D (2011) Nosology and classification of neurotic disorders. In: MT Abou-Saley, C Katona and A Kumar (eds) *Principles and Practice of Geriatric Psychiatry* (3e). John Wiley & Sons, Chichester. pp. 611–15.

2 World Health Organization (1992) *The ICD-10 Classification of Mental and Behavioural Disorders.* World Health Organization, Geneva.

3 Steunenberg B, Twisk JW, Beekman AT *et al* (2005) Stability and change of neuroticism in aging. *J Gerontol Series B: Psychol Sci Soc Sci Online.* **60**: 27–33.

4 Bergmann K (1971) The neuroses of old age. In: DV Kay and A Walk (eds) *Recent Developments in Psychogeriatrics.* Headley Bros, Ashford.

5 Copeland JRM, Dewey ME, Wood H, Searle R, Davidson IA and McWilliam C (1987) Range of mental illness among elderly in the community: prevalence in Liverpool using GMS-AGECAT package. *Br J Psychiatry.* **150**: 815–23.

6 Sheikh JI, Cassidy EL and Swales JI (2002) Acute management of anxiety and phobias. In: JRM Copeland, MT Abou-Saleh and DG Blazer (eds) *Principles and Practice of Geriatric Psychiatry.* John Wiley & Sons, Chichester. pp. 102–3.

7 Kapczinski F, Lima MS, Souza JS *et al* (2009) Antidepressants for generalized anxiety disorder. *The Cochrane Library.* Available online at www.cochrane.org

8 National Institute for Health and Clinical Excellence (2011) *Generalised Anxiety Disorder and Panic Disorder (With or Without Agoraphobia) in Adults: Management in Primary, Secondary and Community Care, CG113.* London. Available at www.nice.org.uk

9 Williams C (2012) *Overcoming Anxiety, Stress and Panic: a Five Areas Approach* (2e). Hodder Arnold, London.

10 Baker R (2011) *Understanding Panic Attacks and Overcoming Fear* (3e). Lion Hudson, Oxford.

11 Butler G (2008) *Overcoming Social Anxiety and Shyness: a Self-Help Guide, Using Cognitive Behavioural Techniques.* Constable and Robinson, London.

12 Hogan B (2007) *An Introduction to Coping with Phobias.* Constable and Robinson, London.

13 Silove D and Manicavasagar V (2009) *Overcoming Panic and Agoraphobia.* Constable and Robinson, London.

14 Black A (1974) The natural history of obsessional neurosis. In: HR Beech (ed.) *Obsessional States.* Methuen, London.

15 Jenike MA (1989) Obsessive-compulsive and related disorders: a hidden epidemic. *NEJM.* **321**: 539–41.

16 Woodman CL, Noyes R, Black DW, Schlosser S and Yagla SJ (1999) A 5-year follow-up study of generalised anxiety disorder and panic disorder. *J Nerv Ment Dis.* **187**: 3–9.

17 Blazer D, George L and Hughes D (1991) The epidemiology of anxiety disorders: an age comparison. In: C Salzman and B Liebowitz (eds) *Anxiety Disorders in the Elderly.* Lawrence Erlbaum Associates, Hillsdale, NJ.

18 Turns DM (1985) Epidemiology of phobic and obsessive-compulsive disorders among adults. *Am J Psychother.* **39**: 360–70.

19 Noyes R, Crowe RR and Harris EL (1986) Relationship between panic disorder and depression. *Arch Gen Psychiatry.* **43**: 146–61.

20 Coryell W (1988) Mortality of anxiety disorders. In: R Noyes and M Roth (eds) *Classification, Etiological Factors and Associated Disturbances of Anxiety Disorders.* Elsevier/North Holland Science Publishers, Amsterdam.

8

Personality disorders and alcohol and substance misuse

INTRODUCTION

People with personality disorders and those who abuse alcohol and other substances are often dismissed as 'cussed' or 'bad, not mad'. These problems do not fit easily into any model, psychological or biological, and can sometimes be disregarded by clinicians. The latter are often under severe pressure to use their time effectively, and may therefore disregard conditions that are perceived as self-inflicted, that are complicated to manage and that do not appear to respond well to treatment. Part of the complexity is due to comorbidity between alcohol and substance misuse, personality disorder and other diagnoses. In old age the prevalence of both alcohol and substance misuse and of personality disorder appears to fall, so that this kind of comorbidity is less of a problem than in younger patients. Some healthcare professionals view personality disorder and alcohol and substance misuse as being completely outside their remit, believing that people with these problems can be dismissed as 'beyond help'. Perhaps there is an element of truth in this attitude, but everyone deserves to have their problems carefully and professionally assessed on an individual basis before premature judgements are made about 'treatability'.

EPIDEMIOLOGY AND PREVALENCE

Personality disorders

One of the earliest comprehensive surveys of mental disorders in old age reported a community prevalence of around 4% for 'character disorders', including non-psychotic paranoid states. More recent estimates of prevalence tend to be in selected samples. For example, in a number of American studies of hospital populations, the prevalence was generally lower than in younger people, and ranged from about 6% to nearly 50%.[1-4] Personality disorder commonly appears alongside another mental illness diagnosis, where it seems to affect the outcome of the main diagnosis.[2,5] In studies in the USA, where it is common to record the main psychiatric diagnosis as an 'Axis 1' diagnosis and the personality disorder as an 'Axis 2' diagnosis, about one-third of elderly patients with depressive disorder have comorbid personality disorder. This is associated with a longer illness and poor social support. Personality dysfunction is commoner in old people with recurrent early-onset depressive disorder than in those with late-onset disorder, and may reflect personality change following earlier episodes of depression, a predisposing personality or even an incompletely recovered depressive syndrome. Avoidant, dependent and compulsive personality abnormalities are most often found in association with depressive illness, and compulsive personality may be more strongly associated with depressive disorder with increasing age.[2,3] There is a long-established relationship between paranoid personality type and social isolation and the development of late-onset forms of paranoid schizophrenia. The effects of increasing age on borderline personality disorder are not clear, but there are indications of a reduction in impulsivity[6] and an increase in somatisation[7] (*see* Chapter 9).

Another group of personality problems that are found in old age are personality changes associated with organic brain disease.[8-10] Relatives report negative personality changes in about two-thirds of patients who develop dementia. These changes may be abrupt or progressive, and are generally reported as negative (e.g. unreasonable, lifeless, childish, cruel or irritable behaviour). They may reflect the demented person's attempts to make sense of their shattered world, as well as being due to direct effects of organic brain damage or secondary to untreated depression. Those dementias that differentially affect the frontal lobes may produce marked disinhibition of sexual or aggressive impulses, sometimes interpreted as personality change. Similarly, strokes that affect certain brain areas may produce some disinhibition and loss of emotional control that may be attributed to personality change.

Alcohol use disorders

The belief persists that alcohol abuse and dependence are rarely, if ever, seen in old age. The current generation of old people drink less alcohol than their younger contemporaries, but this may be misleading for several reasons. First, due to differences in average body composition, old people may need less alcohol to become intoxicated.[11] They may also respond differently to survey methods, and present figures do not rule out the possibility of a cohort effect as our current generation of heavy drinkers grows older. An epidemiological study conducted in London some years ago showed that for women in that area at that time, the prevalence rate for alcoholism continued to rise into the seventh decade, whereas for men it peaked in their fifties.[12] As in other age groups, the epidemiology of alcohol abuse in old age is culturally bound. It is difficult to know whether the relatively low rates found in today's old people represent an age-related decrease in alcohol consumption, a cohort effect, or (perhaps most likely) a combination of both. Period effects are also important, so that the drinking habits of whole populations may change from time to time. Perhaps the most well-known example of this was the era of 'prohibition' in the USA in the early twentieth century. Surveys of heavy drinking as opposed to alcohol abuse or dependence are confounded by the need to vary the definition of heavy drinking according to the age and gender of the population. Generally speaking, the safe drinking limits for the average woman are two-thirds of those for the average man. A similar factor should probably be applied to older people because of the reduced proportion of lean body mass, which results in a smaller volume of distribution for alcohol, which is distributed around the lean body mass rather than in fatty tissues.[11] Ageing brains are probably less able to withstand the toxic effects of alcohol and drug interactions (e.g. with benzodiazepines).[13] These in turn may be more likely because of the increased use of medications in older people. In long-term alcohol abuse, liver and brain damage may complicate the picture. The main conclusion to be drawn from recent studies is that alcohol consumption remains relatively high in the 'young elderly' (65–74 years) age group, but tails off thereafter, although some studies[14] show the highest ever gender-specific rates in women over the age of 75 years. In general, rates are higher in men than in women, but this too may alter as drinking cultures change over time under commercial and other pressures.

Two groups of elderly alcoholics are discernible, namely those chronic alcoholics who have survived into late life and those (often women) who have turned to alcohol for the first time in response to the stresses of ageing (see Case History 2.5 in Chapter 2).

Substance misuse is rare in old age, and has different characteristics to substance abuse in younger adults. Opiate addiction in old age is more likely to be due to the therapeutic use of these drugs than to their being obtained 'on the street'. Similarly, benzodiazepine abuse is likely to be iatrogenic, and barbiturate dependence is still occasionally seen in those who have grown old on repeat prescriptions originally intended to deal with insomnia.

CLINICAL DESCRIPTIONS AND DEFINITIONS

Personality disorder has been succinctly defined as 'a long-standing pattern of maladaptive interpersonal behaviour'.[15] This type of behavioural definition is preferable, since it can enable diagnosis on the basis of observed behaviour without the need to infer underlying motivation. This improves reliability.

'Alcohol dependence'[16] has been defined as a serious medical and psychiatric disorder characterised by the following seven features:

1 narrowing of drinking repertoire
2 priority of drinking over other activities
3 physiological tolerance of the effects of alcohol
4 repeated withdrawal symptoms
5 relief of withdrawal symptoms by further drinking
6 subjective awareness of a compulsion to drink
7 reinstatement of drinking after abstinence.

'Alcohol abuse' can be broadly defined as sufficient alcohol intake to cause harm, whether physical, psychological or social (or more often a combination of all three).

'Substance abuse' in the context of old age can be defined as the continuation of therapy which is no longer helpful and which may cause physical, psychological or social harm. It most commonly arises when patients have been inappropriately started on long-term benzodiazepines as anxiolytics or hypnotics. Patients are often worried that antidepressants may be 'addictive', but there is little evidence of any severe problem with these drugs, although withdrawal symptoms have been described, particularly with paroxetine.

The clinical pictures of personality disorder and alcohol and substance abuse will now be considered separately in more detail.

Personality disorder (*ICD-10*, F60)

Many different personality traits and types have been described by various authors, and interest in their relevance to mental disorder has been revived by the use of multi-axial diagnosis in recent editions of the American Psychiatric Association's *Diagnostic and Statistical Manuals* (*DSM-III* and *DSM-IV*). Although some behaviour which acts as a marker of disorder in younger individuals is less likely to be found in older people, other 'marker' behaviour such as social withdrawal may become more likely because of physical or sensory disabilities or undiagnosed illness, including depressive illness. Social expectations of behaviour also change. An old man who strikes another person is probably less likely to be charged with assault than a young man who carries out the same action. An old woman who behaves histrionically is less likely to be labelled 'hysterical' or 'borderline' than a young woman. We all have socially conditioned expectations about what is 'normal' for people in different age groups and of each gender which influence where we draw the line between 'normal' and 'abnormal' behaviour.

Some personality patterns can be identified that fall short of frank personality disorder. Insecure, rigid and anxiety-prone people have the greatest problems in adapting to old age, and seem especially prone to develop depressive symptoms. Paranoid, isolated people may be at greater risk of developing very-late-onset schizophrenia, but often cope well unless physical or psychiatric symptoms require outside help. Such individuals will often refuse help and may end up living in squalid and unhealthy circumstances. Passively dependent people cope well as long as they have someone to depend on, but they are vulnerable to the loss of a partner or other caring person. A fuller account of personality disorder (and alcohol abuse) can be found in *Seminars in Old Age Psychiatry.*[17]

One study of psychiatric inpatients found that 7% of older patients were given an additional diagnosis of personality disorder, compared with 30% of younger patients. Traits not amounting to 'disorder' were found in 16% of the elderly patients and 4% of the younger group.[18] Around 80% of the diagnoses in elderly people were accounted for by dependent (F60.7), histrionic (F60.4) and compulsive (anakastic F60.5) personality, with dependent personality alone accounting for over half of these cases. In the younger group, the personality diagnoses were distributed more widely between the different personality groups. Personality problems are more common in those with depressive illness in old age, and avoidant, dependent and compulsive traits are particularly likely to occur in these patients, irrespective of age, with some increase in compulsive traits in old age.

Anxious/avoidant (F60.6) personalities are also found, as is illustrated in Case History 8.1. The diagnostic label of anxious (avoidant) personality disorder does little justice to the way in which this woman coped for years with a husband with schizophrenia.

Dissocial (antisocial) personality disorder (F60.2) occurs rarely in older people, but is then often contained within the family, sometimes only emerging when the patient has to go into residential care which is not as tolerant of antisocial behaviour as some families!

Personality and behaviour disorders due to brain disease (F07) occur in dementia and may include some antisocial characteristics. In Alzheimer's disease, changes are often found, and four different patterns have been described:
1 initial change followed by a period of stability
2 continuing change throughout the course of the illness
3 no major change
4 emergence of disturbed behaviour which then regresses as the dementia develops.[9]

In personality change due to brain disorders there is sometimes selective damage which produces a characteristic change in behaviour. Perhaps the best-known example is frontal lobe dementia. In this condition the frontal lobe atrophies in advance of other cortical areas. Sometimes very difficult problems may present as a result (*see* Case History 8.2).

Case History 8.1

MS is a 68-year-old widow. When she was 4 years old her mother died, allegedly as a result of a beating from her husband (although he was never prosecuted). A cause of this beating was that MS was an illegitimate child of her mother's lover, conceived while her father was away during the War. After her mother's death, MS was turned out on the street and taken in by another family. She says that they used to go out drinking a lot. At the age of 17 years she went into hospital with TB, and she later married a man who flew into unexpected rages and was later diagnosed as having schizophrenia. She looked after him for many years, but in the late 1970s he finally went into a hostel. She blamed herself for not looking after him adequately, perhaps reflecting her own feelings of having received inadequate care in childhood, and she had a 'breakdown'. After that she lived a nomadic life staying in boarding houses at various seaside resorts, never very satisfied with her lot, and always anxious and frightened. When she was seen by the psychiatrist she had returned to her home town, and was about to be evicted from the boarding house in which she was living. She had some mild biological signs of depression, and unrealistic expectations that social services could immediately find her permanent accommodation near her sister. After a further journey to another seaside town, she was admitted for treatment of her depression and assessment of what help could be given for her maladaptive responses to stress. She was rehoused after a period of 6 months in hospital during which staff refused to confirm her 'life-script' by rejecting her, despite awkwardness on her part about finding new accommodation. She was followed up in the community by a member of our team, and perhaps at last found the consistent caregiving she had been missing for most of her life.

Case History 8.2

JS was a loving husband and grandfather. For years he had worked on the railways, but at the age of 60 years he was made redundant. Soon after this his wife died unexpectedly from a stroke. He did not seem to be coping well at home, and his daughter and son-in-law invited him to come and stay with them. Almost immediately things started to go wrong, as he was unusually bad-tempered with his 3-year-old granddaughter, and at one point looked as if he was about to strike her. The GP was called and thought that JS might be depressed. In view of the difficult home situation, an urgent visit was requested from the old age psychiatrist. He interviewed the patient's daughter separately and elicited the further distressing information that the patient had been behaving in a sexually over-familiar way towards his daughter. Mental state examination revealed no sign of pervasive depressed mood, but there was some loss of emotional control. Memory seemed to be reasonably well preserved, but the psychiatrist was sufficiently concerned by the picture of frontal disinhibition and the potential risk to the grandchildren to arrange immediate admission for assessment. On the ward the patient's behaviour towards female nursing staff was quite disinhibited, but they managed it firmly. A CT scan confirmed frontal lobe atrophy, and frontal lobe dementia was diagnosed. The family was devastated but wanted to take the patient home to look after him. Because of the potential risk to his grandchildren, the local child protection procedures were invoked, and he was allowed home under controlled circumstances. However, the family could not cope with his behaviour, so he returned to hospital. There his behaviour continued to present considerable problems. Attempts to contain his behaviour by psychological means and medication only just kept the situation manageable. Unfortunately, consistent psychological responses by the nurses to harassment seemed to transfer his over-familiar and sometimes aggressive behaviour to frail female patients. No single-sex unit was available for his management. Medication sufficient to reduce his unwanted behaviour had disabling side-effects and therefore had to be stopped. Eventually he settled in a psychiatric long-stay environment, and although his behaviour became less of a problem as his dementia progressed, it proved impossible to find a nursing or residential home that would take him, in view of his history.

Fortunately, most personality change due to brain disorder is less severe. A group of patients with Alzheimer's disease and vascular dementia were rated by their partners as more out of touch, reliant on others, childish, listless, changeable, unreasonable, lifeless, unhappy, cold, cruel, irritable and mean than mentally healthy partners. Some of these perceived changes may be due to the partner's reaction to the illness, some might be directly determined by organic change, and others might indicate a reaction of the person to the experience of dementia.[10,19]

On the other hand, we all know of individuals who have retained kind and gentle personalities despite having advanced dementia.

Alcoholism and drug-related disorders (FI0–FI9)

Often elderly people with alcohol-related problems present with falls, self-neglect or unexplained confusion. Sometimes they develop a withdrawal delirium after hospital admission that was precipitated by some other problem. Their alcohol intake may be concealed by themselves and either unknown to or concealed by family and friends. Mobility problems may cause them to rely on others for their alcohol supply. These 'others' may be innocent friends or relatives who are an unwitting part of a large supply network, as in Case History 2.5 in Chapter 2, or they may be other alcoholics. If they are close friends or family members who are also alcoholics, then the prognosis for the old person's alcoholism is worsened. If an old person is admitted to hospital and friends or family members come in drunk, then the possibility that the patient also has alcohol problems should be explored. Old people with such problems are especially vulnerable to economic exploitation by other alcoholics, partly because of their frequent dependence on such people for a supply of alcohol and partly because increasing age is a major risk factor for the development of alcoholic dementia, with impaired judgement and disinhibition.

Prolonged excessive alcohol abuse can produce a wide range of complications. These can be broadly classified as biological, psychological and social. Poor nutrition is perhaps the most obvious biological complication. Thiamine deficiency is a particular risk, and may be responsible for the development of Wernicke's encephalopathy, which is fortunately a rare occurrence in alcohol withdrawal delirium (F10.40). Wernicke's syndrome is indicated by the occurrence of delirium with ataxia, nystagmus and disturbance of conjugate gaze, sometimes with evidence of peripheral neuropathy. It constitutes a medical emergency and intravenous (IV) thiamine, 100 mg, should be administered immediately (in hospital, with suitable precautions for anaphylaxis), followed by daily doses of thiamine (orally or IV). Even when Wernicke's encephalopathy does not provide an immediate reminder of the nutritional deficiencies that occur in people who abuse alcohol, attention should always be paid to good nutrition as part of the recovery plan, and dietetic advice is often useful. Untreated Wernicke's encephalopathy can result in a permanent severe amnesic syndrome (F10.6) with memory deficit, relatively well-preserved cognitive function and sometimes some frontal lobe features (Korsakov syndrome). The memory disorder is very characteristic and consists of amnesia often accompanied by confabulation. This entails a severe deficit in the ability to recall memories in an orderly fashion, resulting in fantastical tales that are often based on real memories. For example, a patient on the ward may give a coherent and convincing account of a trip to London on the train the previous night, perhaps based on an experience that really happened 5 years earlier. Unfortunately, confabulation is not diagnostic of Korsakov syndrome, as it is also found (although rarely in so well developed a form) in dementia of other types[20] and in schizophrenia.[21]

Prolonged excessive alcohol consumption damages the immune system, resulting in increased susceptibility to infections such as TB. Alcohol abuse can also produce liver disease, including cirrhosis (which has a particularly poor prognosis in old age).[22] In addition, alcohol abuse is a risk factor for cancer and heart disease, making physical examination and investigation of elderly patients with alcohol problems particularly important.

Excess alcohol intake also carries a risk of drug interactions due to additive sedative effects, reduced or increased metabolism, or complicated consequences of liver damage. Finally, alcohol abuse has a series of sequelae that result from its action on the brain, ranging from acute intoxication through withdrawal syndrome to chronic brain damage, including the Wernicke–Korsakov syndrome, cerebellar degeneration and dementia. Cerebellar degeneration is evidenced by an ataxic gait and problems in the feedback control of motor activity.

More neuropsychiatric consequences include alcoholic hallucinosis (F10.52), with persistent auditory hallucinations (often of a hostile or derogatory nature), and morbid jealousy (F10.5), which usually occurs in men and is characterised by delusions of a partner's infidelity. The latter two disorders rarely arise in old age, but are occasionally seen as newly arising or persistent conditions. Morbid jealousy in particular requires expert management and care planning, since it may be refractory to pharmacological treatment and may be associated with a risk of harm to the partner. In some cases the morbid jealousy only arises when the subject is under the influence of alcohol, and this has obvious implications for prevention.[23] A fuller discussion of alcohol abuse in old people can be found in *Reviews in Clinical Gerontology*.[14] NICE pathways guidance on alcohol-use disorders (http://pathways.nice.org.uk/pathways/alcohol-use-disorders) is also relevant.

Substance abuse in old age is largely a hidden problem. Dependence on benzodiazepines prescribed for anxiety disorders and sleeping tablets of the benzodiazepine group is currently still a significant problem. *The International Classification of Diseases (ICD)* classified mental and behaviour disorders related to sedative or hypnotic use under the general rubric of F13. The conditions we are concerned with fall mostly into F13.1, 'harmful use'. Those atypical depressed patients who respond dramatically to non-selective monoamine oxidase inhibitors may need to continue them indefinitely. In this case, a type of 'dependence' may be a reasonable price to pay for a great improvement in the quality of life. Conventional tricyclic antidepressants and the newer antidepressants do not seem to produce serious physical dependence syndromes, but there is still a risk of relapse of the depression when they are stopped. Mild withdrawal syndromes are reported with SSRIs, especially paroxetine, but can be avoided by careful dose reduction rather than abruptly stopping treatment. As has been indicated above, drug dependence in old people is usually related to prescribed drugs, and both its cause and its cure are in the hands of doctors. Some substances, such as long-acting benzodiazepines (and short-acting benzodiazepines taken more than three times weekly), are associated with increased morbidity from falls and fractures in nursing home populations,[24] even during short-term use. Antipsychotics, sometimes inappropriately prescribed to control behaviour problems in dementia, also cause morbidity (and mortality). Although they do not fall within the definitions usually applied to 'drug abuse', such problems clearly represent abuse of drugs inflicted on patients by medical and other professionals.

UNDERLYING CAUSES

Schizoid and borderline personality types may be genetically related to schizophrenia, although these links are probably less marked in older people. Depressive, avoidant, compulsive and hypochondriacal personality traits may be biologically linked to major affective disorder, but whether this is genetically determined, or a distortion of personality secondary to illness, or whether it represents incompletely treated or recovered illness episodes, is not clear.

A large-scale twin study suggested that (for all age groups) genetic influences were moderate for alcohol abuse, frequency of drug use and illicit drug use, but that prescribed drug use and debilitating drug use were largely environmentally determined by unique person-specific environmental (rather than familial) factors.[25] The same study identified three uncorrelated genetic factors. The first represented social dysfunction associated with drug and alcohol abuse, the second represented a general liability to drug use (illicit or otherwise), and the third appeared to be specific to alcohol abuse.

The tendency to abuse alcohol and a predisposition to personality disorder may in part be genetic, but there is no clear pattern of inheritance and development, and situational factors are probably more important in many cases, especially when they are of late onset. Personality problems are often the result of disturbed relationships in earlier life. However, despite such damage, people will often cope well with life provided that they are not exposed to abnormal stress. Thus aetiology is a mixture of genetics, early life experience and current life situation (*see* Case History 8.1).

DETECTION AND DIAGNOSIS

The detection of personality disorder and alcohol and substance misuse in old people first of all demands that the mental health worker is aware of the possibility. Attitudes expressed by statements such as 'It's all he's got left at his age' can seem to condone excessive drinking by old people. More often, however, it is a hidden problem. Patients will go to considerable lengths to conceal their alcohol problems (and the empty bottles!). Suspicion should be raised whenever there is unexplained self-neglect or falls. The clinician should make even more careful enquiry if other members of the family or household abuse alcohol. Diagnosis may be confirmed by a history from an informant, finding empty bottles, or tracking down the route of supply. Laboratory tests can also be helpful. A simple blood alcohol measurement taken immediately after admission or in the day hospital, raised mean corpuscular volume (MCV) on the blood film without other explanation, and the non-specific but sensitive test of liver damage, gamma glutamyl transaminase (γ-GT), can all help.

Personality disorder diagnoses are rarely made in old people in the UK. The use of a multi-axial diagnostic system such as *DSM-IV* might force us all to be more aware of the less severe examples that we sometimes encounter. One diagnostic problem here is distinguishing the (hopefully temporary) changes in personality caused, for example, by depressive illness from underlying personality disorder.

TREATMENT AND OUTCOME

Personality disorder and comorbidity

When patients with a primary 'Axis 1' diagnosis of functional or organic brain disorder fail to recover with appropriate medical treatment, there may be a tendency to 'blame' an underlying personality disorder. This approach is never helpful. The main thrust of pharmacological management and other physical treatment (e.g. ECT) must be to ensure that the primary illness is as fully treated as possible. Case History 8.3 illustrates this.

Case History 8.3

A 74-year-old woman of previously superior intelligence developed paranoid delusions and hallucinations concerning her neighbours. She initially showed mild cognitive impairment and a poor response to antipsychotics, and prominent depressive symptoms emerged. Antidepressants were added, but side-effects became a problem and her ideas of persecution persisted. Atypical antipsychotics were tried because of the side-effects and poor efficacy of the conventional antipsychotics. Although the florid symptoms subsided, the patient remained suspicious. A review of the history revealed a number of apparent

---

> personality problems, perhaps evidenced by a widely dispersed family. It was tempting to make an Axis 2 diagnosis of personality disorder to explain the patient's treatment resistance. However, the consultant decided to make a further attempt to explore treatability, combining clozapine and an antidepressant. The patient responded well, her persecutory ideas faded and even her cognitive state improved.

This patient could have been dismissed as 'organic' or 'personality disordered' (and, by implication, 'untreatable'). Whenever there is comorbid functional psychiatric illness, the primary psychiatric responsibility is to make sure that it is adequately treated.

In the traditional 'medical model', treatment follows from diagnosis. Personality disorder and alcohol and substance abuse do not fit as easily as some other conditions into the simple disease model epitomised by infective illness, since their boundaries are difficult to define and their causation is commonly complicated. Nevertheless, the first rule of good management is to be alert to the possibility that such conditions may exist, especially as there is some evidence that diagnoses of drug and alcohol misuse in old age may be 'missed',[26] particularly when they present indirectly. If they occur as comorbid conditions with other disorders they may have a profound effect on management. The next responsibility is to ensure that adequate social and psychological management is offered. Because some forms of personality disorder may represent incomplete expression of disorders such as schizophrenia, pharmacological management should not be ruled out. There is some evidence from younger patients that 'borderline' personality disorder may respond to low-dose antipsychotic medication. Medication should rarely, if ever, form the main part of the treatment plan where personality disorder is the main diagnosis. Perhaps more than any other condition, personality disorder highlights the need for strong multidisciplinary teamwork incorporating medical, psychological and social perspectives.

Almost by definition, personality disorder involves relationship problems and therefore social problems. Social relationships develop over the lifespan, from the dependence of childhood to the relative independence and responsibility of adult life. However, in old age all of this may change. Physical or mental frailty may result in dependence on others for support either at home or in institutional care. Relationships between parent and child may be reversed, with the child now exerting authority and control over the diminished older person. Those who have grown old used to living with a compliant partner or alone may suddenly face the unwelcome prospect of group living according to someone else's rules. The amazing fact is that most old people are sufficiently flexible to take these sometimes revolutionary changes in their stride. This adaptation may be at the price of becoming depressed, as is indicated by the high prevalence of depression in those with chronic disability or in residential care. Sometimes a more active rebellion may occur, and this is likely to be labelled as 'personality disorder' or 'behavioural'. In order to manage such problems successfully, it is important to view them as a function of the relationship between the individual and their environment (including other people), and not simply as a function of the personality disorder or 'naughtiness' of the individual.

Successful management of abnormal behaviour that is attributed to personality problems primarily requires patience. The problems must be examined carefully. If there is a residual partially treated depressive illness or other psychiatric illness, then this must be treated as effectively as possible. However, even where there is no comorbidity, or any coexisting disorder has been successfully treated, older people with behaviour problems attributed to personality disorder can often be helped. Some patients may need more time and support than can be offered in a busy modern psychiatric ward, and this is to be regretted. Trust often needs to be established over a period of time, not just with one individual but with several, and the day hospital can be a key setting for this. If problems with dependency are part of the picture, then care must be taken to avoid over-dependency on one individual staff member, and to manage carefully any separations that must occur because of changes of personnel. Consistency between team members and informal caregivers is essential if maladaptive behaviour is to be unlearned. The meaning of the patient's behaviour should be understood and then, over time, they can be offered alternative, more appropriate ways of behaving. In some cases more formal individual or group psychotherapy may be indicated, but sadly it is rarely available to old people in the NHS.

Although there have been no systematic studies of community populations, the impression gained from clinical practice is that the outcome for patients with personality disorder in old age is often better than might be expected. This is probably because many of these patients have developed an ability to cope with life that has been unsettled by illness or other life events. A period of stable, empathetic but firm support can help them to rebuild earlier reasonably successful ways of coping with life's stresses and strains.

Management of substance misuse

The chief remedy for substance misuse is prevention. Doctors, nurses and others concerned with the prescription and administration of potentially addictive medication should be aware of the dangers and should avoid such prescriptions wherever possible, using more appropriate techniques to identify and manage problem behaviours. These will include environmental and social support activities, identification and psychological management of problem behaviours, and proper medical diagnosis so that agitation due to depression or constipation is treated appropriately according to the underlying cause and not with sedatives. If patients have developed long-term dependence on benzodiazepines, a very gradual reduction – usually on an outpatient basis with support from a day hospital and/or members of the community team – can be very successful. During such management it may become evident that an underlying depression or anxiety state for which the treatment was originally prescribed is still present, or symptoms of depression or anxiety may emerge for other reasons. For example, a bereavement reaction that was suppressed by the inappropriate use of benzodiazepines may need to be worked through. These emergent symptoms must be identified and treated appropriately using psychological and/or pharmacological measures as indicated.

A particular problem may arise in terminal care where increasing doses of opiates and other pain-relievers are sometimes used. Generally speaking this is not a problem in the genuinely terminal care situation, where any dependence is a small price to pay for the adequate control of symptoms. However, it does indicate the need for careful management of these conditions by physicians who are skilled in terminal care and who can make appropriate judgements, with the patient's consent, about the benefits and risks of such treatment.

In general, the longer a problem of substance abuse has been present, the more difficult it is to treat. Before recovery is achieved, it is vital to look at other factors, such as social support and activities that could reduce the risk of the behaviour recurring.

Management of alcohol abuse

Alcohol abuse is particularly difficult to treat if it is long-standing or if there are co-alcoholics from whom it is difficult to separate the patient. The extent of the possible medical complications of alcohol abuse means that a thorough physical examination combined with appropriate investigations is essential for managing this disorder. Although outpatient detoxification is generally the rule for younger patients, detoxification of elderly people may often best be conducted in hospital with ready access to assistance from specialist physicians. Alcohol withdrawal is usually carried out under cover of a decreasing dose of benzodiazepine medication. Attention to nutritional status (including parenteral thiamine if there is a risk of the Wernicke–Korsakov syndrome), together with an awareness of the possible emergence of medical complications (e.g. epileptic fits or perforated peptic ulcer), is essential. After this acute phase of management, psychological and social management takes over. This attempts to reduce the motivation to drink alcohol excessively, and to provide alternative social outlets to the pub, club or solitary drinking at home. Alcohol abuse, like personality disorder, demands *multidisciplinary management*, but here, as well as the usual psychiatric, nursing, social and psychological perspectives, it is essential to incorporate appropriate dietetic and specialist medical management. Alcohol-use disorders in younger patients are often treated by specialist services working in collaboration with mental health services. Older people may have difficulty accessing these services, and it is important to ensure either that they are well integrated with older people's mental health services, or that special services are provided that are accessible to older people. Disulfiram medication has sometimes been used, especially in younger patients, but unless administration is supervised, unmotivated patients may simply stop taking it. The risk of side-effects and complications means that it is probably not a treatment of first choice. Withdrawal is usually associated with increased glutamate activity. Drugs such as lamotrigine, memantine and acamprosate that block glutamate activity can reduce withdrawal symptoms when combined with other drugs such as benzodiazepines. Acamprosate should normally be given 1 week before commencing withdrawal, and continued for 2 weeks once withdrawal has started. However, despite the fact that it has been available for some time, a full randomised, placebo-controlled study has still not been undertaken.[27] Psychological approaches to treatment are also important, particularly motivational therapy.[28]

CONCLUSION

Personality disorders and alcohol and substance misuse demonstrate, perhaps more than any other area, the need for an holistic approach to problems in old age. Biological, psychological and social factors intertwine in complex patterns that positively demand a multidisciplinary approach to problem definition and management. Careful problem definition (including a medical and psychiatric diagnosis as well as psychological and environmental considerations) should produce a treatment plan that can be carried through using the resources of the multidisciplinary team. Persistence and re-definition of problems as management progresses are also essential if patients with these often difficult and complex problems are to be helped. Prevention is often better than cure, and in view of the iatrogenic nature of much drug dependence in old age, this should be possible with appropriate education of professionals.

REFERENCES

1   Kay DW, Beamish P and Roth M (1964) Old age mental disorders in Newcastle-upon-Tyne. Part I. A study of prevalence. *Br J Psychiatry.* **110:** 146–58.
2   Pilkonis PA and Frank E (1988) Personality pathology in recurrent depression: nature, prevalence and relationship to treatment response. *Am J Psychiatry.* **145:** 435–41.
3   Fogel BS and Westlake R (1990) Personality disorder diagnoses and age in inpatients with major depression. *J Clin Psychiatry.* **51:** 232–5.

4 Morse JQ and Lynch TR (2004) A preliminary investigation of self-reported personality disorders in late life: prevalence, predictors of depressive severity, and clinical correlates. *Aging Ment Health.* **8**: 307–15.

5 Peselow ED, Sanfilipo MP, Fieve RR and Gulbenkian G (1994) Personality traits during depression and after clinical recovery. *Br J Psychiatry.* **164**: 349–54.

6 Stevenson J, Meares R and Comerford A (2003) Diminished impulsivity in older patients with borderline personality disorders. *Am J Psychiatry.* **60**: 165–6.

7 Trappler B and Backfield J (2001) Clinical characteristics of older psychiatric inpatients with borderline personality disorder. *Psychiatr Q.* **72**: 29–40.

8 Dian L, Cummings JL, Petry S and Hill MA (1990) Personality alterations in multi-infarct dementia. *Psychosomatics.* **31**: 415–19.

9 Petry S, Cummings JL, Hill MA and Shapira J (1989) Personality alterations in dementia of the Alzheimer type: a three-year follow-up study. *J Geriatr Psychiatry Neurol.* **2**: 203–7.

10 Burns A (1992) Psychiatric phenomena in dementia of the Alzheimer type. *Int Psychogeriatrics.* **4 (Suppl. 1)**: 43–54.

11 Vestal RE, McGuire EA, Tobin JD, Andres R, Norris AH and Mezey R (1977) Aging and ethanol metabolism in man. *Clin Pharmacol Ther.* **3**: 343–54.

12 Edwards G, Hawker A, Hensman C, Peto J and Williamson V (1973) Alcoholics known or unknown to agencies: epidemiological studies in a London suburb. *Br J Psychiatry.* **123**: 169–83.

13 Cook PJ, Flanagan R and James IM (1984) Diazepam tolerance: effect of age, regular sedation and alcohol. *BMJ.* **289**: 351–3.

14 Seymour J and Wattis JP (1992) Alcohol abuse in old age. *Rev Clin Gerontol.* **2**: 141–50.

15 Rapp SR, Parisi SA and Wallace CE (1991) Comorbid psychiatric disorders in elderly medical patients: a 1-year prospective study. *J Am Geriatr Soc.* **39**: 124–31.

16 Edwards G and Gross MM (1976) Alcohol dependence: provisional description of a clinical syndrome. *BMJ.* **1**: 1058–61.

17 Wattis J (1998) Personality disorders and alcohol dependence. In: R Butler and B Pitt (eds) *Seminars in Old Age Psychiatry.* Gaskell, London. Available free online via www. rcpsych.ac.uk.

18 Casey DA and Schrodt CJ (1989) Axis II diagnoses in geriatric inpatients. *J Geriatr Psychiatry Neurol.* **2**: 87–8.

19 Buzzola FG, Gorelick PB and Freels S (1992) Personality changes in Alzheimer's disease. *Arch Neurol.* **49**: 297–300.

20 Hirayamam K, Meguro K, Shimada M *et al* (2003) A case of probable dementia with Lewy bodies presenting with geographic mislocation and nurturing syndrome. *No To Shinkei.* **55**: 782–9.

21 Salazar-Fraile J, Tabares-Seisdedos R, Selva-Vera G *et al* (2004) Recall and recognition confabulation in psychotic and bipolar disorders: evidence for two different types without unitary mechanisms. *Compr Psychiatry.* **45**: 281–8.

22 Potter JF and James OWF (1987) Clinical features and prognosis of alcoholic liver disease in respect of advancing age. *Gerontology.* **33**: 380–7.

23 Mirza A, Mirza S, Mirza K, Babu V and Vithayathil E (1995) Morbid jealousy in alcoholism. *Br J Psychiatry.* **167**: 668–72.

24 Cooper JW (1994) Falls and fractures in nursing home patients receiving psychotropic drugs. *Int J Geriatr Psychiatry.* **9**: 975–80.

25 Jang KL, Livesley WJ and Vernon PA (1995) Alcohol and drug problems: a multivariate behavioural genetic analysis of comorbidity. *Addiction.* **90:** 1213–21.

26 McInnes E and Powell J (1994) Drug and alcohol referrals: are elderly substance abuse diagnoses and referrals being missed? *BMJ.* **308:** 444–6.

27 Lingford-Hughes AR, Welch S, Nutt DJ *et al* (2012) *BAP Updated Guidelines: Evidence-Based Guidelines for the Pharmacological Management of Substance Abuse, Harmful Use, Addiction and Comorbidity: Recommendations from BAP.* www.bap.org.uk (accessed 21 June 2012).

28 UKATT Research Team (2005) Effectiveness of treatment for alcohol problems: findings of the randomised UK alcohol treatment trial (UKATT). *BMJ.* **331:** 541.

9

The relationship between physical and mental health

'THIS DOOR SWINGS BOTH WAYS'

In old age, physical illness – particularly if it results in long-term disability – is associated with a higher than average prevalence of anxiety and depression. Of course, acute physical illness can also produce delirium. On the other hand, primary psychiatric and psychological disturbance may result in the patient complaining of physical symptoms. This commonly occurs in the context of a mental illness such as major depression, but may also arise as part of a group of disorders known as the *somatoform disorders* (F45), the most well known of which is probably *hypochondriasis* (F45.2). The complicated interactions between physical and psychiatric symptoms in old age are a great challenge. The traditional manoeuvre of separating body and mind (and not considering the spiritual dimension at all) does not work. Because of this complexity, older people are also unsuited to the kind of over-simplified 'production-line' approach typical of some aspects of modern medicine.

The account which follows will inevitably be over-simplified and may at times appear to support the dichotomising of mental and physical factors. However, we have to consider the whole person in their social and cultural context if behaviour, symptoms and illness are to be understood and managed properly. The spiritual dimension is more subjective and therefore difficult to address in a text such as this. Suffice it to say that religious belief and spiritual experience can be strong determinants of behaviour, and so must be respected and taken into account when assessing and developing management plans for these and other problems that face the mental health worker.

The human organism is a learning organism, and all illness can be viewed as the outcome of interactions between genetic endowment, learned patterns of response, current environment, biology and specific causative agents. For example, an older person may present with the following history.

➤ She is female *(genetic)*.
➤ She had a deprived and abusive childhood *(early learning)*.
➤ She divorced her abusive husband and lives alone *(environment)*.
➤ She tripped on a carpet edge *(environment)*.
➤ She fractured her neck of femur *(biology/genetic risk)*.
➤ She was admitted to hospital for an operation *(environment)*.
➤ She developed pneumonia *(environment/specific cause)*.
➤ She became delirious *(biology, environment)*.
➤ She feared that staff intended to harm her *(early learning)*.
➤ She refused all treatment *(environment/early learning/physical)*.

Often we will only go back one or two steps in the aetiological chain. A psychiatrist who is called to review such a patient might diagnose delirium secondary to pneumonia. However, optimum treatment will depend on nurses who are well enough trained and supported to win the patient's cooperation with treatment for the pneumonia and understand some of the reasons for her distrust. In the longer term it will also depend on making her home safe and perhaps helping her to develop a wider social network. Medically we would also wish to examine her mental state when she has recovered from the delirium for signs of dementia, paranoid illness or depression, and start any appropriate management. Table 9.1 summarises some of the important interactions to be considered.

An inspection of these different factors immediately exposes the problems inherent in any simple model of bio–psycho–social causation. For example, the impairment of function following a stroke can produce disabilities that are only translated into handicaps by the *failure* of an appropriate social response. Moreover, whether directly through biological mediators or indirectly through psychological and environmental mediators, stroke may be associated with depressed mood that renders the patient less accessible to rehabilitation. Should the depression be 'classified' as biological, psychological or environmental? The answer is probably all three, in terms of both causation and management. This is where the multifactorial model mentioned above is particularly useful,

Table 9.1 Biological, psychological and environmental interactions

Biological interactions	*Psychological interactions*	*Environmental interactions*
Genetic predisposition	Psychodynamic factors	Interpersonal environment
Previous illness	Personality	Physical environment
Impairment	Impairment	Handicap
Current causes (e.g. infection)	Current causes (e.g. loss events)	Current causes (e.g. rapid transit into hospital)

for it reminds us again and again that when dealing with older patients (even more than when dealing with younger ones) we should pay attention to all three overlapping and interacting domains.

PHYSICAL SYMPTOMS, 'ILLNESS BEHAVIOUR' AND THE 'SICK ROLE'

Physical discomfort and symptoms are common. Nearly everyone who is reading this sentence will, after a moment's thought, be able to isolate some area of mild discomfort or pain in their own body. Three out of four people (of all ages) have symptoms in any given month which lead them to take action such as medicating themselves, resting in bed or visiting their GP. The pattern we expect is that a symptom will lead to an appropriate course of action.

Each of us will react to perceived illness in a variety of ways, depending on the following:

➤ the nature of the symptoms
➤ the immediate circumstances
➤ our attitudes and beliefs.

This behaviour is sometimes referred to as 'illness behaviour', and is characterised as taking on the 'sick role'. The behaviour and attitudes of others will also affect our reactions. The sick role has certain benefits and costs. For example, if we are ill, others might treat us with tea and sympathy, or take over household tasks. If we have a high temperature, we might retreat to bed, but if we have to sit an important examination, miss our own birthday party or lose wages, we may soldier on. We each weigh up the pros and cons of 'going sick'. Norms for illness behaviour and the sick role are based on cultural and social conventions, and are partially learned within the family. Some people behave in unusual ways that are thought by others to be abnormal. To outsiders, the behaviour may seem to be irrational, selfish or destructive. Individuals who are referred because of the problems that adopting the sick role causes both for themselves and for others present a complex set of problems. Those who want to help them need to understand the gains and losses for each individual at that particular time and in their particular circumstances. It may also be necessary to understand the gains and losses for others involved with the person who is taking on the sick role. The responses of others may be crucial for the maintenance or improvement of these difficulties. For example, one study of married chronic pain patients showed that a reduction of attention by the spouses to their pain behaviour resulted in significantly lower levels of reported pain.[1] The relationship between events, symptoms and behaviours may be hard to elucidate. Changing a long-standing pattern of behaviours and interactions may be extremely difficult.[2]

One of the most important aims of any treatment plan is to enable the patient to satisfy their needs in a way that is acceptable to themselves and others. For example, if the sick role is adopted because it is the only apparent means of gaining visits from the family, then such visits may need to be arranged under other conditions. If this is just not possible, then acceptable alternative sources of company and attention may need to be sought. Often it is difficulty in satisfying just this type of ordinary human need that leads to behaviours which are considered by others to be *manipulative*. Using the sick role to control others without facing arguments or the anxiety of asserting oneself is another possible motive. If such factors are important, then it may be possible to facilitate changes by encouraging the development of social skills, or through marital or family work.

Facilitating self-help behaviour is a common problem if there is little self-help behaviour to start with, and it is tempting for relatives who have only a limited amount of time to do household tasks. There is often a pressure to take over such tasks as a sign of caring. One common constellation of problems concerns the couple who find that they have difficulties in adjusting to retirement. When the wife becomes ill, the couple find a satisfactory resolution to their difficulties in the adoption of a pattern whereby she remains an invalid, while her husband takes over the running of the house. Finally, some relatives are upset to see the patient performing tasks slowly or inefficiently, and may find it difficult to stand back and do nothing.

People may view health problems in a variety of ways. One way of conceptualising this is to divide people into 'normalisers' ('stiff upper lip'), 'psychologisers' (who see everything as being 'in the mind') and 'somatisers' (who explain everything in physical terms). Old people probably somatise more than young ones – that is, they complain of a physical symptom rather than emotional distress. This may be generational, in that they have been less exposed to psychology. Old people are also probably more likely to be assumed to be hypochondriacal (sometimes when they have an undetected underlying physical illness). They are certainly more likely to be suffering from a number of physical symptoms than young people. There is therefore a need when working with the elderly to be familiar with the range of ways in which a complaint about a physical symptom can be understood and treated. In this chapter, we shall not only discuss the range of conditions, but will also focus on psychological models which have been used to explain or treat people suffering from fears of illness and other complaints.

Relationship problems and the social context

As people age, they may become more dependent on their environment and on the people around them. They may have to adapt to reduced income, impaired mobility (due to loss of both physical fitness and transport) and changes in their social and family networks. The importance of increased dependence on family members or caring neighbours should not be underestimated. Younger people are much more able to remove themselves from unsatisfactory or distressing relationships, or to find substitutes. The may also be in a position to exercise control over the terms of the relationship. Elderly people who are experiencing such distress in relationships may be unwilling or unable to remove themselves from the situation, and may be dependent in some important way on the relationships that they find difficult. For some, the dependence in itself may be distressing, particularly if the person has spent half a lifetime since childhood avoiding the experience.

Later in this chapter we shall consider the relationship between physical illness and disability and mental disorder, especially anxiety and depression. However, we shall first discuss the somatoform disorders, and the chapter will end with a general discussion of evidence-based management and some complicated 'real-life' cases.

DIAGNOSTIC CLASSIFICATION: HYPOCHONDRIASIS AND SOMATISATION

The *ICD-10*[3] classification outlines a number of disorders in which beliefs about physical symptoms or illness are features. These include depression (F33.0.01 and F33.1.11), which will be considered later in this chapter with regard to somatisation, and the somatoform disorders (F45), which include somatisation disorder (F45.0), undifferentiated somatoform disorder (F45.1), hypochondriasis (F45.2), somatoform autonomic dysfunction (F45.3), persistent somatoform pain disorder (F45.4), and others (F45.8). The existence of these terms and the range of competing diagnoses highlight the complexity of the relationship between the body, the mind and behaviour.

The somatoform disorders (F45)

The core feature of the group of somatoform disorders is repetitious presentation of physical symptoms, together with requests for medical investigations, in the face of repeated negative findings and reassurances by doctors that the symptoms have no physical basis. When physical illness is present, it is considered insufficient to explain the severity of distress and the extent of concern of the patient. Even if there are clear precipitating life events, the patient does not countenance a link between these and the presentation of physical complaints, although there may be clear symptoms of anxiety or depression. Difficulties in reaching a mutually acceptable understanding of the symptoms can lead to frustration for both doctor and patient. Histrionic behaviour is often a feature, when the patient becomes resentful of their failure to persuade doctors that their illness has a physical basis and requires further investigation.

Somatisation disorder (F45.0)

The main features of this disorder are multiple, recurrent and changing symptoms, usually present for several years before referral into a psychiatric service (over 2 years for a diagnosis). There may be a long history of fruitless investigations and treatments, resulting in a 'fat file'. Reassurance from several doctors has to be unsuccessful for this diagnosis to be made. Symptoms may be attributed to all body parts, but gastrointestinal and skin complaints are among the commonest. Somatisation disorder is associated with disruption of social, interpersonal and family behaviour. Anxiety, depression and secondary dependence on medication may be present and may have to be treated separately. Undifferentiated somatoform disorder (F45.1) is a less clearly defined category in which some of the characteristics of the above are absent.

Hypochondriacal disorders (F45.2)

Hypochondriasis is defined as a persistent preoccupation with the possibility of serious, progressive disease. Patients complain of physical symptoms or of their appearance. Commonplace or normal sensations are interpreted as distressing or abnormal, and there may be a focus on a particular area. The patient may name the disease that they fear. Anxiety and depression are commonly present, and the course of the complaints is chronic but fluctuating. Referral to psychiatric services is often resented, and associated disability is variable. The reassurance of several doctors has no effect. This diagnostic category excludes delusional disorders.

Hypochondriacal disorders are distinguished from somatisation disorders by clarifying the focus of the patient's concern. A somatising patient will ask for removal of the symptoms and comply well with drug treatment, at least for certain periods of time, whereas a hypochondriacal patient will be concerned with the underlying disease from which they feel they are suffering, and may mistrust medication despite making continued requests for investigation. Anxiety and panic disorders may have a similar presentation.

The somatoform disorders also include the following categories, from which old people are not immune.

Somatoform autonomic dysfunction (F45.3)

The patient presents with symptoms as if they are due to a physical disorder of a system or organ under autonomic control (i.e. cardiovascular, gastrointestinal or respiratory system disease). Relatively common types in old people include cardiac neurosis, psychogenic hyperventilation and bowel dysfunction. Two types of symptom are offered, namely those attributable to autonomic arousal (e.g. sweating, palpitations and tremor), and those that are more idiosyncratic, subjective or non-specific. These are referred to a particular organ. There may also be signs of stress. Again, repeated reassurance by doctors is unsuccessful, and no underlying physical disease is found.

Persistent somatoform pain disorder (F45.4)

In this disorder the patient complains of persistent, severe and distressing pain of a degree inexplicable by a physical or physiological process. There are links with current psychosocial problems or emotional conflict, and there is an increase in support or attention.

Other somatoform disorders (F45.8, F45.9)

These categories include symptoms such as disorders of skin sensation, globus hystericus and psychogenic pruritus, limited to a specific system and unrelated to tissue damage (F45.8), and other unspecified disorders (F45.9).

Other diagnostic categories that are relevant to this chapter include the following.

Neurasthenia (F48.0)

This category includes two major variations, namely fatigue after either mental or physical effort. There are often accompanying reports of dizziness, tension headaches and a sense of general instability, while concern about reduced health, irritability, anhedonia and low-level depression or anxiety are common. There may be changes in the duration (hypersomnia) or pattern (disturbance in the early and middle stages) of sleep. The same symptom pattern is found in *chronic fatigue syndrome*, a condition of unknown aetiology that sometimes seems to follow viral illness.

Psychological and behavioural factors associated with disorders or disease classified elsewhere (F54)

This category concerns the presence of psychological or behavioural influences that are thought to have played a significant part in the aetiology of a physical condition. In cases defined as falling within this category, the resulting mental disturbances are minor and do not warrant a diagnostic category in themselves. The physical illnesses commonly associated with this category include asthma, eczema and dermatitis, gastric ulcer, colitis and urticaria.

Finally, we have to consider the rare occurrence of hypochondriasis in psychotic illness, and the much more common occurrence of somatic complaints and hypochondriasis in depressed mood. The relationship between physical illness, disability and social isolation is complicated, and will be considered in more detail later in this chapter.

DEPRESSION AND PHYSICAL ILLNESS

Depressive symptoms are associated with an increased risk of subsequent decline in motor function in older people without overt illness.[4] There is also a general association between gait slowing, heart disease and chronic lung disease on the one hand, and self-reported depressive symptoms and poor life satisfaction on the other. In all conditions except heart disease, the effect appears to be mediated through disability.[5] Depression and depressive symptoms are also associated with poor prognosis in a variety of medical conditions. For medical inpatients, high depression scores on the Hospital Anxiety and Depression (HAD) scale were associated with mortality at 22 months.[6] Another study of outcome among depressed hospitalised patients with physical disability suggested that, nearly 1 year after discharge, depression and disability varied together.[7]

Cardiovascular disease

In community-dwelling older men, coronary heart disease, physical disability and widowhood or divorce have been found to be associated with depression, and in women there are associations between a history of clinical depression and physical disability and depression.[8] Depression was also associated with poorer health status on a variety of measures in primary care patients with heart failure.[9] Even the functional outcome of cardiac surgery may depend more on mood than on the number of arteries stenosed. A study of patients having elective cardiac catheterisation for coronary artery disease showed that, at the time of catheterisation, self-reported physical function differed not only according to the number of arteries stenosed, but also according to observer-rated baseline anxiety and depression quartiles. Deterioration in physical function at 1 year was associated with baseline anxiety or depression, but not with baseline artery status. Surgical or medical treatment appeared to neutralise the effect of coronary stenosis on physical function at 1 year, but not the negative effect of baseline anxiety or depression.[10] Depressed mood was also a predictor of the combined endpoint of transplant or death for outpatients with advanced heart failure.[11]

A study conducted 3 to 4 months after an ischaemic stroke found 'major depression' in over 25% of cases and 'minor depression' in a further 14%. Major depression with *no explanatory factor apart from stroke* was present in nearly 20% of cases. Dependency in daily life following stroke doubled the risk of depression. Previous episodes of depression were also associated with a markedly increased risk of post-stroke depression.[12] Another survey of stroke survivors living in private households used the HAD scale and found high levels (41% of cases) of HAD depression or anxiety and of severe or very severe disability (57%). Not surprisingly, there was a strong association between severe disability and anxiety, and between severe disability and depression. This study had some weaknesses, but it is of interest because the authors also looked at the impact of social contact and found that there was a strong association between social contact and *lower* prevalence of anxiety or depression.[13] Caregivers may also become anxious or depressed after a stroke has occurred in the person they care for. Survivors of stroke and their relatives were asked at 6 months to complete the General Health Questionnaire (GHQ), which is a measure of emotional distress, and the HAD. Over 50% of the carers were in the abnormal range on the GHQ. Caregivers were more likely to be depressed if the patients were severely dependent or emotionally distressed themselves.[14]

The results of intervention studies are not yet available, but the prima facie case for the detection and management of depressed mood in patients with ischaemic heart disease is clear. Old age and liaison psychiatrists should actively encourage and help physicians and surgeons to search for and treat depression in these patients. They are a highly suitable population from the point of view of screening, because the prevalence of depression is relatively high and there is likely to be considerable health gain from detection and treatment. Treatment with cardiac-friendly antidepressants such as the SSRIs (which incidentally may have a potentially useful ability to reduce platelet 'stickiness'), as well as appropriate psychological and social management, is clearly indicated. Treatment of depression in stroke with SSRIs or heterocyclic antidepressants has also been shown to be useful, although their use to *prevent* post-stroke depression has not been established.[15]

Cancer

Cardiovascular disorders are not the only physical illness where important associations are found between depressed mood, physical disease and outcome. After controlling for other known risk factors, depressed mood persisting over 6 years nearly doubled the risk of developing cancer. This risk was consistent across most types of cancer and was not confined to cigarette smokers.[16] There is also a possibility that depressed mood is associated with poorer outcome in patients with cancer, and it has been suggested that this may be mediated through the immune system.

Again, detection and treatment are important for improving the quality of life as well as for any potential benefit in terms of prognosis. In the terminal care setting, the relationship between patient and health professional is perhaps even more important than in other situations. Antidepressants can also help to transform a person who feels helpless and even suicidal into someone who feels more able to cope with the threat and process of dying.

Parkinson's disease

Depression is common in patients with Parkinson's disease. One study found 'major depression' in 16.5% of cases, and dysthymia and other forms of depression in over 25% of cases, not dissimilar overall to the rates found in stroke, but more or less reversed with regard to the proportions of 'major' and other depressions. Reduced abilities in activities of daily living correlated with the diagnosis of depressive disorder. They also correlated with high scores on the observer-rated Hamilton Depression Rating scale.[17] Diagnosis of depression in Parkinson's disease is not easy, since reduced facial expression and bradyphrenia in this disease may be mistaken for the facial appearance of depression and psychomotor retardation seen in depressive disorder. The choice of antidepressant is particularly difficult in patients with Parkinson's disease, because of side-effects and drug interactions. Tricyclics *may* be the drugs of choice, as their anticholinergic effects may be of some benefit in Parkinson's disease, but they may also increase the risk of confusion. SSRIs may also be useful, but some of them have (usually minor) extrapyramidal side-effects that *may* increase parkinsonian symptoms. Sertraline at higher doses has some dopamine reuptake-blocking activity. This is a theoretical reason for using this drug in depressed patients with Parkinson's disease. All antidepressants to a greater or lesser degree may provoke visual hallucinations in Parkinson's disease and may interact with drugs used for the treatment of the disease. This is not an argument for therapeutic nihilism, but for great caution in the use of antidepressant drugs in patients with this condition. This caution should be accompanied by a determination, once antidepressants have been started, to use an adequate dose for an adequate length of time (probably at least 6 weeks) before changing the preparation, unless side-effects or interactions are more disadvantageous to the patient than the prospect of improved mood.

DEPRESSION, DISABILITY AND SOCIAL ISOLATION

Depression is common in old people with a variety of disabling illnesses (and also in those caring for them). It is often associated with increased disability, and the causality may be in both directions. There are also hints of a protective effect against depression through social contacts. This takes us back to the now classic study by Murphy on the social origins of depression in old age.[18] She found an association between severe life events, major social difficulties, poor physical health and the onset of depression. Working-class subjects had a higher incidence of depression, and this was associated with both poorer health and greater social difficulties. Lack of a confiding relationship (associated with lifelong personality traits) increased vulnerability to depression. A more recent large-scale study failed to support some of these findings, but it clearly demonstrated a link between declining health, increasing disability and the onset of depression.[19] Further clarification of the relationship between impairment, disability, handicap, depression and social factors was provided by the 'Gospel Oak' series of studies in London. The prevalence of 'pervasive' depression in this relatively deprived area was 17%. Impairment, disability and particularly handicap were strongly associated with depression. Depression was *over 20 times more common* in the most handicapped quartile compared with the least handicapped one. Adjusting for handicap abolished or weakened most of the associations between depression and social support, income, older age, female gender and living alone.[20] Loneliness was itself also associated with depression.[21]

A follow-up study conducted 1 year later found that the 1-year onset rate for pervasive depression was 12% and the maintenance rate for those initially depressed was 63%. There was a high mortality rate among depressed people. Disablement, especially handicap, was the strongest predictor of onset of depression. Lack of contact with friends was a risk factor for onset of depression. For men, marriage was protective, but for women it was a risk factor. The maintenance of existing depression was predicted by low levels of social support and social participation, rather than by disablement.[22] These studies point to the important interactions between disability, handicap, social isolation and depressed mood. From them we can conclude that measures to reduce handicap and isolation are likely to be important in the management of depression in this context. Antidepressants should be combined with an active strategy to reduce isolation and handicap, perhaps through the use of day hospitals and centres and community therapy services. Evidence is also emerging that regular physical exercise may improve the prospects of recovery from depression.

THE GENERAL MANAGEMENT OF OLD PEOPLE WITH SOMATIC PREOCCUPATION

Step 1: recognise physical or psychiatric illness

The association between somatisation and hypochondriasis and treatable psychiatric or medical illness has been known for many years.[23] The first step in effective management is the identification and treatment of such illnesses. There is a danger of diagnosing 'hypochondriasis' and then discovering clear signs of physical illness that were originally missed because of the way in which the patient presented.

Many old people have one or more chronic illnesses. It is sometimes difficult to determine whether the existing disease may explain new symptoms. Some of the most common illnesses of old age (e.g. cardiovascular disease and arthritis) are not curable, and are protean in their manifestations. They may have profound secondary effects on general levels of fitness and other conditions. Patients may suffer from both physical disease and psychiatric pathology. In addition, they are likely to suffer from a larger number of symptoms related to

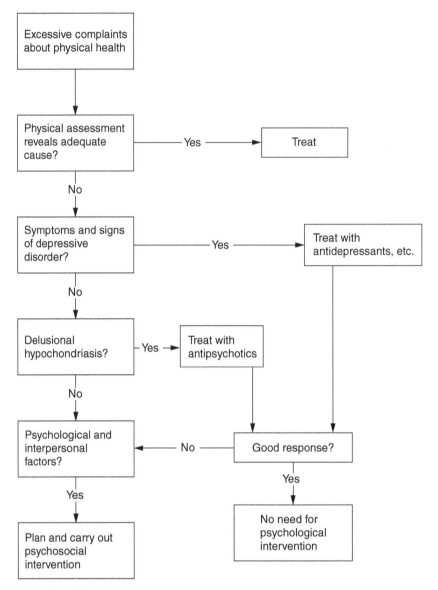

Figure 9.1 Simplified flow chart for deciding on treatment approach in a patient presenting with excessive health anxiety.

major or minor illnesses. Clinicians may become frustrated by their repeated demands, at worst leading to brusque or punitive treatment, or to refusal to investigate complaints, and occasional missed diagnoses. Hypochondriacs can get ill, too (*see* Case History 9.1)!

There is an established association between hypochondriasis and affective disorder. Many years ago, nearly two-thirds of 152 consecutive depressed patients who were admitted to a geriatric unit were found to have hypochondriacal symptoms.[24] The importance of identifying the elderly person who presents with hypochondriasis as part of a depressive illness cannot be over-emphasised. This is not just because there are effective treatments for depression, but also because of the high risk of suicide attempts (over a third in the study referred to above) in depressed elderly people who show hypochondriasis as the dominant symptom. Digestive symptoms, ranging from intense over-concern about constipation to delusions about the cessation of bowel movement and about head and facial pain, are the most frequent hypochondriacal symptoms associated with depression in the elderly.[24,25] Other preoccupations may concern cardiovascular, urinary and genital areas of the body. Complaints about skin and hair (e.g. that handfuls of hair are falling out) seem to occur mainly in women. The doctor needs to assess, through direct questioning, the patient's mood and mental state, looking for the presence of sleep disturbance, depressive thoughts, suicidal ideas, diurnal variation, and loss of energy and interest in life, family, work and hobbies (*see* Chapter 2). The recent, rapid onset of hypochondriacal symptoms in someone who has never previously had such symptoms should be regarded as a possible indicator of affective disorder. If an elderly person has shown lifelong hypochondriacal behaviour with a fondness for unnecessary medication, etc., a depressive episode may be signalled by a dramatic change in the intensity of their concern or in the nature and content of their worries.

Case History 9.1

A 67-year-old woman living with her brother was diagnosed as having pneumonia by one of the authors during a psychiatric home visit requested by the GP, who had assumed that her symptoms were part of her known hypochondriasis. Although there is a danger of reinforcing physical complaints by repeated examinations, the clinician always has to be prepared to consider the emergence of a new physical illness and take the necessary steps.

Step 2: recognise the basis for somatic preoccupation in older people

Although hypochondriasis is defined as severe anxiety about one's health, expressed as a fear of having or a belief that one has a physical illness, many other people may have health anxieties to a lesser extent. Many medical consultations (perhaps even the majority) are made by patients for whom the symptom alone does not fully explain the distress.[26] This may not seem surprising, as even minor illness may significantly disrupt a daily routine and cause a number of 'hassles' at precisely the time when they are most difficult to resolve. Old people often live with health anxieties of varying types and duration. Elderly people who are hypochondriacal sometimes show a degree and type of distressed behaviour which is not only difficult for friends and relatives, but also presents apparently insurmountable problems to the doctor and other professionals. There seem to be a number of related factors that arise during the process of ageing which might account for this.

As individuals age there will be an increasing build-up of minor physical lesions which can become the focus of the hypochondriacal complaint. Not only this, but they will have more direct experience of those close to them suffering serious or terminal illnesses. Such experiences can heighten anxiety both directly, by raising fears of death or helplessness, and indirectly, by increasing isolation from meaningful relationships and activities. If the general level of anxiety is raised, there is a danger that minor aches and pains can be perceived as more extreme or as serious illness. A minor physical lesion may be found at the site of the complaint, or the nature of the complaint may resemble the symptoms of a seriously ill or deceased friend or relative. Social isolation may be encouraging the patient to concentrate on somatic symptoms.

Step 3: psychological and social management

We distinguish here between a psychological approach, which is essential for all, and formal psychological therapy, which should be increasingly available to patients. However, the understanding which is required for an effective psychological approach comes largely from therapeutic work, so the two approaches will be described alongside each other. We also recognise the need for general measures. These include exercise, good nutrition and improving social networks where old people are isolated or dependent on medical contacts for meaning in their lives.

A person's beliefs influence their behaviour, and vice versa. Looking at this interrelationship and its consequences for a person's emotional state forms the basis of cognitive behavioural therapy, the use of which has been expanded into a number of areas, including the treatment of health anxiety and the psychological aspects of illness.[27,28] For treatment purposes, Salkovskis has defined the following three categories of somatic disorders:

1 those people whose presentations include observable and identifiable disturbances of bodily functioning (e.g. irritable bowel, sleep disorder)
2 those for whom the disturbance can be viewed as perceptual, with sensitivity or excessive reaction to normal bodily sensation (e.g. hypochondriasis, somatisation disorder)
3 a mixed group, which includes headache, breathlessness, pain and cardiac neurosis.

When considering a psychological intervention, it is important to estimate the extent to which health anxiety is a major part of the problem. Beliefs about health may have an effect on the patient's understanding of the appropriate treatment and on their compliance with treatment, so the degree of success in dealing with anxieties about health may influence further interventions.

Salkovskis has also listed the factors that maintain health anxieties. These are outlined in Box 9.1. Health anxiety can interact with symptoms. For example, raised anxiety can heighten the experience of pain. When the experience of pain also induces anxiety, a 'vicious circle' of pain increasing anxiety, and anxiety increasing pain, may result. Some people interpret the effects of physiological arousal as symptoms of illness. Figure 9.2 shows a simplified model of this interaction. Thus it can be seen that reducing anxiety directly or indirectly will break this vicious circle and reduce the experience of physical symptoms, which should in turn lead to an abatement of the hypochondriacal complaints. For a more comprehensive approach to psychological strategies for pain, the reader is referred elsewhere.[29]

Box 9.1   Factors that maintain health anxieties

1   Increased physiological arousal, which has effects such as palpitations, sweating or gastrointestinal disturbance.
2   The patient's focus of attention alters so that normal variations in bodily function are seen as new and symptomatic; this may lead to changes in physiological functioning.
3   Avoidance behaviours occur to minimise physical discomfort and to prevent dangerous illness (e.g. avoiding activity in order to prevent a heart attack).
4   Misinterpretations of symptoms, signs and medical communications consistent with the patient's existing beliefs about their condition, which hinder them from accepting reassurance.

Various factors may contribute to the elderly individual's health anxiety (*see* Figure 9.3). These factors must be identified and their relative importance evaluated. Information can be obtained from interviews with the elderly patient, and perhaps also with involved family members or carers. If the patient is reluctant or apparently unable to give much detail about their circumstances, a great deal of information can sometimes be collected by the detailed review of an average day, from waking up in the morning to going to bed at night. Noticing the effects of the symptoms on this average day can provide information about what might be causing anxiety, how the patient copes with their symptoms, and what types of social contacts and interests

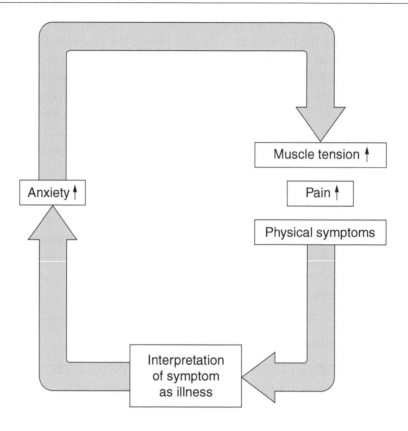

Figure 9.2 Simplified model of hypochondriasis, illustrating the role of anxiety.

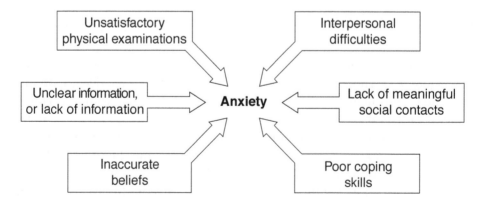

Figure 9.3 Factors that exacerbate anxiety in the elderly person who shows hypochondriasis.

they have. In addition to relaxation procedures, there are techniques such as biofeedback which enable the patient to gain some control over physiological functioning through immediate feedback.

The acceptability of any psychological understanding or technique is of paramount importance. Most techniques require repeated practice. Progressive muscle relaxation is widely used to induce general relaxation. The procedure for this involves learning to discriminate more accurately between tense and relaxed muscles, and increasing control over the relaxation of key muscles. As with all skills, it is more difficult to acquire when someone is in an acute state of anxiety, but it may be useful with old people who have specific or less severe anxiety. An alternative method of relaxation which some elderly people find easier to use involves autogenic imagery. In this approach, a pleasant image (e.g. lying on a beach on a warm summer's day) is brought vividly to mind, producing a feeling of calm. Pre-recorded cassettes or CDs may have some use, but are not a substitute for a personal programme. In all cases, clear explanation, training in self-monitoring and a supportive, gradual approach will aid the development of relaxation skills. Breathing problems are common in old people, and some of these cases are psychogenic, such as hyperventilation. The latter is characterised by shallow, thoracic, rapid breathing, and has been shown to generate unpleasant physiological symptoms within the space of a few minutes.[30] These are often related to anxiety-laden or meaningful events or thoughts. One way of treating hyperventilation is to facilitate relearning of a normal breathing pattern. This involves learning to slow the speed of breathing and use the diaphragm rather than the upper chest. Some people find other techniques (e.g. meditation, yoga, tai chi) useful. These may also effect a general improvement in health because they are forms of regular exercise.

Psychological assessment is often made more difficult because the patient believes that they have a physical illness, and does not welcome the thought of a psychological or psychiatric assessment. The patient's ideas about the assessment itself are important. For example, they may believe that the referral has been made because they have been a nuisance with their complaints, or because the doctor thinks that their complaints are fictitious. In this case, it may be helpful to explain that there are a number of physical illnesses for which psychological approaches can be helpful by, for example, reducing stress and helping the person to cope better with their illness. At the start we seek the patient's views of their condition and present with an open mind as to the nature of the problem and the appropriate treatment, offering the assessment as an assurance that all possible options are being explored. This may allow important information to emerge, including antecedents to the symptoms, such as external events, thoughts or behaviours. With regard to their behaviour when the symptoms are present or becoming worse, patients are asked about their thoughts (including mental images and predictions) and their actions (including withdrawing from social situations, going to bed, telephoning someone for reassurance or help, or watching television to distract themselves). Discussing beliefs about illness in general and about doctors can be useful. Some people also have strategies for protecting themselves by avoiding something (e.g. refusing to go out of the house in cold weather). This may, of course, be totally reasonable, for example in someone with chronic obstructive airways disease or Raynaud's phenomenon.

Patients can be asked to monitor or keep records of their symptoms, the preceding events or thoughts, and the subsequent actions or events, together with their effects. This can provide valuable information about the nature of the problem, which can then be used when designing and implementing treatments. It also provides a record of the degree of symptomatology, so that changes over time can be monitored. Psychological interviews such as this differ from diagnostic interviews because they do not aim for a psychiatric diagnosis, but rather their objective is to achieve a psychological formulation which includes the patient's beliefs and behaviours and their effects.

Although a psychological approach can help in the general management of these disorders, formal psychological treatment can only proceed if it is acceptable to the patient. A great deal of skill is required to make a formulation of the problem and to define treatment goals that satisfy both a psychologically minded therapist and an illness-minded patient. This may mean accepting the reality of the patient's experience, but asking them to try out something new for a limited period. If the approach does not help them after a time, then they are free to go back to their old strategies. In the initial contract, it is explained that the therapist will help the patient to look for and test out alternative reasons for their symptoms, and that medical checks and lengthy discussions of the symptoms will not be part of the treatment (*see* Case History 9.2).

With any patient, change is more likely to occur if there is a therapeutic relationship, in which the patient feels that the professional respects his or her point of view. The patient will probably already have experienced various approaches, including the following:

➤ reassurance ('It's nothing to worry about')
➤ reasoned arguments about the non-physical nature of the symptoms
➤ doubts expressed about the reality of the symptoms ('It's all in your mind')
➤ invalidation of their experience ('People with your illness don't get that').

Falling into one of these traps is not likely to help the patient, nor will telling them that in your view it is a relationship problem, even if you are right! The therapist should only give relevant information in a considered way. It is essential to check that the patient has understood it in the way that the therapist thought they had expressed it. Rather than reassuring the patient that the symptom is not physical, the therapist can collaborate with them in trying to determine what might be happening. Finding out the patient's beliefs and working out ways of testing these with the patient may be a key task. Taking the opportunities presented within sessions, such as the appearance of symptoms in moments of anxiety (perhaps over being late), can be extremely useful for exploring with the patient the role of thoughts, beliefs and anxiety.

Case History 9.2

Mrs ID was a 69-year-old woman who presented with abdominal pains which she was convinced indicated that she had cancer. A depressive hypochondriasis was diagnosed and she showed a dramatic response to antidepressant treatment. Despite this, she stopped taking the treatment and relapsed. Psychological assessment demonstrated some erroneous health beliefs. Despite the GP checking her weight regularly, she was convinced that she was losing weight and that this indicated a serious illness. When she discovered the therapist was interested in finding out what was really happening, she readily agreed to a 'reality test'. She monitored her own weight and brought in the results at each session for the therapist to record. She was told that she always needed to use the same weighing-machine and wear similar clothing, and to expect a 2-pound fluctuation because of varying fluid balance. Within 3 or 4 weeks she agreed that she was not losing weight, and she was able to explore how this unrealistic belief and others like it (e.g. concerning her medication) were adversely affecting her life. Eventually, by becoming more socially active, she developed a close relationship with a man and was helped through her anxiety about becoming sexually active again for the first time since the death of her second husband. There were no further problems with medication compliance.

There are several possible approaches to intervention with patients who complain of physical symptoms for which no organic diagnosis can be made. Apart from medication changes, relaxation and adopting a more healthy lifestyle, it is possible to help the patient to clarify and change their beliefs about their health and the feared outcome. This involves finding out how they acquired these beliefs and then helping them to construct alternative explanations for their observations. For example, a patient may believe that their headache presages a stroke, rather than noticing that it occurs at times of increased tension (e.g. around the time of an extended visit from their much-loved but rowdy grandchildren). It may be necessary to discuss the beliefs which have led them to alter their lifestyle in an attempt to protect themselves or to reduce their symptoms by adopting behaviour such as the following:

➤ spending time in bed with a headache
➤ staying as immobile as possible in order to reduce joint pain.

These 'strategies' may then lead to disabling restrictions to their lifestyle, or to exacerbation of their conditions or their worries. Readers will recognise this approach as the core of such formal therapies as cognitive behavioural therapy. A controlled trial randomised patients with hypochondriasis to three treatment conditions, namely cognitive therapy, behavioural stress management (both 12 sessions) or waiting list. Both active therapies were better than waiting list in improving general mood disturbance, while cognitive therapy appeared to be superior in reducing hypochondriacal complaints.[31] Another trial of 'pure' cognitive and 'pure' behavioural therapy against a 'control period' found them to be equally effective in reducing hypochondriasis.[32] A trial of cognitive behavioural therapy (CBT) versus waiting list in 32 patients over 16 sessions appeared to indicate the usefulness of CBT in this group.

Repeated investigations or visits to the doctor may bring short-term relief, but patients may then ruminate about the reassurance given or the proposed investigation and find something that makes them even more anxious. Whatever the mechanism, the search for reassurance may become protracted. People sometimes suggest that doctors and relatives refuse to offer reassurance. This can be difficult to implement, and it only seems to work if the patient can accept the aims of the strategy.

Social interventions (e.g. arranging 'day care' to reduce isolation), like medical interventions, work best if there is an established, shared understanding with the patient about the nature of the problem, otherwise the patient may dismiss them as irrelevant to what they understand to be the main issue. A critical review of intervention studies for a heterogeneous selection of patients with somatoform disorder[33] concluded that CBT, antidepressants and other non-specific interventions were the most effective approaches.

Step 4: bringing it all together for the benefit of the patient

Barsky[34] has described the following two-stage approach to the hypochondriacal patient:

1 a strategy for medical management
2 a specific (cognitive behavioural) psychotherapeutic approach.

Initial physical examination should be thorough, and it should appear to be thorough to the patient. The clinician needs to recognise that the patient has valid psychological and interpersonal reasons for developing symptoms and seeking medical attention. The clinician should seek a common understanding with the patient of their symptoms, and should not be drawn into arguments about their reality or physical basis. The goal ceases to be to 'cure' the patient's symptoms, and shifts to assisting them in understanding and learning to cope with the symptoms.

Barsky's particular approach to psychotherapy involves group discussions in which cognitive and behavioural exercises are used to teach patients to moderate the following factors that amplify somatic distress and hypochondriacal concerns:

➤ concentration on symptoms
➤ cognitions about symptoms
➤ context of symptoms
➤ mood.

Group exercises can help patients to understand that a certain amount of physical discomfort is normal and does not necessarily signify underlying disease. This approach can be adapted to work with an individual. It is important to explore patients' cognitions about symptoms and disease. These may be very unrealistic (e.g. the 'folk belief' that the third stroke is always fatal). Patients can be helped to understand their symptoms in the context of long-standing physical illnesses or disabilities and social stresses. Information must be kept simple and written down if possible. The use of technical terms should be avoided. Elderly patients may have minor discomfort with impressive labels (e.g. sinusitis or gastritis). These may be misunderstood as being the reason for their hypochondriacal complaints, and their possible implications should be simply explained and clarified. One common area of misunderstanding by staff is the hypochondriacal patient's experience of pain. Patients may still be told that they are 'imagining' the pain because there is no physical lesion, or that the pain is psychological. In fact, pain is a subjective experience and should be accepted as being real for the patient who reports it.

Even when symptoms are part of a *depressive illness*, a psychological approach facilitates the patient's trust and confidence, which will improve compliance with any necessary pharmacological treatment. Many depressed patients with predominant hypochondriasis show particularly poor compliance with physical psychiatric treatments, perhaps because they believe that they are not being treated appropriately. A clear and coordinated management plan is of paramount importance in these cases. At its core should be a consistent response by the psychiatric team, in order to make the acceptance of necessary physical treatment for depression more rather than less likely. Since the GP may receive the bulk of the hypochondriacal complaints, he or she must be fully involved in the psychiatric team's management plan. A pattern of repeated admission and discharge during which the patient never complies adequately with any treatment offered should be resisted. Admission should normally only take place with the agreement of the patient to a clear contract to accept a particular treatment, not because, for example, their partner can no longer cope with the patient's complaints. Case History 9.3 illustrates how difficult the treatment of such a patient can be. A number of approaches were tried, none of which alone proved to be sufficient.

PHARMACOLOGICAL MANAGEMENT

A number of approaches exist for the treatment of patients with health anxieties. Antidepressants are clearly indicated where somatic symptoms are due to or exacerbated by depressive disorder. Many of them also reduce anxiety and may help in cases where anxiety levels are high, even in the absence of serious depression. If an antidepressant is indicated, the choice may depend as much on side-effects as on any other factor (*see* Chapter 5). Good, empathic relationships with patients are essential for helping them to appreciate the need for treatment, and a careful explanation of the physical nature of anxiety and depression may help them to accept that their complaints are not simply being 'dismissed' as 'all in the mind'. Giving medication may in itself lead the patient to worry that there is an underlying serious disease. After all, something has to warrant tablets. The reduction or removal of some long-standing prescriptions can have beneficial effects. Notable in this respect are sleeping medications (hypnotics), which can adversely affect the quality and duration of sleep, and laxatives, which obviously affect bowel function and lead to abdominal pain. The effect of taking such medications over a long period is not limited to side-effects. Without education about the rationale for a sleeping tablet, for example, patients may believe that a full night's sleep is an essential requirement for health. They may continue to be intolerant of reductions in sleep, even over a short period, leading to worries about the problem, demands for an increase or change of prescription, or other strategies which lead to further perceived problems, such as catnapping to make up for 'lost' sleep. Catnapping is one example of a range of lifestyle factors which may affect bodily functioning. These include dietary intake (e.g. fibre affects bowel function, and caffeine affects levels of arousal – the latter effect may increase with age). Exercise has a number of beneficial effects both on general well-being and on bowel function and sleep. Alcohol, nicotine and other drugs can have a number of adverse effects. It may be possible to alter some symptoms significantly by changing these factors.

Case History 9.3

Mrs FV was a 67-year-old married woman who was taken over by our team 1 month after being discharged from a psychiatric ward where incomplete treatment with antidepressants, one application of ECT and attempts at marital therapy had failed. She had a 3-year history of physical complaints apparently precipitated by having her ears pierced, and previous physical investigations included a nose biopsy. Interestingly, her main presenting symptom was of pain in her nose, but other symptoms included ear and mouth pain, chest pain, swollen ankles, athlete's foot and worries about her diabetes, for which she received a daily injection from a district nurse. It was 'catch-22' for the staff involved. On the one hand, Mrs FV demanded help for her physical condition, yet every treatment attempt, whether it was antidepressant medication, painkillers or soothing eardrops, resulted in an apparent exacerbation of her symptoms, possibly because of hypersensitivity to small changes in her bodily state, and then non-compliance. Two admissions ensued, both of which were characterised by lack of compliance, and after her discharge from the second admission the team agreed to resist further admissions until she consented to a full course of ECT. Eventually she agreed and there was a gradual and ultimately marked change in her condition over 11 sessions of ECT. Her complaints diminished, although she still reported some ear and mouth pain, and her level of interest and activity greatly increased. After the sixth session of ECT, marital work was again instituted with the aim of preparing Mr and Mrs FV for a resumption of normal life, as Mr FV had taken over most of his wife's tasks in the home. Ways in which they could both express their affection more directly to each other were also explored, and nursing staff encouraged Mrs FV to be more independent with regard to her physical health by teaching her to self-administer her insulin. Mr and Mrs FV did not wish to attend regularly for marital work after her discharge, but Mrs FV had maintained her improvement at 2-month follow-up. A year later she relapsed following a physical illness, but she readily agreed to come into hospital for a course of ECT and maintenance antidepressants, to which she responded rapidly and completely. Independence and self-respect should be encouraged. In this case, the progression from dependence on a district nurse for her insulin injection to self-administration of her insulin and monitoring of her urine sugar level were important both for Mrs FV's self-esteem and to reduce unnecessary health services input.

SOME MORE 'WORKED EXAMPLES'

The very complexity of managing an elderly patient with physical complaints that are unrelated or only partly related to physical pathology limits our capacity to write in general terms. For this reason we have used a number of case studies to illustrate the need for a wide understanding of these problems and possible solutions. Case History 9.4 illustrates the importance of recognising and managing incompletely resolved bereavement reactions.

Case History 9.4

Mr GM was a sprightly widower in his seventies who was referred for assessment following repeated presentations to his doctor for physical complaints, mainly chest pain and breathing difficulties. After numerous investigations and an operation for a condition he had not noticed but which had been found on examination, he still complained, saying that he was worse than ever. Taking a history revealed that his symptoms had started while his wife was ill, and had improved at times since her death 12 years previously, but had worsened since he had withdrawn from some of the social activities into which he had thrown himself. He had been taught relaxation exercises and breathing exercises, which brought a short-term improvement, probably related to the social aspects, attention and interest. Antidepressant medication was not indicated. Anxieties about his future and loneliness were important factors in his situation. He was offered counselling sessions in which the aim was explicitly to help him to understand and cope with his life situation. For some time he insisted on a medical view of his problems, and he repeatedly sought further investigations, but eventually he began to acknowledge the improvement that the sessions brought him. This led to him being prepared to consider the emotional aspects of his experience, and he talked of his anxieties about being ill, dependent and isolated. For some time he was depressed as he regretted the loss of his wife and not finding another partner. His physical complaints became less important to him, and he began to use health services more appropriately.

In Case History 9.5, a physical illness was combined with health anxiety in a man who found it difficult to tolerate illness and dependency, leading to increased demands for care from his wife. On the other hand, an old person who suffers from a poor social network, a very low level of perceived emotional contact with important family members, or dissatisfaction with the quality of those interactions, can find that the sick role brings with it a sudden and dramatic increase in time, concern and interest from others. Becoming 'well' again can mean a return to the previous unwanted situation. In a few instances, visits from family members can be contingent only upon 'real' physical illness, as the family do not believe in anxiety or depression, nor do they accept any role in the development or maintenance of distressing relationships.

Case History 9.5

Mr NK had always been the dominant partner in his marriage, and made the decisions about household routine, holidays and interior decoration. His wife was rather timid and had looked up to and depended on her husband for many years, to the extent that she rarely left the house without him. After his stroke, the couple had to change their routines. The balance of power within the relationship also had to change, with responsibility for money and dealing with outside agencies falling on Mrs NK. This led to anxiety and resentment on her part, while Mr NK hated the position in which he found himself, and began to accuse her of taking money and deceiving him. Moreover, he refused to dress himself and frequently became distressed by thoughts of his condition and his future death. On referral, work with the couple proved difficult, but after a physical assessment the team members focused on attempts to help Mr NK to understand the nature of his condition, with help from an occupational therapist for assessment and aids. One team member saw Mrs NK to provide support and encouragement for her attempts to develop her skills and an independent life, and to help her to relate to her husband in a less critical way, but without falling in with his demands. Mr NK never accepted his condition with equanimity, but the couple managed to continue to live together.

In Case History 9.6, Mrs OD was able to use the input she was given, but in other cases the whole family may have to be involved in any intervention. A similar phenomenon may occur when a professional becomes involved. For example, one community nurse asked for help when a patient became worse every time he mentioned discharge. Eventually he agreed to a prolonged contract with his patient, but reduced the frequency of sessions over time, so that the patient felt less need to ensure that his visits continued by complaining of symptoms. The patient also eventually improved in this respect with a change in her life circumstances. In some instances, being ill may seem to be the only acceptable way to retain a dependent relationship. Case History 9.7 demonstrates that entrenched patterns of behaviour sometimes overcome attempts to help, even when the underlying issues are recognised and an attempt is made to resolve them.

The analysis of problems and the planned interventions in Case History 9.8 are summarised in Table 9.2.

Case History 9.6

Mrs OD, a 71-year-old widow, was referred some months after a heart attack, at the instigation of her son. Her GP had known her for many years and felt she had used illness as a means of controlling her family in the past. Mrs OD described herself as independent, and said that she did not want to be a burden on her children. At the time of her heart attack, the family had rallied round, each of her three children visiting and contributing to her convalescence. When they attempted to go back to the normal routine, of weekly visits in one instance and less frequent calls from the other two children, both of whom lived some distance away, Mrs OD began to complain of dizziness and breathlessness. She said that she was frightened that she would have another heart attack. These episodes occurred several times towards the end of visits, but also at other times, such as in the middle of the night and on Sunday evenings. Reassurance from her doctor and the specialist did not help. On assessment, there was little reason to suspect that Mrs OD had any physical disability to explain her difficulties. However, she was adamant that she could not undertake a range of activities, such as some household tasks and also socialising at the community centre in the sheltered housing where she lived, because she was afraid that her symptoms would start. She was asked by the psychologist to keep a diary of her symptoms, and when they talked about their appearance, Mrs OD could see how the symptoms coincided with events she found stressful or upsetting. The psychologist talked further with her about the nature of anxiety and how its effects could be interpreted as similar to the earlier physical symptoms. It was clear that the symptoms were serving to keep Mrs OD's children involved. After some time it became possible to discuss with her the cost of having her children under duress, along with the possible benefits of alternatives – mainly reinstating her friendships with her neighbours and the other residents in her complex. A graded series of exercises was agreed to allow Mrs OD to venture outside her home without too much initial anxiety, and once she was out her neighbours welcomed her back. She stopped calling her children at night, she made a good friend of a new resident, and her 'attacks' became less important as she began to enjoy her life again.

Case History 9.7

Mrs BF was referred to the team at 69 years of age, 3 years after the death of her husband, suffering from depression and complaining that she was so ill that she could not look after herself. The event immediately prior to and precipitating referral was the diagnosis of heart disease in her sister. Mrs WY, her much younger sister aged 52 years, lived nearby, and in addition to bringing up her teenage family, running a household and working part-time, she had cleaned Mrs BF's house, done her shopping and washed her laundry. The diagnosis had led to Mrs WY deciding that she had to reduce the number of unnecessary responsibilities and to look after herself better. Mrs BF had responded to the suggestion that she might take back some of her household tasks with increased demands and she became upset. On investigation, there seemed to be no medical reason why Mrs BF should not be completely independent. However, a history taken from herself and her sister suggested that Mrs BF had always been 'delicate' and had been 'spoiled' by her husband, who had done a great deal of the housework himself. For her part, Mrs BF had enjoyed working in their shop, but had never forgiven him for being retired and having to move them to another house. In a meeting arranged with two team members present to attempt to resolve the situation between the two sisters, Mrs WY asserted her independence. Mrs BF was offered both home help and assistance in developing independent living skills. She accepted these reluctantly, but very soon afterwards decided to enter a private residential home, where she enjoyed the company and the attention.

SERVICE CONSIDERATIONS

Communication and education

Our health services were set up with discrete physical illness in mind, and they strongly reinforce the presentation of complaints of physical symptoms. Medical staff time and interventions are only offered on presentation of symptoms. Both patients and medical staff wish for and are happiest with a clear diagnosis of an easily treatable physical illness. The patient may be punitive towards the doctor who dares to suggest an alternative, psychological rationale. Conversely, the doctor may become punitive towards a patient who is 'wasting time' with somatic complaints for which no adequate physical explanation can be found. These are sometimes referred to by the acronym 'MUS' (medically unexplained symptoms). Given that some patients may present with different complaints over the years, it is difficult to know when there is sufficient evidence of a strong psychological component. Yet there are patients who have undergone several serious and costly investigations and treatments that were unnecessary and even harmful, because they were determined that the cause of their distress was physical disease. The earlier identification of such patients by those working both in psychiatry and in general medicine could lead to better treatment.

Case History 9.8

Mrs CF was a 77-year-old divorced woman living on her own who was visited three or four times a week by her caring stepdaughter. Mrs CF's husband, who had left her a number of years previously because of her illness behaviour, lived nearby and had developed dementia. Mrs CF had a long history of taking to her bed as a means of coping, and indeed during her marriage a housekeeper had been employed because of her failure to take on this role. The community nurse asked the clinical psychologist to become involved because of the difficulty she was experiencing in being able to help. Because of the resentment shown by Mrs CF towards the community nurse and the psychiatrist, and the high level of care and involvement shown by her stepdaughter, it was decided that it might be more constructive and effective to decide on a treatment plan which the stepdaughter could implement. She had already developed a planned week which involved sharing her time between her stepmother, her father, her own family and a part-time job! She was particularly concerned about what she regarded as the wasted life that her stepmother was leading and how her preoccupation with her physical state had driven away most of her remaining social contacts. The stepdaughter was extremely pleased to have a specific plan to work from, as she felt that she never knew how best to cope with her stepmother's behaviour. The main points of the plan are presented in Table 9.2, and involved her redistributing her time and care so as to reinforce more appropriate aspects of her stepmother's behaviour. A further aim was to reduce the antagonism which the stepmother's behaviour generated in the stepdaughter. Thus the latter was given verbal strategies which allowed her to state clearly her care for her stepmother, even in the most annoying situations, such as a middle-of-the-night call-out, without reinforcing these aspects of her stepmother's behaviour. Over a 6-week period, on a 10-point rating scale (where 10 represented the worst illness behaviour and 0 represented acceptable illness behaviour) the stepdaughter's average rating per week changed from 7.5 to 5.0, indicating a definite improvement. This was further confirmed by a visit 2 months later by the psychiatrist, who found Mrs CF's mental state 'much improved'. This improvement continued through to follow-up 9 months later, even though the stepdaughter had to reduce the amount of time spent with her stepmother, because of her father's increasing confusion and disability. It is interesting that behavioural change took place more slowly than the change in Mrs CF's verbal behaviour. Thus the stepdaughter noticed her stepmother talking less about her physical state and being aware of and stopping herself in midstream of physical complaints, saying to her stepdaughter, for example, 'But you don't want to hear about that, do you?', prior to her taking up various household tasks again.

Table 9.2 Mrs CF's problems and treatment approach

Problem	Solution
Resents visit by psychiatrist/psychologist	Intervene through caring stepdaughter
Constant talk about physical state	Reduce time and input associated with this
Little normal conversation	Time and interest increased when this is produced
Infrequent self-care and housework	Increase encouragement or reinforcement for attempts/activity
Lack of insight about/constant talk of physical symptoms	When complaints rise above a certain level, stepdaughter leaves, after explaining why
Suicidal/severe illness	Stepdaughter visits, but limits her stay to 1 minute
Behaviour (e.g. phone calls at 2.00 a.m. complaining of 'heart attack')	If there is no evidence of illness, set clear agreed limits

The Royal College of Psychiatrists in collaboration with the Royal College of Nursing, the British Geriatrics Society and the Alzheimer's Society has published guidelines for the development of liaison mental health services for older people.[35] Prevalence rates for somatoform disorders decrease with increasing age, with a prevalence rate of 1.5–13% in people aged 65 years or older, but recognition and diagnosis may be more difficult compared with that in younger people.[36] These factors need to be taken into consideration when planning services.

Physical illness and the way in which the services react may be an important factor in distress. Families may join with an individual in attempting to find satisfactory solutions to life's problems. Some of these attempts may bring additional problems, while the need to deal with social and medical structures can demand enormous persistence, patience and ingenuity.[37]

Educating the psychiatric team in developing a common understanding and approach towards these problems is vital for developing true multidisciplinary teamwork. Communication across service boundaries and education of other health professionals may make for improved practice in the long term.

Coping with persistent complaints

The elderly person who has shown a lifelong pattern of illness complaints and who may often be taking a number of inappropriate and possibly harmful medicines presents particular difficulties for health services. These patients have often either failed to respond to traditional physical/psychiatric treatments, or refused to have anything to do with psychiatry because of the stigma, and because they believe that their problems are physical! It can be almost impossible to discover what psychological factors were present 30 or 40 years ago to cause the problem to develop.

It has been the aim throughout this chapter to present a realistic account of the challenges that face a team working with this particular clinical group. Even so, it may be argued that we have erred on the side of being too optimistic about the prognosis of elderly people who present with anxieties about their health. However, there have been recent developments within health psychology which are useful with regard to the understanding and treatment of such difficulties.

Even with the most effective use of models and skills, there are some people with hypochondriacal complaints whom it is impossible to help. In these cases it is worth remembering the diagram shown in Figure 9.3, which indicates that any increased anxiety is likely to exacerbate the hypochondriacal behaviour. It is then important for the practitioners involved to minimise any additional anxiety that they contribute. Box 9.2 shows a strategy which might be used to try to cope with an elderly person who telephones the GP's surgery 10 times a week complaining of serious illnesses, together with the rationale for each part of the plan. Similar plans can be drawn up to cope with patients who hound the doctor or nurse on the ward, or who talk incessantly about their symptoms and not themselves. Providing such a clear structure may not be a cure, but it helps to limit the damage the patients do to themselves, it opens the way to improvement, and it may reduce the stress experienced by the professionals involved by providing them with a coping strategy.

Box 9.2   Example of a plan for use with a hypochondriacal patient who rings the GP surgery 10 times a week for home consultations

1   One regular visit per week (not following a call). To include 5 minutes of physical examination and firm reassurance. This ensures that the need is met independently of the telephone calls, which are less strongly reinforced.

2   Whenever possible, only one named GP to provide consultations (the GP who is most willing to see the client). This provides consistency and enables the doctor to keep track of the situation.

3   An extra visit is made if 2 days pass without any telephone call from the patient (these criteria to be altered if the situation improves). This reinforces not telephoning.

4   If the GP has to respond to a 'false' urgent call (e.g. the patient feigning a heart attack), the visit should be conducted in a calm manner, examination should be the minimum necessary to exclude a real medical emergency and should be time limited (i.e. 5 minutes or less). The GP should leave as soon as possible with a brief informative comment to the patient (e.g. 'You are not suffering from a heart attack. I have to leave now'). The information is minimal in order to avoid unnecessary reinforcement of the behaviour, and to give the least possible grounds for misunderstanding.

5   The GP's staff are given precise instructions about what information to give during phone calls by the patient. This again reduces potential reinforcement and minimises any possible misinterpretation.

CONCLUSION

We have seen the complicated interactions between psychological, biological and social constructs in explaining the association between depressed mood and physical disorder. Some depressed moods lead to 'hypochondriacal' complaints with little basis in physical pathology. More commonly there is a somatic preoccupation, overvaluing the significance of real but relatively minor physical problems. In the other direction, depressed mood appears to be associated with the development of various physical illnesses, and with poor outcome of physical illness. In addition there is the social dimension, in which isolation and handicap are also associated with depression, and must be managed alongside any pharmacological or psychological intervention for depression if we are to maximise the likelihood of success. The evidence for the existence of the associations between depression, physical ill health, handicap and loneliness is clear. The evidence for the benefit of treatment across the different dimensions is more difficult to obtain. At the moment it certainly seems logical and is consistent with clinical experience gained with individual patients. However, further research would be beneficial for demonstrating conclusively the value of a multidimensional approach to the management of depression in physical illness.

A therapeutic alliance has to be forged with the patient if they are to be persuaded to cooperate with pharmacological treatment or social interventions. In addition, a reasonable balance has to be struck between the investigation of physical complaints and a firm refusal to indulge in over-investigation or speculative symptomatic treatment. The management of depression producing hypochondriacal symptoms includes the basics of good management of depression.

Finally, the probably much rarer condition of somatisation disorder and hypochondriasis not associated with depressed mood must also be recognised. Where anxiety is prominent, antidepressants may help either by their anxiety-moderating effects or because there is a masked depression. Generally, however, if symptoms have been present for many years, a psychotherapeutic assessment may determine whether psychological management (ranging from psychodynamic therapy through cognitive behavioural therapy to environmental manipulation) is justified.

REFERENCES

1 Block AR, Kremer EF and Gaylor M (1980) Behavioural treatment of chronic pain: the spouse as a discriminative cue for pain behaviour. *Pain.* 9: 243–52.

2 Wooley SC, Blackwell B and Winget C (1978) A learning theory model of chronic illness behaviour. *Psychosom Med.* 40: 379–401.

3 World Health Organization (1992) *The ICD-10 Classification of Mental and Behavioural Disorders: Clinical Descriptions and Diagnostic Guidelines.* World Health Organization, Geneva.

4 Penninx BW, Guralnik JM, Ferrucci L, Simonsick EM, Deeg DJ and Wallace RB (1998) Depressive symptoms and physical decline in community-dwelling older persons. *JAMA.* 279: 1720–6.

5 Broe GA, Jorm AF, Creasey H *et al* (1999) Impact of chronic systemic and neurological disorders on disability, depression and life satisfaction. *Int J Geriatr Psychiatry.* 13: 667–73.

6 Herrmann C, Brand-Driehorst S, Kaminsky B, Leibing E, Staats H and Ruger U (1998) Diagnostic groups and depressed mood as predictors of 22-month mortality in medical inpatients. *Psychosom Med.* 60: 570–7.

7 Koenig HG and George LK (1998) Depression and physical disability outcomes in depressed medically ill hospitalized older adults. *Am J Geriatr Psychiatry.* 6: 230–47.

8 Ahto M, Isoaho R, Puolijoki H, Laippala P, Romo M and Kivela S (1997) Coronary heart disease and depression in the elderly: a population-based study. *Fam Pract.* **14:** 436–45.

9 Sullivan MD, Newton K, Hecht J *et al* (2004) Depression and health status in elderly patients with heart failure: a 6-month prospective study in primary care. *Am J Geriatr Cardiol.* **13:** 252–60.

10 Sullivan MD, LaCroix AZ, Baum C, Grothaus LC and Katon WJ (1997) Functional status in coronary artery disease: a one-year prospective follow-up of the role of anxiety and depression. *Am J Med.* **103:** 348–56.

11 Sullivan MD, Levy WC, Crane BA *et al* (2004) Usefulness of depression to predict time to combined endpoint of transplant or death for outpatients with advanced heart failure. *Am J Cardiol.* **94:** 1577–80.

12 Pohjasvara T, Leppavuori A, Siira I, Vataja R, Kaste M and Erkinjuntti T (1998) Frequency and clinical determinants of post-stroke depression. *Stroke.* **29:** 2311–17.

13 Bond J, Gregson B, Smith M, Rousseau N, Lecouturier J and Rodgers H (1998) Outcomes following acute hospital care for stroke or hip fracture: how useful is an assessment of anxiety or depression for older people? *Int J Geriatr Psychiatry.* **13:** 601–10.

14 Dennis M, O'Rourke S, Lewis S, Sharpe M and Warlow C (1998) A quantitative study of the emotional outcome of people caring for stroke survivors. *Stroke.* **29:** 1867–72.

15 Bhogal SK, Teasell R, Foley N and Speechley M (2005) Heterocyclics and selective serotonin reuptake inhibitors in the treatment and prevention of post-stroke depression. *J Am Geriatr Soc.* **53:** 1051–7.

16 Penninx BW, Guralnick JM, Pahor M *et al* (1998) Chronically depressed mood and cancer risk in older persons. *J Natl Cancer Inst.* **90:**1888–93.

17 Liu CY, Wang SJ, Fuh JL, Lin CH, Yang YY and Liu HC (1997) The correlation of depression with functional activity in Parkinson's disease. *J Neurol.* **244:** 493–8.

18 Murphy E (1982) The social origins of depression in old age. *Br J Psychiatry.* **141:** 135–42.

19 Kennedy GJ, Kelman HR and Thomas C (1990) The emergence of depressive symptoms in late life: the importance of declining health and increasing disability. *J Commun Health.* **15:** 93–104.

20 Prince MJ, Harwood RH, Blizard RA, Thomas A and Mann AH (1997) Impairment, disability and handicap as risk factors for depression in old age. The Gospel Oak Project V. *Psychol Med.* **27:** 311–21.

21 Prince MJ, Harwood RH, Blizard RA, Thomas A and Mann AH (1997) Social support deficits, loneliness and life events as risk factors for depression in old age. The Gospel Oak Project VI. *Psychol Med.* **27:** 323–32.

22 Prince MJ, Harwood RH, Thomas A and Mann AH (1998) A prospective population-based study of the effects of disablement and social milieu on the onset and maintenance of late-life depression. The Gospel Oak Project VII. *Psychol Med.* **28:** 337–50.

23 Kenyon FE (1964) Hypochondriasis: a clinical study. *Br J Psychiatry.* **110:** 47888.

24 De Alarcon R (1964) Hypochondriasis and depression in the aged. *Gerontol Clin.* **6:** 266–77.

25 Bradley JJ (1963) Severe localised pain associated with depressive syndrome. *Br J Psychiatry.* **109:** 741–5.

26 Barsky AJ and Klerman GL (1983) Overview: hypochondriasis, bodily complaints and somatic styles. *Am J Psychiatry.* **140:** 273–81.

27 Hawton K, Salkovskis PM, Kirk J and Clark DM (1989) *Cognitive Behavioural Therapy for Psychiatric Problems: A Practical Guide.* Oxford University Press, Oxford.

28 Salkovskis PM (1989) Somatic problems. In: K Hawton, PM Salkovskis, J Kirk and DM Clark (eds) *Cognitive Behavioural Therapy for Psychiatric Problems: A Practical Guide.* Oxford University Press, Oxford.

29 Philips C and Rachman S (1996) *Psychological Management of Chronic Pain.* Springer, New York.

30 Ley R (1985) Agoraphobia, the panic attack and the hyperventilation syndrome. *Behav Res Ther.* **23:** 79–82.

31 Clark DM, Salkovskis PM, Hackmann A *et al* (1998) Two psychological treatments for hypochondriasis. A randomised controlled trial. *Br J Psychiatry.* **173:** 218–25.

32 Bouman TK and Visser S (1998) Cognitive and behavioural treatment of hypochondriasis. *Psychother Psychosom.* **67:** 214–21.

33 Sumathipala A (2007) What is the evidence for the efficacy of treatments for somatoform disorders? A critical review of previous intervention studies. *Psychosom Med.* **69:** 889–900.

34 Barsky AJ (1996) Hypochondriasis. Medical management and psychiatric treatment. *Psychosomatics.* **37:** 48–56.

35 Report of a Working Group for the Faculty of Old Age Psychiatry (2005) *Who Cares Wins. Improving the Outcomes for Older People Admitted to the General Hospital. Guidelines for the Development of Liaison Mental Health Services for Older People.* Royal College of Psychiatrists, London.

36 Hilderink PH, Gollard R, Rosmalen JG and Oudevoshaar RC (2012) Prevalence of somatoform disorders and medically unexplained symptoms in old age populations in comparison with younger age groups: a systematic review. *Ageing Research Reviews.* **28.** (available at www.ncbi.nlm.gov.pubmed/225790 (accessed 28 June 2012).

37 Anderson R and Bury M (eds) (1988) *Living with Chronic Illness: The Experience of Patients and Their Families.* Unwin Hyman, London.

10

The planning and delivery of services

INTRODUCTION

Geriatric medicine in the UK evolved in the optimistic early years of the NHS, and old age psychiatry followed close behind.[1,2] During that time centralised planning was the model adopted by government, not surprisingly in view of its effectiveness in the Second World War. The mission of early old age psychiatrists was to set up good services and to persuade government to recognise them and issue guidance for their national development. In the free-for-all of the 'Thatcher years', national guidance was abandoned and some health authorities chose, for example, not to purchase NHS long-stay beds, although this choice was challenged. Virtually all health authorities reduced the number of such beds available.[3] At the same time other changes, such as the advent of the first generation of drugs to modify the course of Alzheimer's disease, have increased the emphasis on early, accurate diagnosis.

Although the UK took a lead in the development of specialist mental health services for old people, other countries have developed their own models,[4] depending on how health and social care is organised locally. An international survey recently suggested that 12 nations had achieved an acceptable level of service for old people.[5] The authors' experience is chiefly in the UK, and it is mostly experience in that country to which we shall refer, although many of the principles involved can be generalised to other settings. We propose to discuss not only the direct role of old age psychiatrists in planning and delivering services, but also the important educational role of these services.

PLANNING AND PROVIDING SERVICES

Psychiatric services for old people form an important part of a spectrum of care which includes friends and relatives, home care and other social services, the primary health services (including family doctors) and private residential and nursing homes. These services work within a political, ethical and legal framework. To achieve maximum effect, the *clinical* work of a comprehensive psychiatric service for old people should be:

➤ evidence based (including providing good relationships for patients and carers)
➤ focused on severe mental illness
➤ provided through teamwork and collaboration
➤ coordinated
➤ delivered at critical points in the time course of an individual's illness.

It also needs to be able to deliver the following:
➤ coordinated assessment
➤ care planning and management
➤ community treatment and support (including day hospitals)
➤ acute inpatient care of those who temporarily cannot be properly supported in the community.

In addition, most would argue for the retention of some respite and long-stay care facilities,[6] although for political and economic reasons these have tended, in England, to be moved from the free-at-the-point-of-use NHS to private provision supported by means-tested benefits.

Evidence base

The evidence base for the practice of old age psychiatry is good but could be improved. Evidence is generally at its scientifically most valid for treatments that can be assessed using randomised double-blind placebo-controlled trials, mainly the use of medication. Other randomised controlled trials which cannot, by their very nature, be double blind have compared day hospital with acute inpatient care in general psychiatry,[7] although such work has yet to be replicated in older adults. Most of the evidence for the delivery of old age psychiatry services is based on 'before and after' experience[8] or descriptive studies[9,10] that have been more or less systematically evaluated. Relatively unreliable though this evidence is by rigorous scientific standards, it should not be despised. It is the best we have available, and the difficulties of developing adequate methodology and obtaining funding for high-quality service research should not be underestimated.

When considering the evidence base we must remember the importance of *how* we do things as well as *what* we do. Patients and carers value service providers who are genuinely interested in them and who listen empathetically. They generally prefer a sustained relationship with one (or a small number of) team members concentrating on a holistic approach, rather than fragmented task-oriented care from an ever-varying group of task-oriented 'carers'. People value good relationships.

Focus on severe mental illness: epidemiology and the target population

In order to deliver an adequate service there has to be an agreed target population. In the UK it tends to be a geographical catchment area with a defined elderly population. Until 1992, it was reckoned that in the UK one consultant psychiatrist and the associated team of workers could cope effectively with an area containing about 22 000 old people.[11] This assumed a comprehensive service which dealt with all serious mental illness in old people (with the possible exception of those who had grown old in hospital), and not the much rarer pattern of dementia-only service. It also tended to exclude services for younger people with dementia. With the increasing proportion of very old people and the higher expectations placed on services, the Royal College of Psychiatrists revised the number served by one consultant and the associated team to 10 000 old people,[11] a target that has already been achieved in some areas. In addition, the College suggested that, in teaching health districts, where staff have extra educational and research responsibilities, catchment areas should be commensurately smaller. Because of the age-related increase in the prevalence of dementia, it is also helpful when planning and delivering services to know what proportion of the population over 65 years is more than 75 years old.

The population that is served must also be known in order to enable decisions about what personnel and facilities (e.g. day hospital places and inpatient beds) are needed. There are no absolute answers to the 'numbers game'. The most recent recommendations from a consortium led by the Royal College of Psychiatrists[11] are summarised in Box 10.1 and Table 10.1. This guidance, endorsed by the British Geriatric Society and the Royal College of Nursing, among others, also refers to the need for access to translation services, chiropody, speech and language therapy, dietetics and pharmacy advice. It also asserts that additional staffing is needed for memory services, access to psychological therapies and hospital liaison.

Box 10.1   Guidelines for special provision for mentally ill old people (per 1000 members of the population aged > 65 years)[11]

➤ Acute assessment and treatment beds   1–2
➤ Day hospital places (dementia and share of   1–1.5
   non-dementia places)

Table 10.1 Recommended minimum staffing for a UK community mental health team for older people[11] (excluding memory service, psychological therapies and memory assessment services)

Type of staff	WTE*/10 000 over 65 years of age
Consultant psychiatrist	1
Non-consultant doctors	1
Community psychiatric nurses	2.5
Support workers or equivalent	1.0
Occupational therapist	1.0
Social worker	1.0
Physiotherapist	0.5
Clinical psychologist	0.5
Team secretary	1.0
CMHT manager	

*WTE, whole-time equivalent; CMHT, community mental health team.

The truth is that different models of service can provide adequate services from a range of different facilities. What is not in dispute is that *adequate numbers of properly trained and motivated staff are essential.* Sadly, community care has attracted a bad name precisely because these have not been provided. As the large mental hospitals have closed, money has leaked from mental health services (mostly to acute general hospitals) so that community services, in the UK at least, have historically been under-staffed and under-funded. The shifts between provision of different care environments are not absolute. Thus it is not a case of 'hospital care' or 'community care', but rather 'given this amount of hospital care, what community care is needed?', and vice versa. A useful visual model is provided by the image of a line, at one end of which is virtually all community care, while at the other end is virtually all hospital care (*see* Figure 10.1).

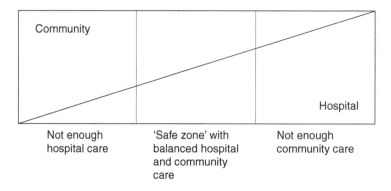

Figure 10.1 The balance between hospital and community care.

The best services operate somewhere in the middle zone, where there is a balance between hospital and community investment. Although this can vary, and to some extent one can compensate for the other, both are essential. Of course, the real picture is much more complicated because factors such as poverty, community cohesion and provision of social care have to be integrated into a multidimensional, multi-agency plan for provision. This is why in the UK effective joint planning and working between health and social services remain a much sought after but never quite attained goal.

A restricted geographical area enables the team to build up relationships with other local workers and to become familiar with the network of facilities that are available locally. In the UK these include general practitioners, district nurses, social workers, home helps and other social and voluntary workers, and the day care, lunch club, carer support and other services, as well as local residential and nursing home facilities.

A population of 10 000 over the age of 65 years would contain at least 500 people with moderate to severe dementia, and a larger number with depression of sufficient severity to impair quality of life significantly. Adding all of the individually rarer causes of mental illness in old age, such as schizophrenia, mania, phobias, anxiety state and alcohol abuse, we can see that there is plenty of work for a mental health team for old people in such a catchment area.

Teamwork and collaboration

Care of the elderly is an area where the traditional distinction between care in the community and hospital-based care is inadequate. Although general practitioners and area social services workers act as the first line of contact for services in the community, secondary care teams are no longer hospital based, and they pride themselves on providing many diagnostic and treatment services to the patient at home. In old age psychiatry an 'integrated' model of the community mental health team has been popular, with the same core team, including the consultant psychiatrist, involved in assessing and managing the patient in the community and being responsible for inpatient or day patient care. There is now an increasing trend for specialisation in inpatient *or* community work in psychiatric services in some old age services. The risks and benefits of this differentiation of function have yet to be assessed. The specialist team needs to work in cooperation with general practitioners and area social services to set up adequate networks of care for old people with mental illness in the community.

The typical specialist team consists of a consultant psychiatrist and one or more doctors in training, as well as community nurses and contributions from one or more social work staff, occupational therapists, physiotherapists, ward and day hospital nurses, and psychologists.

The mixture of different disciplines enriches the culture of the team and makes individual members aware of more therapeutic possibilities than could ever exist for individuals working alone. Not all teams have this richness, and psychologists in particular are often difficult to recruit. The resources available also vary from one area to another, largely as a result of historical accident.[10] Multidisciplinary teams provide an effective way of delivering psychiatric care to old people, but they vary in how they are constituted and the way in which they conduct their business.

A well-functioning multidisciplinary team is characterised by the type of co-working on projects that is a feature of good modern management. The whole team is not involved in looking after every patient, but members know each other well enough to understand the special skills of each discipline and each person, so that they can be called upon when necessary. The team members are often also members of other 'teams' assembled for the care of the patient. The community psychiatric nurse works closely with the diabetic nurse specialist or the terminal care nurse in supporting and treating patients with complicated mixtures of physical and mental illness. At the same time he or she may be asking the psychiatrist to review medication, or asking the psychologist to help with aspects of behavioural management.

Leadership in each case and situation is the responsibility of a specified member of the team, with the consultant often retaining an overall coordinating and leadership role.[12] Thus the community psychiatric nurse may be leading on a particular case as the *keyworker* (or *'care programme coordinator'*), with the consultant psychiatrist being called in to assist as necessary. Different people are happy with different arrangements, but for a team to function well it is essential that management gives team members sufficient autonomy to negotiate some leadership arrangement that works for them, within agreed limits. Problems arise when management hierarchies interfere with team functioning, or when the nominal team leader (usually the consultant psychiatrist) does not possess the necessary leadership skills. The skills of leadership are not easily acquired or generally well taught. Good leaders do not make all of the decisions themselves and then tell others what to do! They recognise that the skills and knowledge contained within the team as a whole are far wider and deeper than that of any individual member (including the leader), and they seek to create a climate in which those skills and that knowledge can be fully used in the provision and development of services.[13,14]

Team building and maintenance are essential activities if the most effective and efficient pattern of multidisciplinary working is to be achieved and sustained. Shared accommodation, democracy about who makes the coffee and who does the washing up, and informal chats over lunch are as important as more formal team development meetings. Coaching is an approach to management that supports team members in working out their own solutions.

It fits well in multidisciplinary teams where different kinds of expertise reside in different team members. The 'GROW' approach advocated by Sir John Whitmore provides a useful framework for team coaching and decisions. After the initial assessment, a series of potential Goals are identified. The Reality around these is explored (with further assessment if appropriate). Options are considered. The Will to act comes next, with specific agreement as to who does what and when.[15]

Each discipline has its own area of expertise. Figure 10.2 is over-simplified, but still gives some idea of the complexity of multidisciplinary working. For example, area A in the doctor's portion of the figure represents such things as medical diagnosis and the prescribing of drugs (although nurse prescribers are now moving into this area!), where the doctor generally has the most appropriate training and skills. A similar area for the ward nurse might be the planned provision of 24-hour care to support patients and at the same time help them to develop their own self-care skills. For the home care manager or social worker, that area might be the detailed planning and provision of support services in the community. Other areas of skill and responsibility overlap with each other (B). Simple examples of this area are the administration of injections and taking blood samples, where both doctors and nurses (and phlebotomists!) may have appropriate training. Yet other areas (C) may be shared by all members of the team. For example, all disciplines might be trained in bereavement counselling. The psychologist on the team may have special

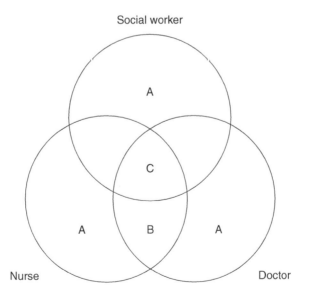

Figure 10.2 Overlaps of skill in the multidisciplinary team.

skills in neuropsychological and behavioural assessment but also share some skills in counselling or psychotherapy with other disciplines. The same mixture of unique and shared skills is also found in occupational therapy, physiotherapy and other disciplines. The exact areas of overlap in any team will depend not only on the boundaries between disciplines, but also on individual training and talent. What is important is that the areas of unique skill or responsibility and of overlap are recognised, and that team members are prepared to accept each other's skills, regardless of their different training backgrounds.

Members of the team must also guard against the tendency to concentrate on the more 'interesting' aspects of their work, while the more mundane tasks are left undone, and they must be secure enough in their own work to be able to listen to constructive criticism from colleagues in their own or other disciplines. If such an ethos can be achieved, mistakes in planning care will be minimised, as all members of the team will be enabled to contribute responsibly. For successful multidisciplinary working, there has to be a sense of trust and mutual respect between team members. Because of the markedly different training between different disciplines, this can be difficult to achieve. There are overlapping areas of expertise, and it is only by discussing case management frankly together that the most appropriate skills can be applied to a particular patient's problems.

The involvement of different organisations and different disciplines in caring for old people with mental illness provides an opportunity for creative collaboration if the workers and their respective organisations can get along together. If they cannot manage to do this, whole groups of elderly people may be left 'out in the cold' as health and social services dispute who is responsible for them. Patterns of working together vary widely from one team to another, and from time to time within a team.

Coordination: the care programme approach

The introduction of the care programme approach (CPA) in the UK followed a number of well-publicised and tragic cases of self-harm or harm to others involving mentally ill people which were blamed on the poor coordination of health and social services. It sought to avoid these tragedies by having a care plan agreed between all of the relevant agencies and the patient and his or her carers. A key worker (or care programme coordinator) was responsible for ensuring that the care plan was delivered, and for arranging regular reviews. The CPA was introduced in a confused way and in parallel to the related process of care management in social services.[16] Most importantly, it was introduced *without adequate resources* to support its delivery, and was seen by many workers in the field to be a cynical attempt to transfer blame from the government to individual key workers who often did not have the resources to deliver proper community care. It combined a role of internal coordination and external liaison that already existed in good teams, and was described in earlier editions of this book with the overarching idea of a single multi-agency plan derived from the care management approach.[17]

A full description of the CPA in the UK was contained in *Building Bridges*,[18] and more recent documents have provided further guidance, including *Refocusing the Care Programme Approach*, published by the Department of Health in 2008 (http://webarchive.nationalarchives.gov.uk/). The essence of the modern CPA is assessment, taking into account all relevant factors, agreement on a care plan by all involved, the appointment of a key worker and a system of regular reviews. *Refocusing the Care Programme Approach* reviewed the CPA process to ensure that national policy is more 'consistently and clearly applied' and unnecessary bureaucracy is removed. Some of the principles include the following:

➤ All individuals receiving treatment, care and support from secondary mental health services are entitled to receive high-quality care based on their individual needs and choices.
➤ The needs and involvement of people receiving services and person-centred care is central to the CPA process.
➤ Individuals with a wide range of needs or who are at high risk should receive a higher level of care coordination.
➤ From 2008, *only* this system of care and support will be called CPA.
➤ Assessments and care plans should address the range of service users' needs.
➤ Whole systems approaches should support CPA. Services and organisations should work together.
➤ The role of the care coordinator is vital. National competencies have been published (*see* below).
➤ Care planning should be focused on improving outcomes for service users and their families.

(For a detailed discussion, including competencies for CPA coordinators, see *Refocusing the Care Programme Approach*, http://webarchive.nationalarchives. gov.uk/)

Most referrals to specialist mental health teams for old people come from primary care, usually from the general practitioner. About 25% of referrals are from other hospital doctors, and some 'community' referrals are really initiated by social services personnel with the approval of the appropriate general practitioner. Until recently the majority of services arranged for an initial assessment of the patient by a senior doctor (consultant or specialist registrar) in the patient's own home.

However, under the pressure to 'modernise' inherent in the National Service Framework for Older People,[19] and in an attempt to match the range of services offered to younger people under the National Service Framework for Mental Health,[20] many services in England have recently undergone rapid changes. A document that acknowledged the shortage of consultant psychiatrists and proposed 'New Ways of Working' (http://webarchive.nationalarchives.gov.uk/) has also been influential in promoting changes. One of these has been the development of a single point of access to the community mental health team (CMHT). This means that in many services more of the initial assessments in the community are done by nurses, social workers and occupational therapists. In some services, medical time is being more concentrated in the hospital. In others an increasing amount of medical support is being put into the community, but as a secondary support to the initial assessment undertaken by other disciplines. Unfortunately, at this stage it is impossible to say whether employing authorities have fully carried through their responsibilities to ensure that individual clinicians and teams have the competencies and resources to deliver what is expected of them. Another recommendation from 'New Ways of Working', to stop defining consultant jobs in terms of catchment area, has, thankfully, not been pursued in old age services.

More differentiated services are also developing. There is an increasing emphasis on memory clinics and memory services (often nurse led).[21] Liaison services to the general hospital are being developed in a variety of ways.[22] In addition, assertive outreach, inreach, community treatment and other models are being tried, sometimes based on day hospital resources. Some services have developed separate teams for those with dementia and those with other mental disorders. These changes seem to have been instituted without extra resources by closing inpatient and day hospital places. Their overall impact has yet to be evaluated.

Formal shared care agreements with general practitioners and pathways for the management of common conditions such as dementia and depression were mandated by the Department of Health. They are a welcome development, but in times of so much change they have not always been implemented whole-heartedly.

In the teams with which the authors are most familiar, initial assessments normally take place within a few hours for urgent referrals, and within a few days for less urgent cases. If the assessment indicates that urgent action is needed, the assessor initiates this immediately. In other cases an initial care plan is drawn up and discussed further at the weekly team meeting where, if continuing involvement is indicated, a key worker is agreed and the process of refining the care plan begins, involving other agencies if necessary. As far as possible the key worker is the focus for any further management decisions, but the consultant also acts as a 'long stop' if decisions need to be made in the key worker's absence. The team meeting also provides an opportunity for members of the team to present ongoing 'cases' with whom they are having particular difficulties for group discussion, and possibly to enlist the help of other disciplines in coping with the problem.

Some patients are assessed as being in need of urgent physical rather than psychiatric attention. These individuals are referred back to the family doctor or to the appropriate medical specialist (usually the physician in geriatric medicine). Many patients who are referred will already be known to local social work staff, who will be invited to participate in meetings where their clients' care plans are reviewed, occasionally taking on the key worker's (care coordinator's) role.

Intervention at critical points: the role of assessment

Assessment at critical points in a patient's mental illness is the key to effective management. The assessment process needs to include biological, psychological and social elements, and is described more fully in Chapter 2. For the community mental health team, critical points occur when the patient needs expert diagnosis, treatment or a coordinated care plan in order to restore health or manage disability, and one or more of these functions are beyond the capability of the primary care team. Assessment may be the point of entry to directly provided services (e.g. inpatient care). Occasionally it will simply be a source of help to the family doctor or other members of the primary healthcare team to whose care the patient will be fully returned after assessment. Most often it will be the beginning of a period of community treatment in which services provided by the old age psychiatry team are married with services provided by the family doctor and social services. An agreed care plan, coordinated by a key worker (or care coordinator) and reviewed at agreed intervals, forms the framework for this collaboration.

The components of this system are very interdependent. In the UK, few opportunities exist for direct access to secondary services. The family doctor effectively acts as a 'gatekeeper' to the secondary services, and problems sometimes arise when family doctors unduly limit access to the community mental health team. At the boundary between health and social services, a shortage of funding for long-term accommodation (which is largely funded in a means-tested manner through social services in the UK) can, for example, lead to 'blocked beds' on the acute wards. This in turn leads to back pressure on the community team striving to look after people at home whose illnesses are of sufficient severity to merit inpatient care. On the other hand, a higher than normal level of community support can enable *some* (but not all) patients to be looked after at home who would otherwise need nursing home or inpatient care. In planning services, therefore, the whole assessment, treatment and support network must be viewed as an interactive system.

In the UK this has traditionally been obstructed by divisions between the NHS, provided by central government, and the social and other services (e.g.

housing), provided by local government. In some areas, 'care trusts' have bridged this divide, although not always successfully. With increasing devolution of political power to govern health services, differences are emerging between the different countries in the UK.

A comprehensive service will also have a training and educational role (*see* pp. 262–264), and should be involved in research, service development and audit, if only at a local level, to ensure that the highest possible quality is achieved for the resources invested.

Community treatment and care, including day hospital care

Community care begins in the patient's home, and that is one of the reasons why community mental health teams for the elderly still favour initial assessment in the patient's home, whether that is a private dwelling or a residential/nursing 'care' home. One of the early insights of geriatric medicine was that hospital was a 'bad place' for old people, and our experience in mental health services for old people fully endorses the view that hospital admission should be avoided whenever the patient can be managed safely and effectively at home. Family and friends are the true 'primary carers', and their role must be recognised and supported. This includes emotional, educational and practical support. Coping with a demented or severely depressed relative at home can be exhausting, and it is important that the carer's needs as well as those of the patient are adequately assessed and, as far as possible, met. Empathetic listening gives emotional support, provided that it is backed up by information about mental illness and services, and by practical help. This practical help may take a number of forms, including the following:

➤ financial allowances (e.g. the 'attendance allowance')
➤ home care and sitting services to relieve the physical burden of care
➤ day care or respite care in local authority-provided accommodation
➤ day hospital care for patients with particular problems of diagnosis or management
➤ intensive short-term community support.

Most old people who live alone receive some support from family and friends. For those who do not, the provision of community care and treatment can be particularly problematic, especially for people with severe dementia, schizophrenia or severe depression. Acute inpatient or residential care is more likely to be needed by these people.

The use of the term 'community care' has been attacked on the grounds that the community generally does not care! Even the term 'care in the community' is misleading, as it does not emphasise the importance of:

➤ *treatment* (psychotherapeutic and pharmacological) for those illnesses that are treatable

➤ *rehabilitation* to reduce residential disability after treatable illness
➤ *planned support* to deal with the disabilities caused by conditions that are essentially progressive and hard to treat, such as some forms of schizophrenia and dementia.

Generally speaking, treatment and rehabilitation are health service responsibilities, and planned support is a local authority responsibility involving housing as well as social services.

Day hospital facilities form part of the community treatment resource. Their importance and how they are used vary from one locality to another. They may serve several different functions. Some are used for the assessment of patients with severe functional mental illness or particular diagnostic or behavioural problems in dementia. Day support for severely demented patients whose relatives want to keep them at home but who need a regular 'break' is now generally provided through social services, but there are still large variations from one area to another. Many day hospitals still carry at least a few long-term support patients with severe dementia whose behaviour cannot be managed in other environments.

Those who are not familiar with mental health services for older people often assume that day hospitals only provide support for patients with dementia. However, many of the patients are suffering from recurrent depressive disorder, and some have paranoid disorders, alcohol abuse or other problems. For them, day hospital treatment may mean that they can avoid the need for inpatient treatment, or it may enable patients to be discharged home sooner and kept in relatively good health despite social isolation and other unfavourable circumstances. The effective functioning of day hospitals depends on the provision of other facilities, such as social services and voluntary day centres, to which those patients who need them can be discharged for 'social' maintenance care. Transport is also a vital factor in day hospitals, as most patients cannot make their own way to the hospital. Transport services need to be arranged so that it is possible for them to wait a while for those who are not ready when the vehicle arrives. Relatives, home helps, district nurses, community nurses and others may need to be enlisted to make sure that the old person does attend the day hospital. In geographically compact areas, day hospitals (whose primary function is assessment, treatment and rehabilitation) may be located together with acute beds in the district general hospital or alongside the community mental health team in a community facility. In some areas with relatively scattered populations, the 'mobile' day hospital has been developed. Staff and equipment travel from the base hospital to a different location each day and run a day hospital in a local church hall, community centre or other suitable facility. This is a useful way of spreading thin resources across a wide geographical area. Other models include the provision of health service staff to augment specialist local authority day centres dealing with dementia, or to provide extended short-term home care as an alternative to admission or day hospital assessment.

Few services approach the guidelines for day places formerly set out by the Department of Health (2 to 3 places for dementia and 0.65 places for functional illness per 1000 members of the elderly population), and many acknowledge that these guidelines were over-generous. Provided that social services and voluntary facilities for day care and other community care are adequate, a smaller number of day hospital places can concentrate on the assessment and treatment of patients with functional illness, including the provision of groups for CBT and other psychological therapies. This prevents or curtails inpatient care. Day hospitals can also focus on the assessment of particular diagnostic or behavioural problems in people with dementia. In our own area, long-term day care is mostly provided by social services, with the Alzheimer's Disease Society playing an increasing role for patients with early-onset dementia, although the hospital service still takes a few patients whom other facilities cannot manage.

Acute inpatient facilities

Services increasingly provide separate wards for assessment of those who are markedly confused and for treatment of other disorders. Separate sleeping and toilet accommodation should be provided for men and women. Ideally, designs should allow some flexibility between the sexes in the use of bed spaces, in the interest of efficiency. Separate day areas are also important for some people, and may be a necessity where cultural factors make sharing accommodation with the opposite sex unacceptable. The location of acute assessment beds is as important as their number. Because of frequent concurrent physical illness and the need for ready access to investigative facilities and close cooperation with geriatric medicine, these beds are best located on a general hospital site where they can be used more efficiently. Former guidelines suggested that about 1.5 beds per 1000 members of the elderly population should be provided for dementia assessment and functional mental illness. The present national average provision for these purposes is not known, but in the mid-1990s there were around 1.1 beds per 1000 elderly. The number of old and very old people continues to increase. More resources (although not necessarily more beds) are needed because of this.

If adequate and rapid access is available to social care, including residential and nursing home places, the present provision of beds may be sufficient. However, in some areas a significant minority of patients have to wait in hospital beds for many months because social services either do not have funds or do not use them efficiently and effectively. There is no clear evidence which of these reasons is most important, but whichever it is, the result is that a proportion of acute hospital beds are blocked.

During the 'internal-market' era of NHS development (in the mid-1990s) it became fashionable to decry 'guidelines' and insist on local solutions. It is certainly true that good social services and community care facilities can produce a reduction in the need for acute inpatient beds and day hospital places, but there will always be an irreducible minimum number of patients for whom inpatient care is the most appropriate management. In the absence of guidelines it is all too easy to neglect the needs of old people who fall into the large gap between health and social services, especially in inner-city areas where the latter are under immense pressure to deliver services on inadequate budgets. The same problems exist in areas of 'elder immigration', where an unusually large proportion of old people in the population puts extra burdens on services.

'Benchmarking' is the modern management substitute for guidelines. It involves the comparison of one's own service with a well-functioning service working in similar circumstances (or more often with some 'average' provision). The problem is that this approach is not yet sufficiently sophisticated, and it could be used to reduce well-functioning services to an unacceptable 'average' level, rather than to improve poor services to an average level. That is why, despite recognising their limitations, we still support the use of some guidelines and quote the 'old' guidelines in this chapter. In England the new NHS Act (2012) will open the way to commercial competition and may lead to fragmentation of services.

Respite care

Respite care can help relatives to continue to cope. It is largely provided through social services. However, some patients have such severe behavioural problems or such complicated medical problems that NHS respite can best meet their needs. Previously some respite care for patients with dementia was offered in social services homes, and care for the severely disabled was offered in psycho-geriatric or geriatric hospital beds, depending on whether the disability was predominantly behavioural or physical. The reduction of beds across the public sector has led to a loss of these services in most areas. In many cases, the private sector has not found it commercially feasible to fill this gap. Hopefully new commissioning arrangements will make enhanced provision of respite care available. Respite care does not help all patients with dementia, as some exhibit increased confusion and hostility during and after a respite admission. This has to be balanced against any benefit in reducing carer strain. 'Respite at home' schemes where staff relieve carers by going into the patient's home are another alternative that needs little capital investment.

Continuing care

Long-stay beds for elderly demented people are now rarely available on the NHS in England. There are now far fewer of these than were available when the first edition of this book was published. Successive governments have promoted the expansion of private long-stay provision at the expense of NHS care. Continuing care facilities are essential for patients with severe dementia who need 24-hour care which cannot always be provided in their own homes. From the end of the Second World War until the mid-1980s, a policy evolved in the UK which broadly divided those with dementia into three groups. Those who were immobile went to NHS geriatric facilities, those who were mobile and without major behavioural problems were looked after at home or in social services 'Part III' accommodation, and those who had major behavioural problems were cared for in psychiatric facilities. The private sector was not interested in these difficult patients.

The Department of Health and Social Security then changed its benefit rules. This encouraged a rapid expansion of private sector provision at public expense. The Audit Commission reviewed the situation and the result, incorporated in the Community Care Act, was a measure to 'cap' this spending by transferring money from the benefit system (in April 1993) into an unspecified but limited fund administered through local government authorities which were expected to assess patients before placing them in residential or nursing homes.

Three basic premises underpinned this change. The first was that making the same authority responsible for residential, nursing and community care would remove perverse financial incentives to move patients (who could be looked after in the community) into residential and nursing home care. The second premise was that people going into care at public expense should be properly assessed. The third (hidden) premise was that by making local authorities responsible, the budget could be controlled and even squeezed without central government having to accept responsibility.

Even before the changes, most people who went into care in the UK apparently needed it. Most patients who were placed from medicine for the elderly or old age psychiatry services were already carefully assessed. An unfortunate effect of the new system has been that many social services departments, for administrative or financial reasons, have been unable to place patients in need of residential or nursing home care quickly from hospital. A multidisciplinary team (including a social worker) may have been involved in keeping a patient at home for several years, and may jointly reach a decision that community care is not viable. Many social services then insist that a new, lengthy and detailed assessment (including a financial assessment of the patient's ability to pay) only starts at that point. Meanwhile, the patient has been admitted to hospital in a crisis and remains there for months until every last detail is resolved. The use of a shared common assessment document (*see* Chapter 2) for all patients who are referred to social services and community mental health services could reduce some of these delays, although the means-testing assessment would still have to be conducted as a separate exercise by the social services.

Agreement over which of those patients who need nursing care should receive it in the health service sector is based upon 'eligibility criteria'. These vary from one area to another, and they generally centre around the need for active medical or psychiatric attention and difficult behaviour, rather than overall levels of disability. Many years ago we collected data on dementia and disability levels in samples from residential, nursing home and psychogeriatric care settings in Leeds.[23] We excluded geriatric care because we could not identify specific 'long-stay' care settings. We estimated the number of patients with dementia and in each disability category in each setting. We found dementia in 97% of residents in hospital and local authority specialist homes for the 'elderly mentally infirm' (EMI), in 93% of residents in registered mental nursing homes, in 80% of people in local authority residential homes and in 59% of residents in private residential care. Dementia was associated with higher overall levels of disability.

Residential and general nursing homes contained a small proportion (12%) of people with low levels of disability, although less than 5% were likely to be capable of 'independent' living. Local authority EMI homes, registered mental nursing homes and psychogeriatric beds only contained patients in the three highest dependency grades, and predominantly in the highest of these.

Only a minority of patients with dementia and high levels of dependency received care from the health service, and this number is probably set to decrease further. In these circumstances the need to use the remaining long-stay NHS resources effectively is obvious, and the Royal College of Psychiatrists, after holding a consensus meeting with other interested parties, produced useful guidelines on the role of psychiatric services in long-term care.[6,24] However, by 2008 even the Royal College of Psychiatrists had abandoned the idea of NHS provision for continuing care of people with dementia.[11]

The healthcare system in the USA is quite different. There is less emphasis on the 'primary care' function of general practitioners, and private facilities provide much of the acute and continuing psychiatric care for old people. These are supported by private health insurance schemes and, for the poor, by social security legislation. More recently, health maintenance organisations have developed to try to contain escalating costs by actively managing the process of healthcare. They have been responsible for innovations such as 'integrated care pathways', which may also be useful in the context of the NHS. At present the USA has some of the finest acute and long-stay facilities in the world, but their availability is even more constrained by geographical and financial considerations than in the UK. We should be cautious when adopting models from the USA. In a World Health Organization survey in the year 2000, the UK was spending 6% of its gross domestic product (GDP) on healthcare and was ranked 18th in terms of overall performance. The USA spent 13.7% of its GDP and came 37th, while France, spending 9.8%, came first. We may have more to learn from France than from the USA.[25]

SOCIAL SERVICES PROVISION

Apart from the family doctor and other members of the primary healthcare team/network, social services are the main partners with the community mental health team in community care. The vast majority of mentally ill old people live at home. If they are lonely or dependent for basic needs on others, then social services provision is often appropriate. Other forms of help have recently been added to the traditional pattern of home care workers, meals-on-wheels and laundry services. The neighbourhood warden is paid by social services to provide a daily human contact for old people who are living alone. Family placement schemes, where families are paid to take in old people, allow caring relatives to have a break. Trained social workers are beginning to take a greater interest in the personal needs of old people and their carers, although legislation diverts much skilled social worker time into childcare. Community services are now more often available in the evenings and at weekends, but there are still often yawning gaps during public holidays, and special out-of-hours services such as night-sitting are only patchily available. There has been a significant move towards private provision of social care services, with social services departments acting in the role of assessors of need and commissioners of services. People in need with private funds now often go straight to private providers and purchase what they need (or want) directly. This is because the process involving social service department assessment is often subject to delays. It is also means tested, so that even after assessment people in need may end up paying for their own services. This presents special problems for people with mental health problems who may not be aware of their needs or the services available. There is the added problem that someone with a depressive illness may receive support rather than a proper assessment and treatment plan. There needs to be much better integration of services, and ways have to be found to achieve this despite pressures in the opposite direction generated by privatisation and commercialisation of services.

Boundaries

Conflict between health and social services often occurs, and it is aggravated by resource problems and different management cultures. There is a need for an educative effort if such cultural differences are to be overcome. In the UK, when old people need medical treatment this is clearly the province of the general practitioner or the hospital authorities. When they need community services such as home care or meals-on-wheels, this is largely a personal or family responsibility, or the responsibility of local government-controlled social services, although district nurses and community psychiatric nurses often contribute. The CPA (*see* pp. 250–253) is designed to ensure that health and social services adopt a coordinated approach.

For those who need residential or nursing home care, the best solution might well be a combined care facility where staff are available to cope with all levels of disability. People admitted to such a facility would be able to stay there for the rest of their life and still receive increased levels of nursing care should they need it. This is the pattern of care that is provided, for example, in some parts of Australia, where residential care facilities often have their own 'nursing home' on the same site. There has been relatively little attempt to provide this type of care systematically in the UK. Divided responsibilities make it difficult to achieve. Local authority housing departments or voluntary bodies are responsible for sheltered housing, social services departments are responsible for purchasing (means-tested) residential care and nursing home care, and the National Health Service is responsible for providing free nursing care. A Royal Commission on long-term care has suggested ways to put this right, but the government did not accept all of its recommendations.

Voluntary provision

Some of the finest initiatives in the care of elderly people with psychiatric disorders are in the 'voluntary' sector. Housing associations provide sheltered housing which will often help to alleviate the loneliness of the depressed old person or enable a husband or wife to continue to look after a demented partner. Groups of relatives of elderly mentally ill people meet for mutual support, and in some areas have arranged sophisticated day-care facilities. Volunteers in 'good neighbour schemes', 'Crossroads' or 'care groups' do shopping or sit with elderly patients at home while relatives take a break. In the USA and Australia, voluntary and charitable bodies, often with church associations, have played a much more prominent role in developing nursing home, residential home and other facilities for the long-term care and support of old people. In the UK there have been some notable initiatives from the Church of Scotland, Methodist Homes for the Aged, and others. The Joseph Rowntree Foundation has recently established a 'retirement community' at Hartrigg Oaks, near York. This aims to provide for all care needs from independent living to full support, but it is likely to be too expensive for most people. For further information on this, see www. jrf.org.uk. Other schemes, such as the family placement scheme in Leeds, are organised by social services with payment to a family to take in old people, usually for a few weeks at a time, while the regular carers take a holiday. Some voluntary bodies have also started to explore the long-neglected spiritual needs of older people and people with dementia.[26,27]

EDUCATIONAL ACTIVITY

We make no apology for mentioning this in a 'practical' textbook. Education is a primary activity for all mental health teams for the elderly. In many centres, this will include the undergraduate and postgraduate training of doctors, nurses and other professional groups within the health service. It will also include offering help in training social services staff and private providers' staff, and working with voluntary bodies in providing input into carers' groups and staff training. More than that, it involves viewing each contact with a patient or carer as an opportunity for education. A third to a half of all consultation time may be spent explaining to the patient (and carer) the nature of the health problem that they appear to have and possible ways of managing this, always encouraging and listening for feedback, so that the management plan is acceptable to both patient and carer and the problems most relevant to patient and carer are addressed.

In educating students we aim to improve their *knowledge*, develop their *skills* and (sometimes) change their *attitudes*. Knowledge is acquired through lectures, reading, seminars, etc. In general, the more 'processing' someone has to do with their knowledge, the better it is understood and consolidated. Thus seminar and 'workshop' models of teaching are generally preferred. Skills are acquired by supervised practice, and attitudes are changed by exposure to people with different attitudes in favourable circumstances. The Royal College of Psychiatrists now mandates the involvement of service users and carers in psychiatric education. There is evidence that a good course in healthcare of the elderly can improve medical students' attitudes as well as their knowledge.[28] The emphasis in medical education has moved away from acquiring detailed knowledge to acquiring basic knowledge, 'learning to learn', and skills in *critical evaluation*. The rapid expansion of medical knowledge encourages the use of computer-assisted methods in order to stay up to date. New knowledge should be acquired 'just in time' rather than 'just in case'.[29]

RESEARCH AND DEVELOPMENT

Research is sometimes thought of as a rather esoteric activity. However, it can be a very practical approach to analysing what services are needed and how they are delivered. The systematic evaluation of alternative patterns of care has always been a weakness in health and social services provision, and it deserves more attention from professional bodies and journals. We tend rather to provide services that seem a 'good idea', increasingly on the basis of political dogma and pressure from private service providers. Some developments, such as 'care planning' and 'case management', are implemented without researching and providing the resources that are needed to ensure their success. Indeed, one systematic review of case management revealed that it increased continuing contact with difficult patients only slightly, but tended to double the admission rate![30] A smaller-scale study concluded that care management had some benefit,[31] and that patterns of care management where the care manager was actively involved with the patient (the 'key worker model') were probably more effective than more remote 'brokerage' models of care management. Both studies highlight the need for more clearly defined research into different patterns of care planning and management.

At an even simpler level of research, hospital doctors can find out what information GPs value in letters about patients, and whether patients prefer to be seen at home or in the clinic.

Components of complicated services can be analysed to see whether there are better ways of achieving the same objectives. This has been done, for example, with regard to domiciliary versus day hospital physiotherapy for post-stroke patients,[32] and for intensive day hospital versus inpatient care for younger psychiatric inpatients.[7] We do not all have the resources or time to develop major research projects of the type that are published in medical journals. However, we can all adopt a progressive and open-minded approach to finding out what people want from our services (as well as what they *need*), and developing those services. This is particularly important at a time when healthcare systems in many countries are coming under financial and political pressure to deliver 'value for money'. Perhaps the motto 'there may be a better way' should be tattooed on all our foreheads. For the benefit of politicians perhaps the line '… but not always the private sector' should be added!

AUDIT AND QUALITY

Another facet of the changes in health services in the UK has been a more self-conscious attitude to audit and quality. If research tells us the best treatments to use, audit tells us whether we are delivering them effectively. Medical audit is essentially a method of education and quality improvement. In our service, the medical staff take a few hours each month to meet together and audit some aspect of our services. We look at issues such as prescribing of antidepressants, assessment of dementia, use of day hospital, and communication on patient discharge, and seek to agree standards against which we then audit our practice. Such audits sometimes reveal that we do not do things as we think they should be done, and repeat audits can then check whether our standards are improving. Some people would argue that without this 'audit cycle' no true audit is being undertaken. However, there is a danger of bureaucratising the process of quality management and trying to agree detailed procedures for everything, which are then monitored from the top down. This approach is worse than useless, as it creates an 'us and them' attitude and does not value the integrity of the individual worker. Management do need indicators that quality is being pursued, but they do not need to be involved in every detail of the process. Audit is also conducted in other disciplines and increasingly in a multidisciplinary setting (clinical audit). Increasingly, in psychiatry, national audits are being developed by the Royal College of Psychiatrists (www.rcpsych. ac.uk/quality/nationalclinicalaudits.aspx) in which local services can participate. In addition, the College has developed a number of Service Quality and Accreditation Projects (www.rcpsych.ac.uk/quality/qualityandaccreditation. aspx). These projects cover a number of areas relevant to old age psychiatry, including the Memory Services National Accreditation Programme (MSNAP).

PLANNING

Business planning

Planning in the National Health Service used to take place in large committees on which practitioners were variably represented. Joint planning with social services involved even larger committees where most members (especially from the social services side) had no contact with service users. After government 'reforms', provider units and trusts adopted a commercial model of business planning with more involvement of the 'coal-face' workers using techniques such as 'SWOT' (Strengths, Weaknesses, Opportunities and Threats) and 'STEP' (Social, Technological, Economic and Political) context analysis to produce annual development plans. Initial enthusiasm for these new approaches rapidly soured when success in the health 'managed market' did not bring extra funds in the same way that it might in a real market, but only increased workloads and debts. Now the NHS in England is moving strongly in the direction of commercial market provision, and NHS organisations that want to compete with private providers will have to sharpen up their business planning. On the other hand, there is no telling whether the markets will be 'rigged' in favour of private (or, less likely, public) providers, or even whether the market experiment will persist.

Nevertheless, a 'bottom-up' approach to planning is far preferable to one that is exclusively 'top down'. (See *Profit Beyond Measure* for an analysis of the Toyota Business Method, a particularly successful industrial application of 'management by means' as opposed to top-down 'management by objectives'.[33]) The wider issues of the health needs of the population are addressed by the commissioners of healthcare, soon to be GP commissioning groups, conducting 'needs assessments' for their populations and purchasing services accordingly. The 'internal market' promised to be an exciting departure from previous cooperative systems of planning, but it led to rapidly increasing management costs without any clear overall benefit in health service delivery. It remains to be seen whether the new 'reforms' will have similar or worse effects (or whether they will lead to the feared fragmentation). One problem was that the expertise of clinicians in the area of needs assessment was often neglected because they were identified with the 'providers' rather than the 'commissioners' of healthcare. However, the main problem (especially in the inner cities) was that the agenda for health authorities was much more about 'cost containment' than about needs assessment.

Designing services

Preoccupation with health service reorganisation in the NHS has taken attention and energy away from the need to design services properly at a local level. Time should be taken to imagine what could be done using existing knowledge and technology.

Principles of good service design include the following:

➤ Local stakeholders, especially those who provide services at the clinical (face-to-face) level, must be involved.
➤ Existing knowledge about local circumstances, the scientific evidence base and good practice elsewhere should be systematically reviewed.
➤ Services should then be designed that provide 'best fit' for particular client groups.
➤ Design should include the promotion of health and the prevention of illness, as well as treatment, rehabilitation and care for those who are ill.
➤ Modern information technology should be used to support the design and operation of services.
➤ Staff roles should be examined and developed. This may include the development of completely new roles. Continuing professional development is essential.
➤ All services should be evaluated and continuous quality improvement should be promoted.
➤ Management should put greater emphasis on supporting clinical services and less emphasis on macro-structural reorganisation.

The era of primary care trusts (PCTs) commissioning within health improvement plans devised locally within the overarching structure of National Service Frameworks was abolished before there was time to evaluate it properly. It remains to be seen whether the new arrangements will be properly evaluated before they are again 'reformed'. An international perspective on service design and delivery is now developing.[34,35] In addition, guidance can be found in the National Service Frameworks for Mental Health and for Older People. The Care Services Improvement Partnership has issued guidance (www.nmhdu.org.uk) that bridges the apparent gap between these documents. An audit and service design tool based on these documents can be found in Appendix 2.

AN ETHICAL FRAMEWORK

Healthcare for old people is a very challenging field for the mental health worker. Ethics are concerned not only with the negative 'thou shalt not' aspects of healthcare, but also with positive obligations to provide care. Similarly, an ethical approach is concerned not only with personal issues, but also with social issues such as the just distribution of healthcare resources.

The value of (old) people

Some would argue that old people are of less intrinsic value than younger people. However, most would accept the person-centred assertion that everyone has equal intrinsic worth. This issue of the value ascribed to older people is of cardinal importance. One of the authors remembers sitting in a planning session when it was asserted that residential care for old people with dementia should be based on units of at least 30 people in the interest of economies of scale. However, younger people with dementia should be looked after in small 'homely' units of no more than six to eight people. When challenged, the person who made this assertion could cite not a shred of evidence that older people fared any better or worse than younger people in larger units. Underlying 'ageist' assumptions were laid bare. These assumptions that older people have less worth than younger people are not uncommon in our 'youth culture' society, and they are exacerbated by a reductionist tendency to measure everything in crude monetary terms. The starting point for any consideration of the ethics of medical care in old age must be that old people, even old people with dementia, are fully human and should be valued as such and not devalued by being treated as subhuman commodities to be traded for profit. Some ethical issues are considered in this section. Others, including the issue of consent, are considered in the section on the legal framework.

Euthanasia

Euthanasia literally means an 'easy death'. The more specific term 'physician-assisted suicide' is being increasingly used. This stresses the fact that the physician is merely assisting by carrying out the autonomous decision of the patient. The whole issue is the subject of heated debate, and for individuals with dementia the difficulties are compounded by the issue of the patient's competence.

First we shall deal briefly with the arguments for and against euthanasia itself. At one pole of the debate are those who strongly believe that the principle of autonomy is of such importance that people who want to die should be allowed to kill themselves or even be assisted in ending their life. To some extent this view was reflected in the 'decriminalisation' of suicide many years ago. Another element in the decision to decriminalise suicide was the view (upheld by research) that many of the people who commited suicide were suffering from mental illness (mainly depression). This was held to influence their judgement, so that they could not be held criminally responsible.

At the other pole of the ethnical debate are those who maintain that all human life is of the highest value, and who do not accept any circumstances in which killing is right. This group would not even accept the view that killing can be justified by war. Most people sit somewhere in between these two positions. In 1994, the House of Lords Select Committee on Medical Ethics considered the issues and decided that it was best not to legalise euthanasia, but the pressure from 'right to die' campaigners continues.

After any absolute moral imperative, perhaps the strongest argument against legalisation is the 'slippery-slope' argument that if euthanasia is legalised in certain carefully defined cases, the practice will gradually spread to include more and more categories of people. Once the line of respect for human life is crossed, it is argued, voluntary euthanasia in controlled circumstances will inevitably lead to pressure for involuntary euthanasia for those who are an economic burden and who are perhaps (if they suffer from dementia) considered by some to be no longer human. The type of argument that was heard in the abortion debate about when a fetus becomes a 'person' could be applied in reverse, to the question of when a patient with dementia loses their personhood. The evidence from the Netherlands, where euthanasia has been practised for some time, lends some support to the 'slippery-slope' argument[36,37] and to the possibility that patients whose judgement is clouded by reversible mental illness are being allowed to choose euthanasia rather than treatment for depression.[38] There are, of course, many more arguments on both sides than can be accommodated in this brief account, and the reader is referred to Wennberg's *Terminal Choices*[39] for a balanced consideration of the moral and spiritual arguments from a Christian point of view.

The issue of competence to make such 'terminal choices' raises particular difficulties in people who suffer from dementia. This problem is not really resolved by the idea of an 'advance directive' made before a person develops dementia. An advance directive in terms of avoiding 'heroic treatment' could be a matter of overriding importance in reaching a decision about interventions to preserve life in a person with dementia and coincidental life-threatening illness. However, an 'advance directive' in favour of euthanasia would be impractical as well as (currently) illegal. Who would decide when the required level of dementia had been reached? What if the person's preconceptions about dementia were wrong? What if they had changed their mind?

The ethics of early diagnosis

Another area of ethical difficulty is the genetic testing of individuals to determine their risk of developing dementia. In the case of the autosomal-dominant inheritance of Huntington's chorea, genetic testing is offered with counselling. However, in the case of Alzheimer's disease, the American College of Medical Genetics advised against genetic testing of the apolipoprotein E genotype on the grounds of lack of sensitivity and specificity. This advice would almost certainly change if a more accurate test became available. Here the 'autonomy' argument would probably (rightly) hold sway, especially as useful treatments for Alzheimer's disease begin to be developed.

The ethics of research in people with dementia

Here the tradition has been to accept that non-therapeutic research should not be conducted on those whose ability to give consent is in question. However, therapeutic research raises different questions. It is doubtful whether some patients with even mild or moderate dementia could fully understand the intricacies of randomised double-blind placebo-controlled trials. This might exclude them from participation in clinical trials. A pragmatic approach is usually taken. The trial (having of course received ethical approval) is explained to the patient as far as possible, and to a relative or other caregiver in more detail. The patient and carer are given written information and time to consider it. Patients are only included in the trial if they consent and their relatives are also in agreement. This is by no means a perfect solution, since it is unlikely that patients fully understand what they are consenting to, and in UK law the relative has no right to consent on behalf of an incompetent patient unless they have an appropriate 'lasting power of attorney' (*see* p. 273) in England and Wales or its equivalent in Scotland or other jurisdictions. Nevertheless, it seems to be an acceptable and necessary compromise if research into the treatment of a devastating group of diseases is to continue. The current position is that people with dementia might be included in research when they do not have the capacity to give their informed consent. However, this can only be lawfully carried out under the Mental Capacity Act (2005) if an appropriate body, usually an Ethics Committee, is satisfied that the following conditions have been met:

➤ The research must be safe.
➤ The research must relate to a condition that the person has.
➤ There must be reasonable grounds for believing that the research could not be carried out successfully only in patients with capacity.
➤ The benefit to the person must outweigh the risks or burden to the person. If the research is intended to improve scientific knowledge, the risk to the person should be negligible.

A full summary can be found on the Alzheimer's Society website, *Volunteering for Research into Dementia* (2010), Fact sheet 409 (www.alzheimers.org.uk), as well as in the Mental Capacity Act (2005) (www.legislation.gov.uk).

THE LEGAL FRAMEWORK

Legal aspects of management

We are indebted to Shabir Musa, Arun Devasahayam and Jayanthi Devi Subramani, who wrote a chapter for *Practical Management of Dementia* (2nd edition), on which this section is based.

INTRODUCTION

This section has been written with detailed reference to the law in England and Wales. Although details differ in different jurisdictions, the same principles apply. People suffering from dementia exhibit various clinical features, including decline in cognition, intellectual functioning, reasoning ability, judgement and insight. People with other severe mental illnesses may also have their capacity to make decisions for themselves affected. Several legal issues arise in relation to management. Capacity is the central issue in many cases. The Mental Capacity Act 2005, Mental Health Act 1983 and Deprivation of Liberty Safeguards provide statutory principles and a framework which helps to support and protect people suffering from mental illness (including dementia), and their carers.

CAPACITY

Capacity is the 'ability to make a decision'. Capacity is a legal concept, and it is defined in personal law (the part of law that deals with the matters pertaining to a person and their family) as 'a status' which determines whether they may make binding amendments to their rights, duties and obligations, such as getting married, entering into contracts, making gifts and writing a valid will. For the purpose of the Mental Capacity Act, a person lacks capacity in relation to a matter if, at the material time, they are unable to make a decision or communicate the decision because of an impairment of, or a disturbance in the functioning of, the mind or brain.[40]

In English law, an adult has the right to make decisions affecting their own life, whether the reasons for the choice are rational, irrational, unknown or even non-existent. This right remains even if the outcome of the decision might be detrimental to the individual. However, such a right to self-determination is meaningful only if the individual is appropriately informed, has the ability (capacity) to make the decision and is free to decide without coercion.[41] An adult is presumed to have the capacity until the contrary is proven, and a person who legally lacks capacity remains in that state until the contrary is proven.

Medical practitioners are frequently asked to give opinions about individuals' capacity. Psychiatrists are usually consulted about capacity issues in complex cases, and when someone is suspected of or is suffering from a mental disorder such as dementia. In disputed cases of capacity, the courts make the final decision.

MENTAL CAPACITY ACT 2005

The Mental Capacity Act 2005 for England and Wales came into force in October 2007. The Act affects people aged 16 or over and provides a statutory framework to empower and protect people who may lack capacity to make some decisions for themselves.[42] The Act covers a wide range of decisions made, or actions taken, on behalf of people lacking capacity. These can be decisions about day-to-day matters, such as what to wear, or what to buy when doing the weekly shopping, or decisions about major life-changing events such as whether the person should move into a care home or undergo a major surgical operation. The Act also stipulates decisions which cannot be made by others even though a person lacks capacity. Some of these decisions concern family relationships, such as consenting to marriage or civil partnership, sexual relationship, divorce or dissolution of a civil partnership. Other decisions include voting rights, unlawful killing and assisted suicide.

The Mental Capacity Act is underpinned by five statutory principles (*see* Box 10.1). These are intended to support, protect and assist people who may lack capacity to make particular decisions. They are not intended to restrict or control these people's lives. When the principles are followed and applied to the decision-making framework, they will help people to take appropriate actions in individual cases. The principles are also intended to help people to find the right solutions in difficult and uncertain situations.

Box 10.1   Mental Capacity Act 2005: five statutory principles

➤ A person must be assumed to have capacity unless it is established that they lack capacity.

➤ A person is not to be treated as unable to make a decision unless all practicable steps to help them to do so have been taken without success.

➤ A person is not to be treated as unable to make a decision merely because they make an unwise decision.

➤ An act done, or decision made, under this Act for or on behalf of a person who lacks capacity must be done, or made, in their best interests.

➤ Before the act is done, or the decision is made, regard must be had to whether the purpose for which it is needed can be as effectively achieved in a way that is less restrictive of the person's rights and freedom of action.

ASSESSMENT OF CAPACITY

To help to determine one's ability to make decisions, the Mental Capacity Act sets out a two-stage test to assess capacity.

Stage 1

Does the person have an impairment of the mind or brain, or is there some sort of disturbance affecting the way their mind or brain works? (It does not matter whether the impairment or disturbance is temporary or permanent.)

Stage 2

If so, does that impairment or disturbance mean that the person is unable to make the decision in question at the time when it needs to be made?

A person is unable to make a decision if they cannot meet the criteria listed in Box 10.2.

Box 10.2   Definition of 'inability to make a decision'

A person is unable to make a decision if they cannot:
➤ understand information about the decision to be made
➤ retain that information in their mind
➤ use or weigh that information as part of the decision-making process *or*
➤ communicate their decision (by talking, using sign language or any other means).

Special efforts should be made when assessing capacity of a person with cognitive impairment or other serious mental illness. Before the assessment, it is helpful to collect background information about the person. The presence of a friend or relative might make the person feel at ease and might help them to understand the information. However, their right to confidentiality should be respected. Relevant information should be provided in a simple and clear fashion. Too much information might confuse them. The time of the day and the place where the assessment takes place might help or hinder decision making. The information may need to be repeated several times in some situations. Enough time should be given for the person to arrive at their decision. For people with communication difficulties, every effort should be made to find alternative ways to help them in the decision-making process. For example, interpreters, sign-language specialists, pictures and written materials should be used as appropriate.

BEST INTERESTS

Many different people may be required to make decisions or act on behalf of a person who lacks capacity to make decisions for him- or herself. Under the Act, they are referred as 'decision maker'. Depending upon the situation they could be nurses, doctors, carers, attorneys or deputies appointed by the Court of Protection. The Act requires the decision makers to make decisions in the best interest of the person who lacks capacity. As a matter of good practice it is advisable to obtain a second opinion from another doctor in cases where a complex decision is contemplated.

When arriving at the person's best interests, consideration should be given to:

➤ the past and present wishes of the person
➤ the need to maximise the person's participation in the decision
➤ the views of others as to the person's wishes and feelings
➤ the need to adopt the course of action that is least restrictive to the person's freedom.

There are two circumstances when the best interests principle will not apply. The first is where someone has previously made a valid advance decision to refuse medical treatment while they had the capacity to do so. Their advance decision should be respected when they lack capacity, even if others think that the decision to refuse treatment is not in their best interests. The second is participation in research when they lack capacity to consent.

POWERS OF ATTORNEY

A power of attorney is a deed by which one person (the 'donor') gives another person (the 'attorney') the authority to act in the donor's name and on his or her behalf. It is possible to choose more than one attorney. If more than one attorney is chosen, then they could act either jointly (that is, they must all act together and cannot act separately) or jointly and severally (that is, they can all act together but they can also act separately if they wish).

There are two types of powers of attorney, ordinary power of attorney and lasting power of attorney (the terms used vary in Scotland and other jurisdictions).

Ordinary power of attorney

Ordinary powers of attorney are created for a set period of time in cases where the donor is going abroad or is unable to act for some other reason and wishes someone else to have the authority to act on his or her behalf. The ordinary power of attorney can be specific or general. If it is specific, the attorney only has the authority to do the things specified by the donor in the power. If it is general, the attorney has the authority to do anything that the donor can lawfully do with his or her property and affairs.

The test of capacity, which a person must satisfy in order to make an ordinary power of attorney, is that the donor understands the nature and effect of what he or she is doing. Although the legal form completed by the donor is usually simple, it is generally advisable to seek legal advice. There is no requirement to register the ordinary power of attorney. An ordinary power of attorney ceases to have effect if the donor becomes mentally incapable – for example, if they develop significant dementia. The donor or the attorney can cancel the ordinary power of attorney at any time.

Lasting power of attorney

The lasting power of attorney (LPA) replaced the enduring power of attorney (EPA) in England and Wales in October 2007. There are two types of LPA: personal welfare LPA and property and affairs LPA. The Mental Capacity Act stipulates what the LPAs are and how they should be used.

Procedure

The donor must follow the right procedures for creating and registering the LPA for it to be valid. They can only make an LPA if they have the 'capacity' to do so. There are separate statutory forms for the personal welfare LPA and the property and affairs LPA.

For an LPA to be valid, the following conditions must be met.

➤ The donor must sign a statement confirming that they have read the prescribed information (or that somebody has read it to them).

➤ The document should state the names of people (not any of the attorneys) who should be notified when an application to register the LPA is being made. However, the donor could choose not to name anyone to be notified.

➤ The attorneys must sign a statement saying that they have read the prescribed information and that they understand their duties, in particular the duty to act in the donor's best interests.

➤ The document must include a certificate completed by an independent person certifying that, in their opinion, at the time the LPA is made:
  – the donor understands the purpose of the LPA and the scope of the authority under it
  – no fraud or undue pressure is being used to induce the donor to create the LPA, *and*
  – there is nothing else that would prevent the LPA from being created.

The LPA must be registered with the Office of the Public Guardian (OPG) before it can be used. The donor can register the LPA when they are still capable, and the attorney can register it at any time. All EPAs which were in existence in October 2007 must be registered with the OPG for them to be valid.

Personal welfare LPA

The personal welfare LPA allows someone to choose one or more people to make decisions on their behalf with regard to their personal welfare and healthcare. This includes consenting or refusing medical treatments and decisions about where to live. If the donor wants the attorney to make decisions about life-sustaining treatment, they should express this specifically on the form. The attorney cannot consent on behalf of the donor about a treatment for which the donor has made a valid advance decision. The attorney of a personal welfare LPA cannot make decisions about property and financial affairs.

Property and affairs LPA

The property and affairs LPA allows someone to choose one or more people to make decisions about their property and affairs (including financial matters). If there are no restrictions stipulated on the LPA, the attorney(s) can make any decisions about the finances, such as buying or selling property, operating bank accounts, managing investments, receiving income, inheritance and any entitlement on behalf of the donor.

Court-appointed deputy

The Mental Capacity Act 2005 provides for a system of court-appointed deputies to replace the old system of receivership. Deputies will be able to take decisions on welfare, healthcare and financial matters as authorised by the Court of Protection. The Court will not give authority to the deputies to make decisions about life-sustaining treatment. They will only be appointed if the Court cannot make a one-off decision to resolve the issues and no valid LPA is in place. Usually deputies are necessary when a series of decisions need to be made regarding property and financial affairs. If the only income of a person who lacks capacity is social security benefits and they have no property or savings, there will usually be no need for a deputy to be appointed. This is because the person's benefits can be managed by an *appointee*, appointed by the Department for Work and Pensions to receive and deal with the benefits of a person who lacks capacity to do this for themselves. Deputies for personal welfare are needed in situations when someone has to make a series of welfare decisions over time and it would not be beneficial or appropriate to require all these decisions to be made by the court, or there is a history of serious family disputes that could have a detrimental effect on the person's future care unless a deputy is appointed to make necessary decisions.

INDEPENDENT MENTAL CAPACITY ADVOCATE (IMCA)

An IMCA is someone appointed by the local authority or NHS organisation to support a person who lacks capacity and who has no one to speak on their behalf, such as family or friends. IMCAs are involved when decisions are being made about serious medical treatment, when deprivation of liberty is being considered or when a change in the person's accommodation to the one provided by the NHS or a local authority is proposed. They are also to be involved whenever a person who lacks capacity with no unpaid carers remains in hospital for more than 28 days or in a care home for more than 8 weeks. The IMCA makes representations about the person's wishes, feelings, beliefs and values, at the same time as bringing to the attention of the decision maker all factors that are relevant to the decision. The IMCA can challenge the decision maker on behalf of the person lacking capacity, if necessary.

ADVANCE DECISIONS

If an individual is found to lack capacity, then reference should be made to any advance decisions the person may have made. The Mental Capacity Act sets out guidance when someone has made an advance decision to refuse treatment. Advance decisions are declarations whereby competent people make known their views on what should happen if they lose the capacity to make decisions for themselves. This allows people to state which treatments they would or would not want if they become seriously ill and no longer have the mental capacity to make decisions. Advance decisions can take a variety of forms, ranging from general lists of life values and preferences to specific requests or refusals. They can be written or oral. Advance decisions about refusing life-sustaining treatments should be written, signed and witnessed. They should also clearly state that the decision applies even when life is at risk.

The test for capacity to make an advance statement about medical treatment is similar to that for capacity to make a contemporaneous medical decision. In order for an advance statement to be valid, the patient must have been competent when the statement was made, must have been acting free from pressure and must have been offered sufficient, accurate information to make an informed decision. It is recommended that advance statements be updated regularly, usually every 3 years, to indicate that they truly reflect the person's current views.

OFFICE OF THE PUBLIC GUARDIAN

The Public Guardian has several duties under the Act, and is supported in carrying these out by an Office of the Public Guardian (OPG). The OPG registers LPAs and the EPAs. It also supervises the deputies appointed by the

Court of Protection and provides information to help the Court to make decisions. The OPG is an agency of the Ministry of Justice and works with other agencies, such as the police and social services, to respond to any concerns raised about the way in which an attorney or deputy is operating. A Public Guardian Board scrutinises and reviews the way in which the OPG discharges its functions.

COURT OF PROTECTION

The Mental Capacity Act provided for a new Court of Protection to make decisions in relation to 'property and affairs' and 'health and welfare' of someone who lacks capacity. It also has power to make declarations about whether someone has the capacity to make a particular decision. The Court has the same powers, rights, privileges and authority in relation to mental capacity matters as the High Court. It is a superior court of record and is able to set precedents.

The Court of Protection has the powers to:

➤ decide whether a person has the capacity to make a particular decision
➤ make declarations, decisions or orders on financial or welfare matters affecting people who lack capacity
➤ appoint deputies to make decisions for people who lack capacity
➤ decide whether an LPA or EPA is valid
➤ make decisions on cases concerning objections to registering an LPA or EPA
➤ remove deputies or attorneys who fail to carry out their duties
➤ make decisions on cases relevant to Deprivation of Liberty Safeguards
➤ decide whether an advance decision is valid.

APPOINTEESHIP

The appointeeship system enables another individual, known as an appointee, to receive and administer social security benefits and allowances on behalf of a mentally incapable person. Appointeeship is governed by Regulation 33 of the Social Security (Claims and Payments) Regulations 1987. Medical evidence of the claimant's inability to manage their own affairs may be requested.

The Secretary of State can revoke an appointment at any time, and there is no right of appeal against the Secretary of State's refusal to appoint a particular individual as appointee or against the revocation of such an appointment. Appointees have no authority to deal with the claimant's capital. If the Court of Protection appoints a deputy to manage property and affairs, it is likely that the deputy will take over the appointee's role.

CAPACITY TO MAKE A WILL

A will is a document in which the maker (called the 'testator' if he is a man and the 'testatrix' if she is a woman) appoints an executor to deal with their affairs when they die and describes how their estate is to be distributed after their death.[43] The degree of understanding which the law requires a person making a will to have is known as *testamentary capacity*. Testamentary capacity should be present both when giving instructions for the preparation of the will and at the time of execution or signing of the will. A greater degree of mental capacity is likely to be required when making a complex will compared with a simple will.

The criteria listed in Box 13.3 should be assessed when deciding whether an individual has testamentary capacity.

Box 13.3   Testamentary capacity

An individual who is making a will should:
➤ understand the nature of the act and its effects
➤ understand the nature and extent of the property being disposed
➤ be able to distinguish and compare potential beneficiaries
➤ be free from an abnormal state of mind.

A person with mental disorder may legitimately make a will, provided the mental disorder does not influence any of the criteria relevant to the making of the will. Old age psychiatrists and GPs are most likely to be asked to give their opinion as to testamentary capacity in cases of presumed or established dementia. Solicitors are advised that, when drawing up a will for an elderly person or someone who is seriously ill, they should ensure that the will is witnessed or approved by a medical practitioner. The medical practitioner should record his or her examination and findings. The capacity to revoke a will is the same as the capacity to make a will in the first place. A will is automatically revoked when the person gets married.

Statutory wills

If a person is both (a) incapable, by reason of mental disorder, of managing and administering his or her property and affairs, and (b) incapable of making a valid will, an application can be made to the Court of Protection for a statutory will to be drawn up and executed on the person's behalf. The Court requires medical evidence of both types of incapacity. The Court is obliged to make a will, consistent with the one the patient would have made for him- or herself, within reason, and with competent legal advice.

MENTAL HEALTH ACT 1983

In 2007, several amendments were made to the Mental Health Act 1983 (MHA). Patients with dementia may become subject to various sections of the MHA.[44] For a detailed account of all the possible sections of the MHA that are applicable to patients with dementia, the reader is referred to the *Mental Health Act Manual*.[45] A brief account of the commonly applied sections of the MHA is provided below.

Section 5(2): Doctor's holding power

An informal inpatient who wishes to leave hospital may be detained for up to 72 hours if the doctor believes an application should be made for compulsory admission under the MHA. This requires a single medical recommendation by the doctor in charge of the patient's care, or his or her nominated deputy. It is usual to consider a change to a Section 2 or 3 order as soon as possible.[46]

Section 2: Assessment order

Criteria

Section 2 provides that a person may be detained under the MHA for a period of up to 28 days on the grounds that the person:

➤ is suffering from a mental disorder of a nature or degree that warrants their detention in hospital for assessment (or for assessment followed by treatment) for at least a limited period *and*

➤ ought to be so detained in the interests of their own health or safety or with a view to the protection of others.

Procedure

The Section 2 procedure requires the following.

➤ Application by the patient's nearest relative or an approved mental health professional (AMHP), who must have seen the patient within the last 14 days. The AMHP should, so far as is practicable, consult the nearest relative.

➤ Medical recommendations by two doctors, one of whom must be approved under Section 12 of the MHA. If the medical recommendations are performed separately, they should be done within 5 days of each other.

Section 3: Treatment order

Criteria

Section 3 provides that a person may be detained under the MHA for an initial period of up to 6 months on the grounds that:

➤ the person is suffering from a mental disorder of a nature or degree which makes it appropriate for them to receive medical treatment in hospital
➤ it is necessary for the health or safety of the person or for the protection of other persons that they should receive such treatment, and it cannot be provided unless the patient is detained under this section
➤ appropriate medical treatment is available.

Procedure

The Section 3 procedure requires the following.
➤ Application by the patient's nearest relative or an AMHP. The AMHP must, if practicable, consult the nearest relative before making an application, and cannot proceed if the nearest relative objects.
➤ Medical recommendations similar to those for Section 2. In addition, the recommendations must state the particular grounds for the doctor's opinion, specifying whether any other methods of dealing with the patient are available and, if so, why they are not appropriate.

When making recommendations for detention under Section 3, doctors are required to state that appropriate medical treatment is available for the patient. Preferably, they should know in advance of making the recommendation the name of the hospital to which the patient is to be admitted. However, if that is not possible, their recommendation may state that appropriate medical treatment will be available if the patient is admitted to one or more specific hospitals (or units within a hospital). The order may be renewed on the first occasion for a further 6 months, and subsequently for a year at a time.

Section 7: Guardianship order

The purpose of guardianship is to enable patients to receive community care where it cannot be provided without the use of compulsory powers. It provides an authoritative framework for working with a patient, with a minimum constraint, to achieve as independent a life as possible within the community.

Procedure

The application, medical recommendations, duration and renewal are similar to those for Section 3 of the MHA. The guardian is usually the local social services authority. Sometimes a private individual is appointed as the guardian. The guardian has a number of powers, and these are detailed in Box 10.4.

The guardian can use this power to convey the patient to the required place of residence. There is no power to force entry into the patient's home if the patient refuses access. For guardianship to be successful, a degree of cooperation is required from the patient.

Box 10.4   Powers of guardianship

The guardian has three specific powers:
➤ they have exclusive rights to decide where the patient should live
➤ they can require the patient to attend for treatment, work, training or education at specific times and places (but they cannot use force to take the patient there)
➤ they can demand that a doctor, an AMHP or another relevant person has access to the patient at the place where the patient lives.

DEPRIVATION OF LIBERTY SAFEGUARDS

People who suffer from a disorder or disability of mind and who lack capacity to consent to the care or treatment should be cared for in a way that does not limit their rights or freedom of action. In some cases, members of this vulnerable group need to be deprived of their liberty for either treatment or care, because it is necessary in their best interests and to protect them from any harm.

The Deprivation of Liberty Safeguards, which came into force in England and Wales in April 2009, provide a legal framework to authorise deprivation of liberty where this is necessary to provide care and treatment for people lacking capacity.[47] These safeguards were introduced to make the English and Welsh law compatible with the European Convention on Human Rights, and the MCA 2005 has been amended to include them. The safeguards apply to people in England and Wales who have a mental disorder and lack capacity to consent to the arrangements made for their care or treatment, but for whom receiving care or treatment in circumstances that amount to a deprivation of liberty may be necessary to protect them from harm and appears to be in their best interests.

The European Court of Human Rights (ECtHR) has drawn a distinction between the deprivation of liberty of an individual (which is unlawful, unless authorised) and restrictions on the liberty of movement of an individual. The difference between deprivation of and restriction upon liberty is merely one of degree or intensity, and not one of nature or substance.[48]

The following factors, which are not exhaustive, may indicate that deprivation of liberty is taking place:
➤ restraint is used, including sedation, to admit a person to an institution where that person is resisting admission
➤ staff exercise complete and effective control over the care and movement of a person for a significant period
➤ staff exercise control over assessments, treatment, contacts and residence
➤ a decision has been taken by the institution that the person will not be released into the care of others, or permitted to live elsewhere, unless the staff in the institution consider it appropriate

➤ a request by carers for the person to be discharged to their care is refused
➤ the person is unable to maintain social contacts because of restrictions placed on their access to other people
➤ the person loses autonomy because they are under continuous supervision and control.

The deprivation of liberty process involves two key bodies, namely a managing authority and a supervisory body.

Managing authority

The managing authority has responsibility for applying for authorisation of deprivation of liberty for any person who may come within the scope of the Deprivation of Liberty Safeguards. It is either the hospital trust or the manager of the care home, depending upon where the relevant person is.

Supervisory body

The supervisory body is responsible for considering requests for authorisations, commissioning the required assessments and, where all of the assessments agree, authorising the deprivation of liberty. Where the Deprivation of Liberty Safeguards are applied to people in hospitals or to people in care homes, the supervisory body is the local authority.

There are two types of authorisation, namely standard and urgent. A managing authority must ask the supervisory body for a standard authorisation when it appears likely that, at some time during the next 28 days, someone will be accommodated in circumstances that amount to a deprivation of liberty. Where this is not possible, the managing authority can give an urgent authorisation and then obtain standard authorisation within 7 days. This can be extended for a further 7 days, by the supervisory body, in exceptional circumstances.

There are six assessments that must be conducted before a supervisory body can give an authorisation:
➤ age assessment
➤ no refusals assessment
➤ mental capacity assessment
➤ mental health assessment
➤ eligibility assessment
➤ best interests assessment.

These assessments must be completed within 21 days of a request for a standard deprivation of liberty authorisation, or when an urgent authorisation has been given, before that urgent authorisation expires.

Age assessment

This is to confirm that the relevant person is over 18 years of age.

No refusals assessment

This is to confirm that the Deprivation of Liberty Safeguards authorisation does not conflict with any other existing authority for decision making for that person. It can include any valid advance decisions to refuse treatment made by the relevant person, and any valid decision made by the attorney of LPA or by the deputy appointed by the Court of Protection.

Mental capacity assessment

The purpose of the mental capacity assessment is to establish whether the relevant person lacks capacity to decide whether or not they should be accommodated in the relevant hospital or care home to be given care or treatment.

Mental health assessment

The purpose of the mental health assessment is to establish whether the relevant person has a mental disorder within the meaning of the MHA. This is not an assessment to determine whether the person requires mental health treatment. This assessment must be done by a Deprivation of Liberty Safeguards-trained registered medical practitioner.

Eligibility assessment

This assessment relates specifically to the relevant person's status, or potential status, under the MHA. The eligibility assessment can be done by a Deprivation of Liberty Safeguards-trained, Section 12-approved doctor or the best interests assessor, who is also an AMHP.

A person is not eligible for a deprivation of liberty authorisation if they:

➤ are detained as a hospital inpatient under the MHA
➤ are subject to a guardianship order or a community treatment order under the MHA, and accommodating them in a particular care home would conflict with the requirement imposed on them by their guardian or by the conditions of their community treatment order
➤ meet the criteria for an application for admission under Sections 2 or 3 of the MHA.

Best interests assessment

The purpose of the best interests assessment is to establish whether:

➤ it is in the best interests of the relevant person to be deprived of their liberty

➤ it is necessary for them to be deprived of their liberty in order to prevent harm to themselves *and*

➤ deprivation of liberty is a proportionate response to the likelihood of the relevant person suffering harm and the seriousness of that harm.

The best interests assessment may be undertaken by an AMHP, social worker, nurse, occupational therapist or chartered psychologist, and they should have successfully completed the training that has been approved by the Secretary of State to be a best interests assessor.

There must be a minimum of two assessors. The mental health and the best interests assessments cannot be done by the same person.

If all of the assessments conclude that the relevant person meets the requirements for authorisation, then the supervisory body can give a deprivation of liberty authorisation for up to 12 months. Deprivation of liberty should last for the shortest period possible. The best interests assessor should only recommend authorisation for as long as the relevant person is likely to meet all of the qualifying requirements.

The supervisory body may attach conditions to the authorisation as recommended by the best interests assessor, and may add other conditions. It is the responsibility of the supervisory body to appoint a representative for the relevant person. The representative represents and supports the relevant person in all matters relating to the Deprivation of Liberty Safeguards, including, if appropriate, triggering a review, using an organisation's complaints procedure on the person's behalf or making an application to the Court of Protection.

A standard authorisation can be reviewed at any time when it is felt that the relevant person no longer meets the criteria for deprivation of liberty. This review is carried out by the supervisory body.

DEMENTIA AND DRIVING

It is the duty of the driving licence holder or the applicant to notify the Driver and Vehicle Licensing Authority (DVLA) of any medical condition which may affect safe driving.[49] The DVLA must be notified as soon as a diagnosis of dementia is made. In early dementia when sufficient skills are retained, and progression is slow, a licence may be issued subject to annual review. A formal driving assessment may be necessary. It is extremely difficult to assess driving ability in those with dementia.

There are some circumstances in which the licence holder cannot, or will not, inform the DVLA of a significant medical condition which may affect safe driving. Under these circumstances the General Medical Council has issued clear guidelines. These are as follows.

➤ The DVLA is legally responsible for deciding if a person is medically unfit to drive. It needs to know when driving licence holders have a condition that may, now or in the future, affect their safety as a driver.

➤ Therefore, where patients have such conditions, doctors should make sure that the patients understand that the condition may impair their ability to drive. If a patient is incapable of understanding this advice – for example, because of dementia – the doctor should inform the DVLA immediately. The doctor should explain to patients that he or she has a legal duty to inform the DVLA about their condition.

➤ If the patient refuses to accept the diagnosis or the effect of the condition on their ability to drive, the doctor can suggest that the patient seeks a second opinion. The patients should be advised not to drive until the second opinion has been obtained.

➤ If patients continue to drive when they are not fit to do so, every reasonable effort should be made to persuade them to stop. This may include telling their next of kin.

➤ If the patient continues to drive contrary to medical advice, the doctor should disclose relevant medical information immediately, in confidence, to the medical adviser at the DVLA.

➤ Before giving information to the DVLA, the doctor should inform the patient of his or her decision to do so. Once the DVLA has been informed, the doctor should also write to the patient, to confirm that a disclosure has been made.

When the DVLA is notified about any relevant medical condition, the medical adviser can take several possible courses of action. They may request more information about the patient's current state of health from the GP or hospital doctor. The patient may be requested to undergo a medical examination by a doctor appointed by the DVLA. In some circumstances, the medical adviser may require the patient to be examined by a clinical psychologist. If a decision to revoke the driving licence is taken, this is communicated to the patient by letter. The individual has the legal right to appeal against the decision, but such appeals are rarely successful. Although this issue rarely arises in other serious mental illness apart from dementia, the same principles apply

CONCLUSION

The emphasis of this book has been on the practice rather than the theory of psychiatry of old people. We have tried to cover these practical aspects thoroughly and to give appropriate references for those who wish to pursue them. Our aim has been to show that proper psychiatric care of mentally ill old people is immensely worthwhile and rewarding. We have pointed to political and managerial issues as well as purely psychiatric issues, as we believe that proper care for old people is dependent on the political, managerial and economic commitment to provide it. We hope that you have found the book useful and thought provoking, and that you have enjoyed reading it as much as we have enjoyed writing it.

REFERENCES

1 Wattis JP (2002) The pattern of psychogeriatric services. In: JR Copeland, MT Abou-Saleh and DG Blazer (eds) *Principles and Practice of Geriatric Psychiatry* (2e). John Wiley & Sons, Chichester.

2 Wattis JP (2002) Development of health and social services in the UK in the twentieth century. In: JR Copeland, MT Abou-Saleh and DG Blazer (eds) *Principles and Practice of Geriatric Psychiatry* (2e). John Wiley & Sons, Chichester.

3 Alzheimer's Disease Society (1993) *NHS Psychogeriatric Continuing Care Beds: A Report*. Alzheimer's Disease Society, London.

4 Draper B, Melding P and Brodaty H (eds) (2005) *Psychogeriatric Service Delivery*. Oxford University Press, Oxford.

5 Reifler BV and Cohen W (1998) Practice of geriatric psychiatry and mental health services for the elderly: results of an international survey. *Int Psychogeriatrics*. **10**: 351–7.

6 Royal College of Psychiatrists (1997) Statement on continuing care for older adults with psychiatric disorders. *Psychiatr Bull*. **21**: 588.

7 Creed F, Black D and Anthony P (1989) Day hospital and community treatment for acute psychiatric illness: a critical appraisal. *Br J Psychiatry*. **154**: 300–10.

8 Burns A, Arie T and Jolley D (1995) The first year of the Goodmayes psychiatric service for old people. *Int J Geriatr Psychiatry*. **10**: 927–32.

9 Wattis JP, Wattis L and Arie TH (1981) Psychogeriatrics: a national survey of a new branch of psychiatry. *BMJ*. **282**: 1529–33.

10 Wattis JP (1988) Geographical variations in the provision of psychiatric services for old people. *Age Ageing*. **17**: 171–80.

11 Royal College of Psychiatrists (2008) *Raising the Standard*. Royal College of Psychiatrists, London.

12 Wattis J, Macdonald A and Newton P (1999) Old age psychiatry: a specialty in transition results of the 1996 survey. *Psychiatr Bull*. **23**: 331–5.

13 Harvey-Jones J (1989) *Making it Happen: Reflections on Leadership*. Fontana, London.

14 Wattis JP and Curran S (2011) *Practical Management and Leadership for Doctors*, Radcliffe, London.

15 Whitmore J (2002) *Coaching for Performance*. Nicholas Brealey Publishing, London.

16 Burns T (1997) Case management, care management and care programming. *Br J Psychiatry*. **170**: 393–5.

17 Onyett S (1995) Responsibility and accountability in community mental health teams. *Psychiatr Bull*. **19**: 281–5.

18 Department of Health (1995) *Building Bridges: A Guide to Arrangements for Inter-Agency Working for the Care and Protection of Severely Mentally Ill People*. Department of Health, London.

19 Department of Health (2001) *National Service Framework for Older People.* DoH, London. http://webarchive.nationalarchives.gov.uk/

20 Department of Health (1999) *National Service Framework for Mental Health.* DoH, London. http://webarchive.nationalarchives.gov.uk/

21 Timlin A, Gibson G, Curran S and Wattis JP (2005) *Memory Matters: A Report Exploring Issues Around the Delivery of Anti-Dementia Medication.* University of Huddersfield, Huddersfield.

22 Holmes J, Bentley K and Cameron I (2002) *Between Two Stools: Report of a UK Survey on Psychiatric Services for Older People in General Hospitals.* University of Leeds, Leeds. *See also* 'Who Cares Wins': www.rcpsych.ac.uk

23 Wattis JP, Hobson J and Barker G (1992) Needs for continuing care of demented people: a model for estimating needs. *Psychiatr Bull.* **16:** 465–7.

24 Wattis JP and Fairbairn A (1996) Towards a consensus on continuing care for older adults with psychiatric disorder: report of a meeting on 27 March 1995 at the Royal College of Psychiatrists. *Int J Geriatr Psychiatry.* **11:** 163–8.

25 Kmietowicz Z (2000) France heads the WHO's league table of health systems. *BMJ.* **320:** 1687.

26 Treetops J (1992) *A Daisy Among the Dandelions: The Churches' Ministry with Older People: Suggestions for Action.* Faith in Elderly People Project, Leeds.

27 Froggatt A (1994) Tuning in to meet spiritual needs. *Dementia Care.* **2:** 12–13.

28 Smith CW and Wattis JP (1989) Medical students' attitudes to old people and career preferences: the case of Nottingham. *Med Educ.* **23:** 81–5.

29 Weed L (1997) New connections between medical knowledge and patient care. *BMJ.* **315:** 231–5.

30 Marshall M, Gray A, Lockwood A and Green R (1997) *Case Management for Severe Mental Disorders.* Cochrane Library Update Software, Oxford.

31 Holloway F, Oliver N, Collins E and Carson J (1995) Case management: a critical review of the outcome literature. *Eur Psychiatry.* **10:** 113–28.

32 Young JB and Forster A (1992) The Bradford community stroke trial: results at six months. *BMJ.* **304:** 1085–9.

33 Johnson HT and Bröm A (2000) *Profit Beyond Measure.* Nicholas Brealey Publishing, London.

34 Draper B, Melding P and Brodaty H (2005) *Psychogeriatric Service Delivery: An International Perspective.* Oxford University Press, Oxford.

35 International Psychogeriatric Association Service Delivery Bibliography. www.ipa-online.org

36 Olde Scheper TM and Duursma SA (1994) Euthanasia: the Dutch experience. *Age Ageing.* **23:** 3–6.

37 van der Wal G and Dillman RJ (1994) Euthanasia in the Netherlands. *BMJ.* **308:** 1346–9.

38 Ogilvie AD and Potts SG (1994) Assisted suicide for depression: the slippery slope in action? *BMJ.* **309:** 492–3.

39 Wennberg RN (1989) *Terminal Choices: Euthanasia, Suicide and the Right to Die.* Wm B Eerdmans, Grand Rapids, MI.

40 Mental Capacity Act 2005. Available at: www.legislation.gov.uk/ukpga/2005/9/contents

41 Grisso T (1986) *Evaluating Competencies: Forensic Assessments and Instruments.* Plenum, New York.

42 *Mental Capacity Act 2005 – Code of Practice* (2007) The Stationery Office, London.

43 British Medical Association and Law Society (2010) *Assessment of Mental Capacity: a practical guide for doctors and lawyers* (3e). BMA, London.

44 Mental Health Act 2007. Available at: www.legislation.gov.uk/ukpga/2007/12/contents

45 Jones R (2008) *Mental Health Act Manual.* Sweet & Maxwell Ltd, London.

46 *Mental Health Act 2007 – Code of Practice.* London: The Stationery Office; 2008.

47 *Deprivation of Liberty Safeguards – Code of Practice* (2008) The Stationery Office, London.

48 *HL v United Kingdom* (2004) 40 EHRR 761, ECtHR.

49 Driver and Vehicle Licensing Authority (2009) *At a Glance Guide to the Current Medical Standards of Fitness to Drive for Medical Practitioners.* DVLA, Swansea.

Old age service development

Assessment of *service principles* (based on World Health Organization/World Psychiatric Association [WHO/WPA] Consensus Statement)

Principle and description	Where we are now	Where we want to be in 2–3 years' time
Comprehensive: should take into account all aspects of a patient's physical, psychological and social needs and be patient centred.		
Accessible: user-friendly, readily available, minimising geographical, cultural, financial, political and linguistic obstacles to obtaining care.		
Responsive: listens to and understands the problems brought to its attention and acts promptly and appropriately.		
Individualised: focuses on individuals in their family and community context. Care tailored and acceptable to individual and family, aiming where possible to keep individuals at home.		
Transdisciplinary: going beyond traditional professional boundaries to optimise the contributions of people with a range of personal and professional skills. Collaborates with other agencies to provide a comprehensive range of community services.		
Accountable: accepts responsibility for assuring the quality of service; it delivers and monitors performance with patients and families; is ethically and culturally sensitive.		
Systemic : flexibly integrates all available services to ensure *continuity of care*, and coordinates all levels of service provision. (In the NHS this can be interpreted as all parts of health and social services working together with the voluntary sector to provide a gap-free service.)		

Assessment of how far *care needs* are met (based on WHO/WPA Consensus Statement)

Care need and description	Where we are now	Where we want to be
Prevention: cardiovascular risk, lifestyle, social interaction, support in times of trouble, continued physical and intellectual activity, recognising care needs.		
Early identification: population awareness and availability of early expert assessment of possible mental health problems; screening in high-risk populations.		
Comprehensive medical and social assessment and diagnosis: this should take into account all areas of need, and social, physical and mental health, and be carried out in an appropriate environment, often initially in the patient's home but also involving outpatient, day or inpatient settings when needed.		
Management (more than just treatment): a coherent and comprehensive plan addressing all areas of need, the needs of any carers as well as medical/psychiatric treatment and follow-up.		
Continuing care, support and review of individual and carers: practical, comprehensive and regular support and review for patient and carers.		
Information, advice and counselling: ready access to understandable and accurate information about all aspects of disease, treatment and services. Good sharing of information between services.		
Regular breaks (respite): breaks from caring to sustain those burdened by long-term care, often in social care day or residential settings.		
Advocacy: legal, financial and other rights must be protected and managed.		
Residential care: quality residential care for those who cannot be managed at home.		
Spiritual and leisure needs: addressed in all settings.		

Assessment of *components* of service (based on WHO/WPA Consensus Statement)

Descriptors of service components	Where we are now	Where we want to be
Community mental health teams (all disciplines?)		
Inpatient services		
Day hospitals		
Outpatient services		
Hospital respite care		
Continuing hospital care		
Liaison services		
Primary care collaboration		
Community and support services		
Preventive programmes		

Descriptors of service components	Where we are now	Where we want to be
Memory services (NSF OP/EB)		
Community treatment (NSF MH)		
Intermediate care, includes mental health (NSF OP/EB)		
Assertive outreach (ISF MH)		
Crisis intervention (NSF MH)		
Behavioural and psychological interventions (NSF MH/EB)		
Support to residential and day care settings (NSF OP/EB)		
Mental healthcare for people in general hospitals (NSF OP/EB)		
Special groups: early-onset dementia, learning disabilities, older prisoners (NSF OP/EB)		

EB, Everybody's Business; NSF MH, National Service Framework for Mental Health; NSF OP, National Service Framework for Older People.

NSFs can be accessed via the Department of Health website www.dh.gov.uk The WHO/WPA Consensus Statement can be accessed via the WHO website at www.who.int/mental_health/media/en/19.pdf

Additional information

USEFUL WEBSITES

Action on Elder Abuse: www.elderabuse.org.uk
Age UK: www.ageuk.org.uk
Alzheimer's Society: www.alzheimers.org.uk
British Geriatrics Society: www.bgs.org.uk
Cochrane Library: www.thecochranelibrary.com
Department of Health: www.gov.uk
Faculty of the Psychiatry of Old Age, Royal College of Psychiatrists:
http://www.rcpsych.ac.uk/workinpsychiatry/faculties/oldage.aspx
Medicines and Healthcare Products Regulatory Agency (MHRA (including the
Committee on Safety of Medicines)): www.mhra.gov.uk
Mental Capacity Act (2005): www.legislation.gov.uk
Mental Capacity Act (2005) (Code of Practice, 2008): www.gov.uk
National Institute for Mental Health in England: www.mhhe.heacademy.ac.uk
National Institute for Health and Clinical Excellence (NICE): www.nice.org.uk
NHS Direct 111. www.nhsdirect.nhs.uk
Royal College of Psychiatrists: www.rcpsych.ac.uk
United States Food and Drug Administration (USFDA): www.fda.gov

ADDITIONAL WEBSITES

British Association for Psychopharmacology: www.bap.org.uk
Care Quality Commission: www.cqc.org.uk
British Psychological Society: www.bps.org.uk
British Association of Social Workers: www.basw.co.uk
Driver and Vehicle Licensing Agency (DVLA): www.dft.gov.uk/dvla
Memory Services National Accreditation Programme (MSNAP), Royal College
of Psychiatrists: www.rcpsych.ac.uk
Carers UK: www.carersuk.org

Index

CPD with Radcliffe

You can now use a selection of our books to achieve CPD (Continuing Professional Development) points through directed reading.

We provide a free online form and downloadable certificate for your appraisal portfolio. Look for the CPD logo and register with us at: **www.radcliffehealth.com/cpd**

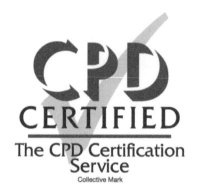